Musculoskeletal MRI-Ultrasound Correlation

Editor

JAN FRITZ

MAGNETIC RESONANCE IMAGING
CLINICS OF NORTH AMERICA

www.mri.theclinics.com

Consulting Editors
SURESH K. MUKHERJI
LYNNE S. STEINBACH

May 2023 • Volume 31 • Number 2

ELSEVIER

1600 John F. Kennedy Boulevard • Suite 1800 • Philadelphia, Pennsylvania, 19103-2899

http://www.mri.theclinics.com

MAGNETIC RESONANCE IMAGING CLINICS OF NORTH AMERICA Volume 31, Number 2
May 2023 ISSN 1064-9689, ISBN 13: 978-0-323-93953-9

Editor: John Vassallo (j.vassallo@elsevier.com)
Developmental Editor: Arlene Campos

Magnetic Resonance Imaging Clinics of North America (ISSN 1064-9689) is published quarterly by Elsevier Inc., 360 Park Avenue South, New York, NY 10010-1710. Months of issue are February, May, August, and November. Business and Editorial Offices: 1600 John F. Kennedy Blvd., Ste. 1800, Philadelphia, PA 19103-2899. Customer Service Office: 3251 Riverport Lane, Maryland Heights, MO 63043. Periodicals postage paid at New York, NY and additional mailing offices. Subscription prices are $408.00 per year (domestic individuals), $783.00 per year (domestic institutions), $100.00 per year (domestic students/residents), $455.00 per year (Canadian individuals), $1021.00 per year (Canadian institutions), $573.00 per year (international individuals), $1021.00 per year (international institutions), $100.00 per year (Canadian students/residents), and $275.00 per year (international students/residents). International air speed delivery is included in all *Clinics* subscription prices. All prices are subject to change without notice. **POSTMASTER:** Send address changes to *Magnetic Resonance Imaging Clinics*, Elsevier Health Sciences Division, Subscription Customer Service, 3251 Riverport Lane, Maryland Heights, MO 63043. Customer Service (orders, claims, online, change of address): Elsevier Health Sciences Division, Subscription **Customer Service, 3251 Riverport Lane, Maryland Heights, MO 63043. Tel:1-800-654-2452 (U.S. and Canada); 314-447-8871 (outside U.S. and Canada). Fax: 314-447-8029. E-mail: journalscustomerservice-usa@elsevier.com (for print support); journalsonlinesupport-usa@elsevier.com (for online support).**

Reprints. For copies of 100 or more of articles in this publication, please contact the Commercial Reprints Department, Elsevier Inc., 360 Park Avenue South, New York, NY 10010-1710. Tel.: 212-633-3874; Fax: 212-633-3820; E-mail: reprints@elsevier.com.

Magnetic Resonance Imaging Clinics of North America is covered in the *RSNA Index of Imaging Literature, MEDLINE/PubMed (Index Medicus),* and *EMBASE/Excerpta Medica.*

Contributors

CONSULTING EDITORS

SURESH K. MUKHERJI, MD, MBA, FACR
Clinical Professor of Radiology and Radiation
Oncology, University of Illinois, Robert Wood
Johnson Medical School, Rutgers University,
Faculty, Otolaryngology–Head and Neck
Surgery, Michigan State University, National
Director of Head and Neck Radiology, ProScan
Imaging, Carmel, Indiana, USA

LYNNE S. STEINBACH, MD, FACR
Emeritus Professor of Radiology on Full Recall,
Department of Radiology and Biomedical
Imaging, University of California San Francisco,
San Francisco, California, USA

EDITOR

JAN FRITZ, MD, PD, RMSK
Associate Professor, Department of Radiology,
Chief, Division of Musculoskeletal Radiology,

NYU Grossman School of Medicine, NYU
Langone Orthopedic Hospital, New York, New
York, USA

AUTHORS

RONALD S. ADLER, MD, PhD
Professor of Radiology, NYU Grossman School
of Medicine, New York, New York, USA

MARYAM RASHED AL-NAIMI, MD
Consultant Radiologist, Aspetar Orthopedic
and Sports Medicine Hospital, Doha, Qatar

**MARIA PILAR APARISI GÓMEZ, MBChB,
FRANZCR**
Department of Radiology, Auckland City
Hospital, Auckland, New Zealand; Department
of Radiology, IMSKE, Valencia, Spain

THOMAS M. ARMSTRONG, FRCR
Consultant Musculoskeletal Radiologist, Royal
Free Hospitals NHS Foundation Trust, London,
United Kingdom

JAVIER ARNAIZ, MD
Consultant Radiologist, Aspetar Orthopedic
and Sports Medicine Hospital, Doha, Qatar

ALBERTO BAZZOCCHI, MD, PhD
Diagnostic and Interventional Radiology,
IRCCS Istituto Ortopedico Rizzoli, Bologna,
Italy

NIDHI BHATNAGAR, MD
Principal Consultant and Head, Department of
Radiology, Max Multispeciality Centre, New
Delhi, India

MARCELO BORDALO, MD, PhD
Chief of Radiology, Aspetar Orthopedic and
Sports Medicine Hospital, Doha, Qatar

CHRISTOPHER J. BURKE, MBCHB
NYU Langone Orthopedic Hospital, New York,
New York, USA

AVNEESH CHHABRA, MD, MBA
Division of Musculoskeletal Imaging,
Department of Radiology, Department of
Orthopedic Surgery, UT Southwestern Medical
Center, Professor of Radiology and Orthopedic
Surgery, Dallas, Texas, USA; Adjunct Faculty,
Johns Hopkins University and Walton Centre
for Neuroscience, United Kingdom

STEVEN P. DANIELS, MD
Department of Radiology, NYU Grossman
School of Medicine, New York, New York, USA

SWATI DESHMUKH, MD
Harvard Medical School, Beth Israel
Deaconess Medical Center, Boston,
Massachusetts, USA

FATEMEH EZZATI, MD
Associate Professor, Division of Rheumatic
Disease, Department of Internal Medicine, UT
Southwestern Medical Center, Dallas, Texas,
USA

BENJAMIN FRITZ, MD
Department of Radiology, Balgrist University
Hospital, Faculty of Medicine, University of
Zurich, Zurich, Switzerland

JAN FRITZ, MD, PD, RMSK
Associate Professor, Department of Radiology,
Chief, Division of Musculoskeletal Radiology,
NYU Grossman School of Medicine, NYU
Langone Orthopedic Hospital, New York, New
York, USA

ANDREW J. GRAINGER, FRCR
Consultant Musculoskeletal Radiologist,
Radiology Department, Cambridge University
Hospitals NHS Foundation Trust,
Addenbrookes Hospital, Cambridge,
Cambridgeshire, United Kingdom

GIUSEPPE GUGLIELMI, MD
Department of Radiology, Hospital San
Giovanni Rotondo, Italy; Department of
Radiology, University of Foggia, Foggia, Italy

JACQUES H. HACQUEBORD, MD
Clinical Associate Professor, Department of
Orthopedic Surgery, NYU Grossman School of
Medicine, New York, New York, USA

APARNA KOMARRAJU, MD
Harvard Medical School, Beth Israel
Deaconess Medical Center, Boston,
Massachusetts, USA

SIRISHA KONERU, MBBS, DO
Musculoskeletal Radiology Fellow, NYU
Grossman School of Medicine, New York, New
York, USA

THEODORE T. MILLER, MD
Professor of Radiology, Department of
Radiology and Imaging, Hospital for Special
Surgery, New York, New York, USA

VINH T. NGUYEN, MD
Clinical Associate Professor, Department of
Radiology, NYU Grossman School of
Medicine, New York, New York, USA

PARHAM PEZESHK, MD
Associate Professor, Division of
Musculoskeletal Imaging, Department of
Radiology, UT Southwestern Medical Center,
Dallas, Texas, USA

EMMA ROWBOTHAM, FRCR
Consultant Musculoskeletal Radiologist,
Chapel Allerton Hospital, Leeds Teaching
Hospitals NHS Trust, NIHR Biomedical
Research Centre Leeds, Leeds, United
Kingdom

MEGHAN E. SAHR, MD
Assistant Professor of Radiology, Department
of Radiology and Imaging, Hospital for Special
Surgery, New York, New York, USA

MOHAMMAD SAMIM, MD
NYU Langone Orthopedic Hospital, New York,
New York, USA

ADAM SINGER, MD
Radiology Partners/Northside Radiology
Associates

THEODOROS SOLDATOS, MD
Iasis Diagnostic Centre, Kalamata, Greece

KEVIN SUN, MD
Harvard Medical School, Beth Israel
Deaconess Medical Center, Boston,
Massachusetts, USA

JIM S. WU, MD
Harvard Medical School, Beth Israel
Deaconess Medical Center, Boston,
Massachusetts, USA

EDUARDO YAMASHIRO, MD
Consultant Radiologist, Aspetar Orthopedic
and Sports Medicine Hospital, Doha, Qatar

Contents

periarticular fluid collections, tendon tears and impingement, and neurovascular impingement, often with features indicating the causative etiology. MR imaging assessment requires technical modifications to reduce metal artifact, such as multispectral imaging, and optimization of image quality, and a high-performance 1.5-T system. US images periarticular structures at high-spatial resolution without interference of metal artifact, permitting real-time dynamic evaluation, and is useful for procedure guidance. Bone complications (periprosthetic fracture, stress reaction, osteolysis, and component loosening) are well depicted on MR imaging.

Early diagnosis of arthritis is of paramount importance to slow the progression of disease and joint destruction. Because of temporal dissemination of the clinical and laboratory manifestations of the inflammatory arthritis and overlap of the findings, diagnosis can be challenging in early stages of the disease. This article highlights the utility of advanced cross-sectional imaging, including color-Doppler ultrasound, diffusion-weighted MR imaging, and perfusion MR imaging in the domain of arthropathy so that the reader can apply these principles and techniques in their practices for timely and accurate diagnosis and improved multidisciplinary communications for better management of such conditions.

 Video content accompanies this article at http://www.mri.theclinics.com.

Multimodality imaging of the brachial plexus is essential to accurately localize the lesion and characterize the pathology and site of injury. A combination of computed tomography (CT), ultrasound, and MR imaging is useful along with clinical and nerve conduction studies. Ultrasound and MR imaging in combination are effective to accurately localize the pathology in most of the cases. Accurate reporting of the pathology with dedicated MR imaging protocols in conjunction with Doppler ultrasound and dynamic imaging provides practical and useful information to help the referring physicians and surgeons to optimize medical or surgical treatment regimens.

Elbow pain is very common and can be due to many pathologic conditions. After radiographs are obtained, advanced imaging is often necessary. Both ultrasonography and MR imaging can be used to evaluate the many important soft-tissue structures of the elbow, with each modality having advantages and disadvantages in certain clinical scenarios. Imaging findings between the two modalities often correlate. It is important for musculoskeletal radiologists to understand normal elbow anatomy and how best to use ultrasonography and MR imaging to evaluate elbow pain. In this way, radiologists can provide expert guidance to referring clinicians and best guide patient management.

MAGNETIC RESONANCE IMAGING CLINICS OF NORTH AMERICA

FORTHCOMING ISSUES

August 2023
MR Angiography: From Head to Toe
Prashant Nagpal and Thomas M. Grist, *Editors*

November 2023
Clinical Value of Hybrid PET/MRI
Minerva Becker and Valentino Garibotto, *Editors*

February 2024
MR Perfusion
Max Wintermark and Ananth Madhuranthakam, *Editors*

RECENT ISSUES

February 2023
MR Imaging of the Adnexa
Erica B. Stein, Kim L. Shampain, and Kim Shampain, *Editors*

November 2022
Postoperative Joint MR Imaging
Luis Beltran, *Editor*

August 2022
MR in the Emergency Room
John Conklin and Michael H. Lev, *Editors*

SERIES OF RELATED INTEREST

Advances in Clinical Radiology
Neurologic Clinics
PET Clinics
Radiologic Clinics

VISIT THE CLINICS ONLINE!
Access your subscription at:
www.theclinics.com

PROGRAM OBJECTIVE

The goal of *Magnetic Resonance Imaging Clinics of North America* is to keep practicing physicians up to date with current clinical practice by providing timely articles reviewing the state of the art in patient care.

TARGET AUDIENCE

All practicing physicians and healthcare professionals who provide patient care utilizing findings from Magnetic Resonance Imaging.

LEARNING OBJECTIVES

Upon completion of this activity, participants will be able to:
1. Review current trends and updates in MRI studies, including WHO classifications.
2. Discuss correlations of MRI and US in images.
3. Recognize best practice and preferred imaging study/studies for muscle injuries.

ACCREDITATION

The Elsevier Office of Continuing Medical Education (EOCME) is accredited by the Accreditation Council for Continuing Medical Education (ACCME) to provide continuing medical education for physicians.

The EOCME designates this journal-based CME activity enduring material for a maximum of 10 *AMA PRA Category 1 Credit*(s)™. Physicians should claim only the credit commensurate with the extent of their participation in the activity.

All other healthcare professionals requesting continuing education credit for this enduring material will be issued a certificate of participation.

DISCLOSURE OF CONFLICTS OF INTEREST

The EOCME assesses conflict of interest with its instructors, faculty, planners, and other individuals who are in a position to control the content of CME activities. All relevant conflicts of interest that are identified are thoroughly vetted by EOCME for fair balance, scientific objectivity, and patient care recommendations. EOCME is committed to providing its learners with CME activities that promote improvements or quality in healthcare and not a specific proprietary business or a commercial interest.

The planning committee, staff, authors and editors listed below have identified no financial relationships or relationships to products or devices they or their spouse/life partner have with commercial interest related to the content of this CME activity:

Ronald S. Adler, MD, PhD; Maryam Rashed Al-Naimi, MD; Maria Pilar Aparisi Gómez, MBChB, FRANZCR; Thomas Armstrong, PhD; Javier Arnaiz, MD, PhD; Alberto Bazzocchi, MD, PhD; Nidhi Bhatnagar, MBBS, MD; Marcelo Bordalo, MD, PhD; Christopher J. Burke, MBChB; Steven P. Daniels, MD; Swati Deshmukh, MD; Fatemeh Ezzati, MD; Benajmin Fritz, MD; Andrew J. Grainger, FRCP, FRCR; Giuseppe Guglielmi, MD; Lynette Jones, MSN, RN-BC; Aparna Komarraju, MD; Sirisha Koneru, MBBS, DO; Kothainayaki Kulanthaivelu, BCA, MBA; Theodore T. Miller, MD; Vinh T. Nguyen, MD; Parham Pezeshk, MD; Emma L. Rowbotham, MB Bchir, MRCS, FRCR; Meghan E. Sahr, MD; Mohammad Samim, MD; Adam Singer, MD; Theodoros Soldatos, MD, PhD; Kevin Sun, MD; Jim S. Wu, MD; Eduardo Yamashiro, MD

The planning committee, staff, authors, and editors listed below have identified financial relationships or relationships to products or devices they or their spouse/life partner have with commercial interest related to the content of this CME activity:

Avneesh Chhabra, MD, MBA: Consultant: ICON Medical, TREACE Medical Concepts Inc.; Speaker: Siemens; Advisor/Researcher: ImageBiopsy Lab Inc.

Jan Fritz, MD: Researcher: Siemens AG, BTG International, Zimmer Biomed, DePuy Synthes, QED, and SyntheticMR; Advisor: Siemens AG, SyntheticMR, GE Healthcare, QED, BTG, ImageBiopsy Lab, Boston Scientific, and Mirata Pharma; Patent Beneficiary: Siemens Healthcare

Jacques H. Hacquebord, MD: Consultant: Synthes, Tissium, Checkpoint Therapeutics

UNAPPROVED/OFF-LABEL USE DISCLOSURE

The EOCME requires CME faculty to disclose to the participants:
1. When products or procedures being discussed are off-label, unlabelled, experimental, and/or investigational (not US Food and Drug Administration [FDA] approved); and
2. Any limitations on the information presented, such as data that are preliminary or that represent ongoing research, interim analyses, and/or unsupported opinions. Faculty may discuss information about pharmaceutical agents that is outside of FDA-approved labelling. This information is intended solely for CME and is not intended to promote off-label use of these medications. If you have any questions, contact the medical affairs department of the manufacturer for the most recent prescribing information.

TO ENROLL

To enroll in the *Magnetic Resonance Imaging Clinics of North America* Continuing Medical Education program, call customer service at 1-800-654-2452 or sign up online at http://www.theclinics.com/home/cme. The CME program is available to subscribers for an additional annual fee of USD 270.00.

METHOD OF PARTICIPATION

In order to claim credit, participants must complete the following:

1. Complete enrolment as indicated above.
2. Read the activity.
3. Complete the CME Test and Evaluation. Participants must achieve a score of 70% on the test. All CME Tests and Evaluations must be completed online.

CME INQUIRIES/SPECIAL NEEDS

For all CME inquiries or special needs, please contact elsevierCME@elsevier.com.

Foreword

Musculoskeletal Ultrasonography–MR Imaging Correlation

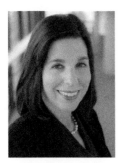

Lynne S. Steinbach, MD, FACR
Consulting Editor

Over the last few decades, it has been exciting to see how MR imaging and ultrasound have made leaps and bounds in diagnosis, characterization, and treatment of musculoskeletal disorders. These imaging techniques that do not contain ionizing radiation can be used separately but are often complementary. Many imagers are learning about the potential of this area, including how and when to perform these studies as well as how to interpret them. This issue elucidates the application of ultrasound and MR imaging for musculoskeletal imaging with cutting-edge material and visuals.

You can expect to see details about MR imaging and ultrasound for imaging of muscle, peripheral nerves, the brachial plexus, sarcomas and other soft tissue masses, painful total hip arthroplasty, rheumatologic disorders, and acute and chronic joint disorders. These subjects have been enhanced with state-of-the-art images.

Thanks to those who participated in this project for your excellent work that will enlighten our fellow imagers. Special thanks to Jan Fritz, Editor of this issue of *Magnetic Resonance Imaging Clinics of North America*. Dr Fritz, who is Associate Professor and Chief of the Division of Musculoskeletal Radiology at NYU, has done a great job of choosing the best authors to spread the word, including himself. These individuals have been recognized as having world-class expertise in their subject.

I predict that readers will constantly refer to this valuable synopsis on the use of ultrasound and MR imaging for musculoskeletal imaging. Put this reference prominently on the shelf in your reading room or make a note of it for online reading wherever you interpret and perform studies.

Lynne S. Steinbach, MD, FACR
Department of Radiology and Biomedical Imaging
University of California
San Francisco, 505 Parnassus
San Francisco, CA 9413-0628, USA

E-mail address:
lynne.steinbach@ucsf.edu

Magn Reson Imaging Clin N Am 31 (2023) xi
https://doi.org/10.1016/j.mric.2023.01.010
1064-9689/23/© 2023 Published by Elsevier Inc.

Preface

Musculoskeletal Ultrasonography–MR Imaging Correlation: A Key Component for Best Practice

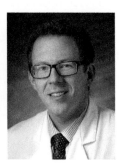

Jan Fritz, MD

Editor

Ultrasonography and MR imaging are commonly used in musculoskeletal radiology to evaluate bones, joints, ligaments, muscle-tendon units, nerves, and vessels. Each imaging modality has advantages and limitations in various body parts and parts of musculoskeletal radiology, whereas in some parts, either modality may be applied gainfully in a similar fashion. Neither ultrasonography nor MR imaging uses ionizing radiation, making either perfectly suitable for any age group or serial examinations.

Ultrasonography is useful for examining superficial central and extremity muscles, tendons, and ligaments, dynamic evaluations, and blood flow assessments without injecting a contrast agent. Ultrasound is widely available, portable, and can be performed quickly at the sideline, bedside, and in the office, making it a formidable good option for acute injuries and bedside evaluation.

MR imaging, on the other hand, is particularly useful for visualizing the bones, joints, and soft tissues in great detail and is often the modality of choice for evaluating the spine, shoulder, pelvis, and intra-articular derangements, including ligament tears and articular cartilage injuries.

Ultrasonography is often more cost-effective than MR imaging when evaluating an accessible focal condition, whereas MR imaging is often more cost-effective when evaluating large and deeper anatomic regions with broader differential diagnostic considerations and for more complex conditions. However, the cost-effectiveness of either imaging modality depends on various factors, including the availability of equipment and expertise and the local health care system and reimbursement policies.

Overall, the effectiveness of ultrasonography and MR imaging in musculoskeletal radiology will

Magn Reson Imaging Clin N Am 31 (2023) xiii–xiv
https://doi.org/10.1016/j.mric.2023.01.001
1064-9689/23/© 2023 Published by Elsevier Inc.

depend on the specific indication, the expertise and dedication of the operator, and the quality of the obtained images.

Musculoskeletal ultrasonography and MR imaging are complex and require a profound knowledge of anatomy, physiology, pathology, injury patterns, treatments, and healing and recurrence patterns. While either can be studied with dedicated ultrasound and MR imaging literature and teacher files, the high-quality correlation reviews of ultrasound and MR imaging appearances of various conditions and specialties in this issue may be especially valuable to advance practical skills, interpretations, and best practice.

I am grateful to Dr Lynne S. Steinbach for entrusting me with editing this issue and to each author for their expert contributions, enormous detail, high accuracy, and superb illustrations.

Jan Fritz, MD
Division of Musculoskeletal Radiology
Department of Radiology
NYU Grossman School of Medicine
660 1st Avenue, 3rd Floor, Room 313
New York, NY 10016, USA

E-mail address:
jan.fritz@nyulangone.org

Imaging of Muscle Injuries

MR Imaging—Ultrasound Correlation

Marcelo Bordalo, MD, PhD*, Javier Arnaiz, MD, Eduardo Yamashiro, MD,
Maryam Rashed Al-Naimi, MD

KEYWORDS

• MR imaging • Ultrasound • Muscle • Musculotendinous • Strains • Tears • Injuries

KEY POINTS

• Muscle injuries can be located at musculotendinous junction, myofascial junction, and at the intramuscular tendon (intratendinous).
• Ultrasound (US) evaluation of muscle tears provides high spatial resolution and is a valuable tool in this assessment.
• MR imaging is mainly indicated in the following situations for muscle injury assessment: evaluation of a high-performance athlete, potential surgical indications, differential diagnosis with other conditions, and evaluation of deep located or proximal muscle groups.
• Connective tissue damage during a muscle injury is related to longer recovery times.

INTRODUCTION

Traumatic muscle injuries are one of the most common problems faced by athletes, accounting for up to 31% of sports-related professional injuries.[1,2] These injuries cause up to 37% of time lost in competitions in professional athletes and 20% in amateur athletes, leading to significant economic and social consequences.[3,4] For that reason, there is enormous effort in developing diagnostic and treatment strategies for muscle injuries to accelerate the return to sports and decrease the recurrence rate. In elite sports, the main goal is to optimize the return of the athlete to training and competition without increasing the risk of recurrent injury or worsening the initial injury.

Initial injury assessment is clinical and can define prognosis and adequate treatment to decrease recovery time. It has been shown that imaging assessment may contribute to injury prognosis, treatment guiding, and predicting the return-to-play time.

Ultrasound (US) and MR imaging are the most frequent imaging modalities used to assess sports muscle injuries. In this review, the authors discuss the types of muscle injuries, terminology, classification, indications, and clinical relevance of US and MR imaging in muscle injury assessment, with a correlation between both methods.[5]

Muscle Anatomy

The striated skeletal muscle presents 2 histologically different components: the contractile and elastic muscle fibers and the less elastic connective tissue.[6] This connective tissue is composed of tendon prolongation within and at the periphery of the muscle body. The contact zones between the muscle fibers and the connective tissue are the weak zones of the muscle in traction and are the location of most indirect muscle tears.

The connective tissue is composed of the *endomysium* (surrounding each muscle fiber), the *perimysium* (surrounding a muscle fascicle, which is the set of muscle fibers), and the *epimysium* (the muscle fascia or aponeurosis) (**Fig. 1**).

Types of muscle injuries and terminology
Mechanisms of muscle injuries can be direct or indirect. A direct injury is caused by an external blunt

---

Radiology Department, Aspetar Orthopedic and Sports Medicine Hospital, Al Waab Street, Zone 54, PO Box 29222, Doha, Qatar
* Corresponding author.
E-mail address: marcelo.bordalo@aspetar.com
Twitter: @marcelobordalo (M.B.)

Magn Reson Imaging Clin N Am 31 (2023) 163–179
https://doi.org/10.1016/j.mric.2023.01.002

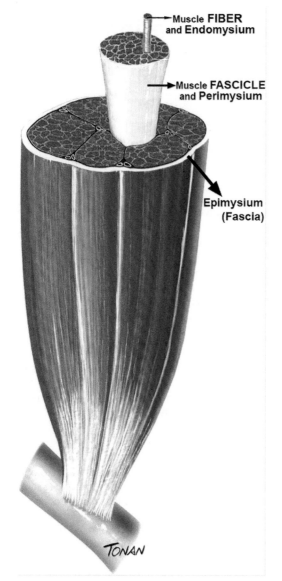

Muscle **FIBER** and Endomysium

Muscle **FASCICLE** and Perimysium

Epimysium (Fascia)

TONAN

Fig. 1. Muscle anatomy. Each muscle fiber is surrounded by the endomysium. A set of fibers form the muscle fascicle, which is surrounded by the perimysium. The muscle fascia is the epimysium.

force with muscle contusion or laceration. Recently, indirect injuries were classified as functional and structural. Functional injuries represent fatigue-induced or neurogenic damages, such as delayed-onset muscle soreness (DOMS). Structural injuries are defined by a tear of a muscle fiber, usually during eccentric contraction of the muscle-tendon unit, leading to a myotendinous tear or tendon avulsion.

There is a high degree of variability in the terminology of muscle injuries, which can lead to differences in study results and conclusions. For

example, the term *strain* is widely used and represents a biomechanical rather than a structural injury. The term *tear* is more indicated for describing structural damage and therefore the loss of muscle fiber continuity.[7]

The site of the muscle injury can be located (1) at the peripheral aspect of the muscle, called *myofascial*; (2) within the muscle belly, without tendon involvement called *musculotendinous*; and (3) with tendon involvement called *intratendinous* (**Fig. 2**). It is important to highlight that to be classified as an intratendinous tear, the intramuscular tendon must be partially or completely torn, whereas in the musculotendinous tear, the intramuscular tendon has normal continuity and signal, although these types of tears most commonly occur surrounding the musculotendinous junction. Tears that affect the intramuscular tendon have a worse prognosis in terms of recovery time, and imaging has an important role in this diagnosis.[8,9]

Classification

There are several imaging classification systems for muscle injuries (**Table 1**).[4,7,9–11] The classic 1 to 3 classification system lacks diagnostic accuracy and provides limited prognostic information.

Grade 1 injury is defined as an edematous pattern without muscle disruption on MR imaging. US can be negative or show ill-defined areas of increased echogenicity (**Fig. 3**). Grade 2 is defined as an area of focal fiber disruption (**Fig. 4**), and grade 3 is defined as complete disruption of the musculotendinous unit with fluid (hematoma) filling the gap created by the tear (**Fig. 5**). However, the presence of intramuscular hematoma can also occur in muscle contusions and grade 2 tears. Dynamic evaluation of muscle tears on US is useful to evaluate the presence of fiber disruption.

The Munich consensus on the classification of muscle injuries included grades according to the cause of the injury.[7]

The British Athletics Muscle Injury classification is based on the extent and location of injury (myofascial junction, intramuscular, and tendinous), introducing the differentiation between injuries involving solely the muscle fibers and injuries involving connective tissue (intramuscular tendons).[9] It has been shown that connective tissue injuries directly affect injury prognosis. The strength of this classification system lies in providing prognostic information based on the lesion site, length, and tendon involvement.

Adequate staging of the muscle injury is crucial to avoiding underestimation of the injury and consequent recurrent muscle tear because of a premature return to play.

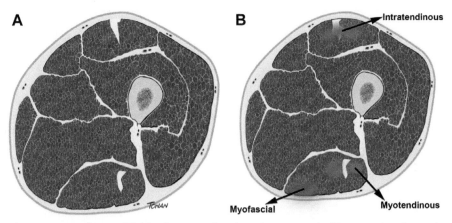

Fig. 2. Muscle anatomy and tears. (*A*) Muscle connective tissue is composed of intra- and perimuscular extension of the tendons (*arrows*). (*B*) Muscle injuries occur at the periphery of the muscle (myofascial), the muscle belly (myotendinous), and the intramuscular tendon (intratendinous). Most commonly, the myotendinous type occurs at the intramuscular myotendinous junction, without affecting the tendon itself.

Importance of connective tissue involvement

Connective tissue acts as a scaffold for muscle support. Injuries of the tendon, intermuscular, and perimuscular aponeurosis lead to biomechanical dysfunction. Connective tissue is an anatomic and functional support for the muscle. Therefore, connective tissue damage during a muscle injury is correlated with a longer recovery time and duration of painful symptoms compared with a strictly muscular injury[12–14] (**Fig. 6**).

Clinical management based on imaging results

Most of the muscle injuries are low-grade tears (0 and 1) and, when confirmed by imaging methods, evolve favorably with the disappearance of hyperechoic (on US) and hypersignal changes (on MR imaging) on some days.[8,15,16] The T2 hypersignal may persist for approximately 6 months and do not provide clinical value even as athletes resume training in the absence of any painful symptoms or restrictions. The clinical value of these persistent signal changes and whether they indicate a higher risk of recurrence remain unknown.

A negative MR imaging does not exclude a clinically relevant muscle injury. Some studies demonstrated a discrepancy between clinical symptoms (functional injuries) and imaging (anatomic injuries). The diagnosis and clinical management are based on clinical history, examination, and imaging.[4,17]

Imaging Method: Ultrasound

Current US technology allows visualization of muscle fascicles and perimysium at a spatial resolution of less than 200 μm, which is higher than MR imaging resolution.[18] High-frequency linear probes (>10 MHz) are mainly used to visualize muscle tears. In some cases, in patients with abundant adipose tissue or thick muscle mass, low-frequency convex probes can be used. High-frequency transducers provide higher spatial resolution, which allows differentiation between distinct tissues. Therefore, at higher frequencies, there will be a greater absorption of US waves, which makes it more difficult to visualize deep tissues.[19,20] Advances in hardware and software technology, such as the use of tissue harmonic imaging, postprocessing algorithms of the returned signal, or high-frequency probes up to 20 MHz, make it possible to improve tissue contrast to better visualize muscle architecture. Extended field of view imaging allows better demonstration of large lesions.

On US, the muscle fascicles appear as hypoechogenic linear structures, and the perimysium appears as hyperechogenic strips between the fascicles (**Fig. 7**). During contraction, muscle fascicles shorten and thicken, and connective tissue remains unchanged, giving the muscle the appearance of a more hypoechogenic structure.[21]

Our imaging protocol initiates with visualization of the site of a suspected lesion (painful site suggested by anamnesis) on the long and short axes, continuing with probe movement on the muscle belly from its origin to the distal insertion. Visualization of the proximal and/or distal enthesis, myotendinous junction, and fascia is also important. Comparative assessment with the asymptomatic contralateral side may be helpful and is a great advantage of US evaluation. The tear can be dynamically detected during muscle contraction or passive mobilization to better define the extent of the injury and tear grading (**Fig. 8**). US evaluation of a muscle tear must ideally be

Table 1
Classification systems for muscle injuries

Classification System	Peetrons (2002)—US	Modified Peetrons (2012)—MR Imaging	Munich (2013)—US/MR Imaging	BAMI (2014)—MR Imaging
Grading	Grade 0: normal appearance	Grade 0: normal MR imaging	Grade 0: Normal MR imaging	Grade 0: normal MR imaging—grade 0a or characteristic MR imaging features of DOMS (grade 0b)
	Grade 1: focal/diffuse bleeding, lesions < 5% of muscle volume or cross-sectional area	Grade 1: edema without architectural distortion	Grade 1A: fatigue-induced muscle disorder—normal MR/US	Grade 1a: MR imaging HSI myofascial border: <10% extension into muscle belly, longitudinal length <5 cm
			Grade 1B: DOMS—normal US/MR or edema only	Grade 1b: MR imaging HSI < 10% of cross-sectional area of the muscle, longitudinal length < 5 cm
	Grade 2: partial rupture—lesions from 5% to 50% of the muscle volume or cross-sectional diameter	Grade 2: partial tear with architectural distortion	Grade 2A: spine-related neuromuscular disorder—normal US/MR or edema only	Grade 2a: MR imaging HSI myofascial border extending into muscle, 10%–50% of cross-sectional area of the muscle at the maximal site, longitudinal length 5–15 cm
			Grade 2B: muscle-related neuromuscular disorder—normal US/MR or edema only	Grade 2b: MR imaging intramuscular HSI, 10%–50% of muscle cross-sectional area at the maximal site, longitudinal length 5–15 cm
				Grade 2c: MR imaging HSI extends into the tendon, <50% of maximal tendon cross-sectional area, <5 cm of tendon cross-sectional area
	Grade 3: complete muscle rupture with retraction	Grade 3: complete muscle or tendon rupture	Grade 3A: minor partial muscle tear—fiber disruption on high-	Grade 3a: MR imaging HSI myofascial border, >50% of cross-sectional area at the

	resolution MR imaging. Intramuscular hematoma Grade 3B: moderate partial muscle tear—fiber disruption on US/MR, probably including some retraction, with fascial injury and intermuscular hematoma		maximal site, longitudinal length >15 cm Grade 3b: MR imaging HSI >50% of cross-sectional area of the muscle, longitudinal length >15 cm Grade 3c: MR imaging HSI extends into the tendon, >5 cm longitudinal length of tendon, >50% of cross-sectional area of tendon Grade 4: complete discontinuity of the muscle, with retraction Grade 4c: complete discontinuity of the tendon with retraction
	Grade 4: (Sub)total muscle tear/tendinous avulsion—subtotal/complete discontinuity of muscle/tendon on US/MR. Possible wavy tendon morphology and retraction. With fascial injury and intermuscular hematoma Contusion: direct injury. US/MR diffuse or circumscribed hematoma		
Anatomic site of the injury	Not defined by image	Not defined by image	a. Myofascial b. Intramuscular c. Intratendinous

Abbreviation: HIS, high signal intensity.

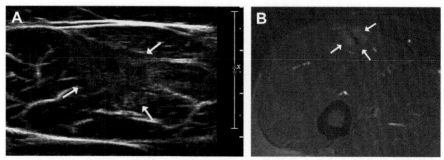

Fig. 3. Grade 1 muscle tear—US/MR correlation. A 21-year-old male soccer player with a proximal indirect injury of the thigh while training 4 days ago. (A) US transverse image of the rectus femoris demonstrates ill-defined hyperechogenicity in the myotendinous junction (*arrows*). The intramuscular tendon evaluation is difficult. (B) Axial T2-weighted fat-saturated MR imaging of the rectus femoris shows mild edema at the myotendinous junction, with normal aspect of the intramuscular tendon.

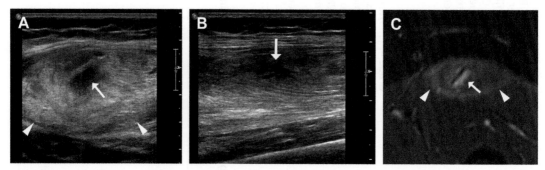

Fig. 4. Grade 2 muscle tear—US/MR correlation. A 34-year-old male soccer player with proximal indirect injury of the thigh 5 days ago. US transverse (A) and longitudinal (B) images of the proximal thigh demonstrates well-defined hyperechogenicity in the myotendinous junction of the rectus femoris (*arrowheads*) with a small anechoic area adjacent to central tendon (*arrow*), better demonstrated on the longitudinal image (*arrows*) and compatible with partial fiber detachment (grade 2 tear). (C) Axial T2-weighted fat-saturated MR imaging shows the grade 2 muscle tear surrounding the central tendon (*arrow*) with peripheral muscle edema (*arrowheads*).

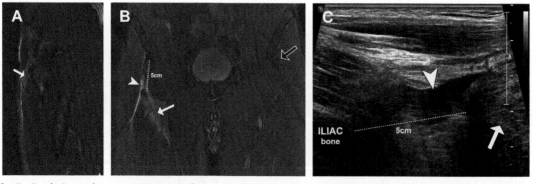

Fig. 5. Grade 3 muscle tear—US/MR correlation. Sagittal (A) and coronal (B) T2-weighted MR imaging of the right proximal thigh with fat saturation. Longitudinal US image (C) of the right thigh. A 36-year-old male soccer player with a complete proximal tear of the conjoint rectus femoris tendon at the myotendinous junction (*white arrows*) with a 5.0 cm gap from the proximal tendon origins at the pelvis with small amount of fluid (*arrowheads*). On (B) note the normal left origin of the direct tendon head of the rectus femoris (*black arrow*).

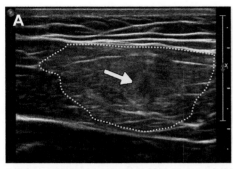
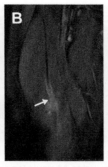
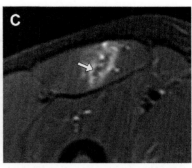

Fig. 6. Muscle tear with connective tissue involvement—US/MR correlation. US transverse image (*A*) of the right thigh depicts a tear of the intramuscular tendon of the rectus femoris (*arrow*) with associated surrounding muscle fiber disruption, represented by hyperechogenicity and loss of fibrillar pattern (*dotted line*). Coronal (*B*) and axial (*C*) T2-weighted MR imaging shows a tear of the central intramuscular tendon (*arrows*) with edema of surrounding muscle fibers.

performed 48 to 72 hours after the injury because there is a risk of false positive or tear underestimation before this time.[22]

US features of muscle injuries are loss of fascicular pattern with fiber disruption, hypoechoic and/or hyperechoic focal areas within the muscle, and focal or complete fiber discontinuity (**Fig. 9**). Usually, fiber discontinuity occurs at the myofascial junction or around the myotendinous junction; however, it can occur at any location within the muscle. After a direct or indirect tear, there is interstitial hemorrhage that appears as a hyperechoic area with poorly defined margins. In the case of high-grade tears, an intramuscular hematoma will develop, appearing as a variable echogenicity zone, depending on the time of the lesion.[23] In the acute stage (until 48 h), the hematoma seems hyperechoic (**Fig. 10**). As it undergoes progressive liquefaction and resorption, it becomes iso- and hypoechoic with internal debris (**Fig. 11**). In chronic stages, a focal hyperechoic scar may form (**Fig. 12**).

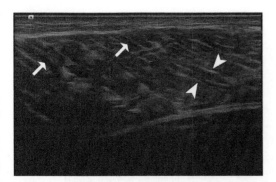

Fig. 7. Normal US of muscle fibers. US longitudinal image of the calf in an asymptomatic volunteer. The perimysium appears as hyperechoic strips (*arrowheads*) and the muscle fascicles as hypoechoic linear structures in between (*arrows*).

Power or color Doppler evaluation can demonstrate hyperemia surrounding the tear due to granulation tissue formation, which is useful in follow-ups to differentiate chronic tears from recent retears (**Fig. 13**). The hyperemia is secondary to angiogenesis surrounding the tear, appears 3 to 8 days after the injury, and disappears at approximately 12 weeks.[15] Power Doppler persistence suggests that a tear remains active; however, there is no evidence between a positive Doppler and healing and return-to-play time. Thus, clinical examination is still needed.

Imaging Method: MR Imaging

Although MR imaging does not have the same spatial resolution as US, it is more sensitive for low-grade muscle injuries (especially for deeply located muscles), has higher tissue contrast, and is more reproducible. However, US in experienced hands is comparable to MR imaging in the detection of muscle injuries.[14,24]

MR imaging's most classic feature of muscle injury is diffuse, ill-defined high signal intensity change (called "edema") on fluid-sensitive sequences. When edema is found around the musculotendinous junction, we may have the classic "feathery" appearance[25,26] (**Fig. 14**). Fiber discontinuity is seen as a focal area of well-defined high signal intensity (**Fig. 15**). A special type of tear is the rectus femoris intramuscular degloving tear,[27] in which the inner bipennate portion of the indirect musculotendinous complex is detached from the outer unipennate portion (**Fig. 16**). Muscle injuries may also occur far from the musculotendinous junction and at the peripheral myofascial junction[5] (**Figs. 17–19**). Muscle tears within the muscle belly and far from connective tissue attachments (myotendinous or myofascial junctions)

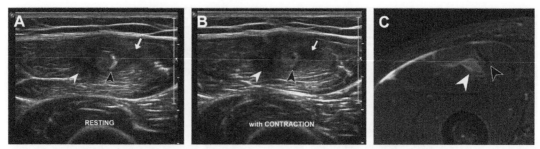

Fig. 8. Role of muscle contraction on US evaluation with MR correlation. US transverse images of the thigh resting (*A*) and with contraction (*B*) thigh muscles. Musculotendinous junction tear of the rectus femoris. The central intramuscular tendon is normal (*black arrowheads*). Ill-defined hypoechoic area adjacent to central tendon (*white arrowheads*) that, with muscle contraction, becomes anechoic, demonstrating there is fiber discontinuity. There is also another anechoic area adjacent to central tendon (*white arrows*) that increases in size with muscle contraction. Correlation with (*C*) axial T2-weighted fat suppressed MR imaging shows central tendon is normal (*black arrowhead*) and muscle fibers disruption (*white arrowhead*). The other area with fiber tears visualized with muscle contraction on US is not depicted at the MR imaging.

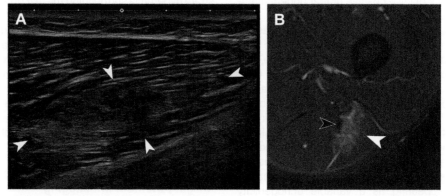

Fig. 9. Muscle tear on US with MR correlation. Soccer athlete with an injury for 4 days. US longitudinal image of the long head of the biceps femoris muscle (*A*) with musculotendinous ill-defined area of hyperechogenicity with loss of the fibrillar pattern (*white arrowheads*), indicating a muscle tear. Correlation with axial T2-weighted MR imaging with fat suppression (*B*) shows edema at the musculotendinous junction (*white arrowhead*), with normal aspect of the intramuscular tendon (*black arrowhead*).

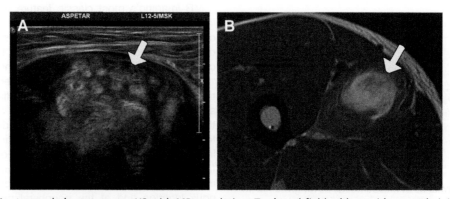

Fig. 10. Acute muscle hematoma on US with MR correlation. Track and field athlete with a muscle injury 1 day ago. US transverse image of the vastus medialis muscle (*A*)—a well-defined hyperechoic area (*arrow*) with interweaving hypoechoic areas. On the correlated axial T2-weighted MR imaging (*B*), an intramuscular hematoma is seen (*arrow*).

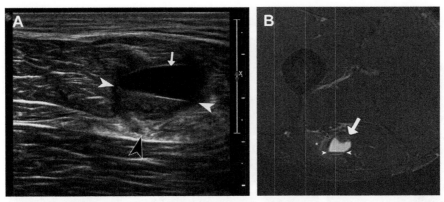

Fig. 11. Subacute muscle hematoma on US with MR correlation. Handball athlete with muscle injury 8 days ago. US transverse image of the semitendinosus muscle (*A*) shows an intramuscular anechoic fluid collection (*arrow*) with fluid-fluid level and debris (*arrowheads*), consistent with hematoma, adjacent to a normal intramuscular tendon (*black arrowhead*). Correlation with an axial T2-weighted MR imaging (*B*): intramuscular hematoma at the musculotendinous junction, adjacent to intramuscular tendon (*black arrowhead*), with fluid-fluid level (*white arrowheads*) and surrounding muscle edema (*asterisk*).

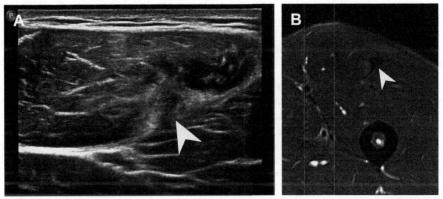

Fig. 12. Muscle scar—US/MR correlation. Soccer athlete with previous muscle injury and hematoma formation 4 months prior. US transverse image of rectus femoris (*A*) shows well-defined "triangle-shaped" tissue at the myofascial junction of the muscle (*arrowhead*). On MR imaging (*B*), the area corresponds to a fibrotic scar (*arrowhead*).

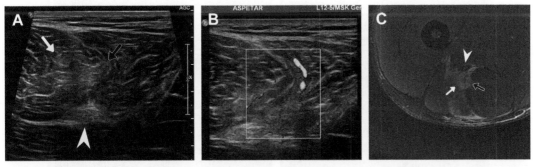

Fig. 13. Muscle tear—US Doppler/MR correlation. Soccer athlete with a muscle injury 5 days prior. US transverse image of the hamstrings (*A*): ill-defined hyperechoic area at the semitendinosus (*white arrow*) and semimembranosus (*black arrow*) muscles. Sciatic nerve is adjacent to the tear (*arrowhead*). On Power Doppler evaluation (*B*), there is Doppler signal present at the tear, indicating angiogenesis. On MR imaging (*C*), same findings are seen on the muscles, with edema surrounding the sciatic nerve (*arrowhead*).

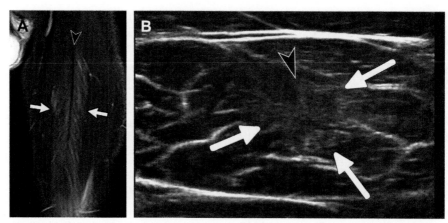

Fig. 14. Feathery appearance on MR imaging with US correlation. (*A*) Coronal T2-weighted fat-suppressed MR imaging of the thigh shows muscle fiber edema at the rectus femoris musculotendinous junction (*arrows*), surrounding the normal central tendon (*black arrowhead*). US image (*B*) shows ill-defined hyperechoic muscle tear (*arrows*) surrounding a normal central tendon (*black arrowhead*).

are very rare and mostly related to direct trauma (contusions) (**Fig. 20**).

Ultrasound or MR Imaging: Which Modality Should Be Used?

US and MR imaging offer excellent spatial and contrast resolution to perform a detailed evaluation of muscles and connective tissue. US has some advantages over MR imaging: higher spatial resolution, low cost, accessibility, fast examination, and dynamic evaluation. In addition, US can thoroughly evaluate muscle and connective tissue, which can be masked by edema on MR imaging. US is, however, less sensitive than MR imaging for low-grade muscle injuries and more operator dependent.

MR imaging is considered to be the reference method for muscle injury assessment because of its excellent contrast resolution, multiplanar spatial resolution, and especially for deep-located and proximal injuries, which are hardly accessible by US.[5,8] MR imaging also allows the evaluation of both soft tissue and bone. Some investigators consider MR imaging the examination of choice to confirm and assess the extent and severity of muscle tears. MR imaging has an important role in the follow-up of muscle tear severity and in the return-to-play evaluation, although this role remains controversial.

There is very little evidence in the literature concerning the clinical relevance of US evaluation of acute muscle injuries. It has been shown that US is less sensitive than MR imaging for diagnosis of soleus muscle tears.[28] However, studies show agreement between US and MR imaging on hamstring evaluation of acute injuries.[8,14] The location and extent of injuries described on US were associated with increased recovery times.

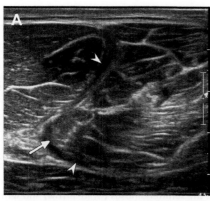
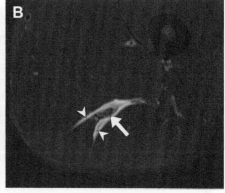

Fig. 15. Muscle fiber detachment with MR/US correlation. (*A*) Axial T2-weighted fat-suppressed MR imaging. (*B*) US transverse image shows a tear of the long head of the biceps femoris tendon (*arrows*) with muscle fiber retraction and fluid surrounding the muscle belly (*arrowheads*).

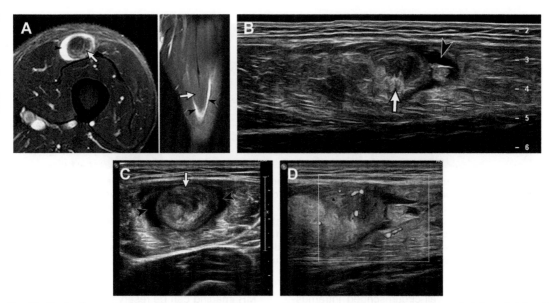

Fig. 16. Degloving rectus femoris injury with MR/US correlation. Soccer player with 1-day muscle injury. Axial and coronal T2-weighted fat-suppressed MR imaging (*A*) shows fiber detachment and retraction of inner bipennate (*arrows*) from outer unipennate portions of rectus femoris, with fluid involving the bipennate portion (*arrowheads*). A nice correlation with longitudinal (*B*) and transverse (*C*) US images is seen, with fiber detachment and retraction of the inner bipennate portion (*arrows*) and fluid surrounding the inner portion (*arrowheads*). On (*D*), there is an increase in power Doppler signal surrounding the tear.

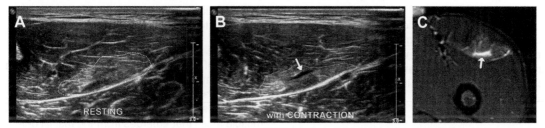

Fig. 17. Myofascial tear with US contraction and MR correlation. Muscle injury in a soccer player for 3 days. US transverse images of rectus femoris without (*A*) and with (*B*) muscle contraction. Hyperechoic area and loss of fibrillar pattern without unequivocal fiber discontinuity (*dotted lines*) at the posterior myofascial junction. After patient performs muscle contraction, a linear anechoic area of fiber discontinuity appears (*arrow*). MR correlation (*C*) shows fiber discontinuity (*arrow*) at the myofascial junction, with surrounding muscle edema.

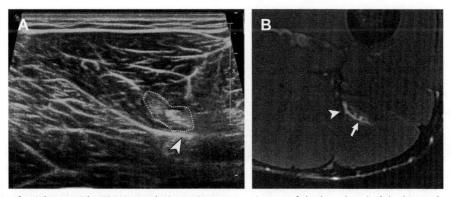

Fig. 18. Myofascial tear with MR/US correlation. US transverse image of the long head of the biceps femoris muscle (*A*) shows hyperechoic area of muscle fibers at the myofascial portion (*dotted lines*), with normal aspect of connective tissue (*arrowhead*). MR correlation (*B*) depicts fiber discontinuity with high signal intensity of the muscle fibers (*arrow*) and normal aspect of the conjoint tendon (*arrowhead*).

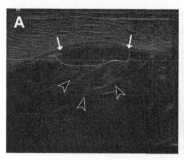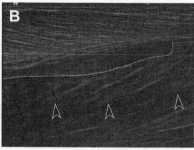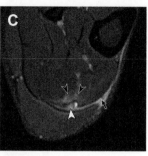

Fig. 19. Myofascial tear of the soleus/gastrocnemius complex with US/MR correlation. Marathon runner with acute muscle injury for 5 days. Transverse (*A*) and longitudinal (*B*) US images of the soleus/gastrocnemius complex show a posterior soleus fascia tear (*white arrows*) with adjacent muscle fiber hypoechogenicity of the soleus (*dotted lines*) and surrounding muscle hyperechoic ill-defined areas (*black arrowheads*), without loss of fibrillar pattern. MR correlation (*C*) shows tear of the posterior fascia of the soleus with adjacent muscle fiber disconti-nuity (*white arrowhead*) and surrounding mild muscle edema (*black arrowheads*). There is small amount of fluid in the intermuscular space with the medial gastrocnemius (*black arrow*).

In the case of a well-circumscribed intramus-cular hematoma, US-guided aspiration can be performed, followed by compression to avoid or minimize the recurrence of the hematoma. Fluid aspiration may decrease healing time, prevent the occurrence of a hypertrophic scar, and limit the appearance of calcifications and ossifications.[24,29]

If clinical diagnosis is evident and the lesion is of low clinical grade, no imaging study is warranted. In case of clinical doubt with a more advanced injury or to aspirate a hematoma, the US will ideally confirm within 2 or 3 days. It is particularly effective for superficial tears.

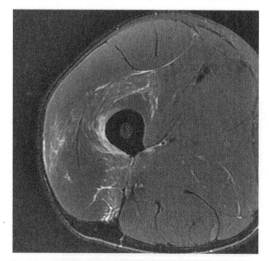

Fig. 20. Muscle contusion. Soccer player with a direct muscle injury at the lateral aspect of the thigh for 5 days. Axial T2-weighted MR imaging with fat sup-pression shows ill-defined diffuse muscle edema at the vastus lateralis and intermedius muscles without connective tissue injury.

MR imaging can be reserved for the evaluation of a muscle injury in these situations: high-performance professional athletes (because of financial and logistic reasons), for potentially surgi-cal indications (eg, complete tendinous ruptures); in case of chronic pain, for differential diagnosis with other nontraumatic conditions; and to over-come US limitations on muscle injury evaluation (deep located and proximal muscle groups).

Muscle herniation

Rupture of the muscle fascia can occur with consequent herniation of the muscle in the subcu-taneous tissue.[30] This type of muscle injury is especially seen with dynamic US evaluation as a muscle mass that emerges from the fascial defect during contraction.[31] On MR imaging, there is a protuberant mass with normal muscle signal and architecture. The fascia defect can be identified if the hernia is large enough and if there is sufficient contrast with the subcutaneous fatty tissue (**Fig. 21**).

Morel–Lavallée lesion

The potential consequence of high-energy trauma is a Morel–Lavallée lesion. This condition is caused by the detachment of the fascia from the overlying subcutaneous tissue by excess shear stress with a consequent accumulation of hemolymphatic fluid collection that classically occurs in the lateral aspect of the proximal thigh and knee.[32,33]

Morel–Lavallée lesions can be easily identified through US or MR imaging.[34–36] On US, a hypere-choic (acute phase) or anechoic (subacute phase) compressible collection at the interface between subcutaneous fat at muscle fascia was observed. On MR imaging, the lesion has a heterogeneous T2 signal in the acute phase and a T2 hypersignal signal in the subacute phase (**Fig. 22**). Contours

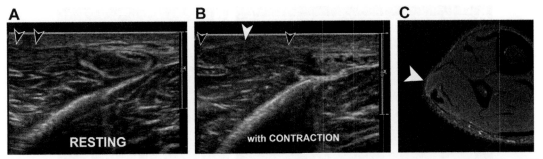

Fig. 21. Muscle herniation—US/MR correlation. Transverse US images of the peroneus longus muscle without (A) and with (B) muscle contraction. Discontinuity of the superficial muscle fascia (*black arrowheads*) with herniation of muscle tissue toward the subcutaneous fat during muscle contraction (*white arrowhead*). Axial MR T2-weighted fat suppressed MR imaging (C) performed with plantar flexion shows the fascial rupture with muscle herniation (*white arrowhead*).

are ill defined in the acute phase and better delimitated as the lesion becomes subacute and chronic. US-guided aspiration can be performed to decrease the volume of fluid collection; however, recurrence is very common due to the impossibility of performing a compression bandage on the pelvis and the highly exudative nature of this lesion.[37]

Delayed-onset muscle soreness
DOMS is an overuse muscle injury related to unusual, prolonged, or very intense physical activity, with progressive pain developing 24 to 72 hours after a specific activity. It is considered a less severe muscle injury because the fibers are not torn and is related to edematous infiltration. Symptoms usually resolve in 7 to 14 days.

MR imaging signs are similar to a grade 0 or 1 injury with patchy or diffuse muscle edema on fluid-sensitive sequences and may present an increase in muscle volume. Different from low-grade muscle tears, there is no "feathery" appearance on DOMS.[38]

On US, there is diffuse hyperechogenicity, muscle volume increase, and hyperemia on color or power Doppler, with preserved muscle fiber architecture[39] (**Fig. 23**).

Chronic exertional compartment syndrome
Chronic exertional compartment syndrome (CECS) is characterized by chronic and recurrent pain induced by physical activity, usually in athletes, related to an increase in intramuscular pressures with a decrease in muscle perfusion and ischemic pain. Pain develops in a muscle compartment after the start of exercise and usually decreases with rest.[40] The gold standard for the diagnosis of CECS is the measurement of intracompartmental pressure, with an increase in pressure after exercise initiation.[41] However, this is an invasive procedure in which a needle is introduced in the affected muscle compartment.

Imaging, especially MR imaging, can be performed to diagnose CECS.[42,43] Our protocol is composed of MR acquisition before and immediately after exercise. After initial MR acquisition,

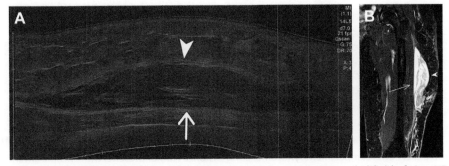

Fig. 22. Morel-Lavallée—US/MR correlation. High-energy trauma in a cyclist. Extended field of view US image (A) shows a hypoechoic fluid collection at the interface between deep subcutaneous tissue (*arrowhead*) and muscle fascia (*arrow*). MR correlation (B) demonstrates the same findings, consistent with a Morel-Lavallée lesion. (*Courtesy of* Dr. Marcos Felippe de Paula Correa, M.D., Sao Paulo, Brazil.)

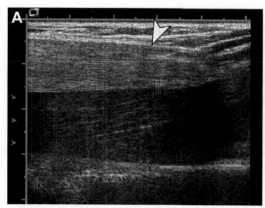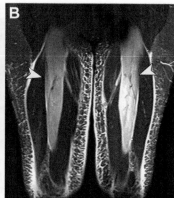

Fig. 23. Delayed-onset muscle soreness (DOMS)—US/MR correlation. Pain at the posterior thigh 3 days after gym workout. Longitudinal US image of the semitendinosus muscle (*A*) with diffuse complete muscle hyperechogenicity with preserved fibrillar pattern (*arrowhead*). MR imaging correlation (*B*) shows bilateral diffuse complete semitendinosus muscle edema (*arrowheads*).

we ask the patient to perform the same exercise responsible for the onset of pain in our training facility (close to MR imaging magnet) and to stop when pain develops. Usually, there is a progressive increase in the T2 signal on the affected muscle compartment after exercise. An increase in muscle T2 values of 20% before and after exercise is considered positive for CECS. T2 mapping is useful to quantify the increase in T2 values[44] (**Fig. 24**).

US is less sensitive than MR for CECS assessment and can demonstrate an increase in muscle volume after exercise. Doppler US is usually not useful in the diagnosis of CECS.[45]

Calcifications and Myositis Ossificans

A muscle tear may evolve to intramuscular calcifications or myositis ossificans. Calcifications most frequently occur after direct muscle injury or are associated with neuromuscular diseases.[30,46]

Myositis ossificans can be intramuscular or periosteal and are not associated with any previous history of muscle tears in 40% of cases.[30] In the inflammatory phase, there is an inordinate proliferation of stem cells that causes intramuscular peripheral marginal bone proliferation, usually 2 to 4 weeks after injury. On US, 3 concentric zones are described: a peripheral hypoechoic zone that surrounds the lesion, a middle hyperechoic zone that corresponds to the calcifying front, and a central hypoechoic zone that corresponds to the central fibroblastic stroma.[47] In the inflammatory phase, MR imaging also demonstrates a peripheral hypersignal and well-defined zone with surrounding ill-defined muscle edema and may be mistaken for a sarcoma or muscle abscess in this phase. US and plain radiographs/computed

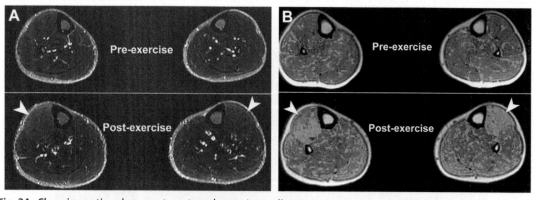

Fig. 24. Chronic exertional compartment syndrome. Long-distance runner presents with chronic anterior leg pain after 5 to 10 km running. (*A*) Axial T2-weighted fat-suppressed MR imaging with (*B*) T2-mapping acquisition of both legs performed before and after exercise (patient was asked to run in a treadmill and to stop when pain develops). After exercising, there is increase of volume and T2 signal on extensor muscle compartments bilaterally (*arrowheads*), consistent with chronic exertional compartment syndrome.

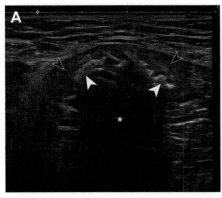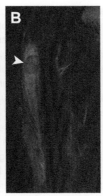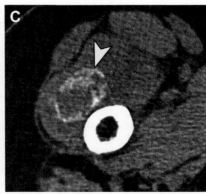

Fig. 25. Myositis ossificans—US/MR/CT correlation. (*A*) Axial US image of vastus lateralis muscle demonstrates intramuscular echogenic structure (*white arrowheads*) with posterior acoustic shadowing (*), consistent with muscle calcification or ossification. There is hypoechogenicity of muscle fibers surrounding the ossification (*black arrowheads*). (*B*) Coronal T2-weighted MR imaging with fat suppression of the thigh shows an intramuscular round nodule with intermediate signal and a rim of low signal (*white arrowhead*) with significant surrounding muscle edema. (*C*) Axial computed tomography (CT) image of the thigh confirms an intramuscular ossification (*white arrowhead*), consistent with myositis ossificans.

tomography may be useful to show peripheral ossification. Imaging methods show a centripetal evolution and a peripheral edge of ossification that progresses toward the center. On US, ossification seems as a hyperechogenic structure with posterior acoustic shadowing (**Fig. 25**).

Retears

Muscle tear recurrence may be an injury that does not progress properly within the usual timeframe or a repetitive lesion favored by too early resumption of physical activity, insufficient rehabilitation, incomplete recovery, or poor healing. Recurrence rates vary from 9% to 44%.[4,17,48,49] Scar tissue has elasticity and stiffness properties different from those of normal tissue and may increase the risk for retear; however, this remains controversial.

Return to Play

It is controversial whether imaging methods can predict the return-to-play time. It has been shown that a negative MR imaging is a good prognostic factor, and the return-to-play time is 7 to 10 days after the injury.[17] In the case of a positive MR imaging, there is no sufficient evidence to predict a return-to-play time. It seems that high-grade injuries have a longer recovery time than low-grade injuries, and an injury affecting the connective tissue has a worse prognosis than a lesion affecting only the muscle fibers; however, less biased studies with larger case series are warranted to confirm this.

SUMMARY

In summary, US and MR imaging are important tools for evaluation of muscle injuries and have good correlation with each other. Although it is controversial whether imaging studies can provide prognostic information, injuries extending to intramuscular connective tissue are associated with longer recovery and return-to-play times and must be described by the radiologist in the reports.

CLINICS CARE POINTS

- Muscle injuries can be myofascial, musculotendinous, or intratendinous.
- Intratendinous tears have a longer recovery time.
- US is less sensitive than MR imaging for low-grade muscle injuries and more operator dependent.
- MR imaging is indicated for the evaluation of a muscle injury in high-performance professional athletes, for potentially surgical indications, differential diagnosis with other nontraumatic conditions, and deep located and proximal muscle groups.

DISCLOSURE

The authors have nothing to disclose.

REFERENCES

1. Ekstrand J, Hägglund M, Waldén M. Epidemiology of muscle injuries in professional football (soccer). Am J Sports Med 2011;39(6):1226–32.

2. Junge A, Engebretsen L, Mountjoy ML, et al. Sports injuries during the Summer Olympic Games 2008. Am J Sports Med 2009;37(11):2165–72.

3. Elliott MC, Zarins B, Powell JW, et al. Hamstring muscle strains in professional football players: a 10-year review. Am J Sports Med 2011;39(4):843–50.

4. Ekstrand J, Healy JC, Waldén M, et al. Hamstring muscle injuries in professional football: the correlation of MRI findings with return to play. Br J Sports Med 2012;46(2):112–7.

5. Crema MD, Yamada AF, Guermazi A, et al. Imaging techniques for muscle injury in sports medicine and clinical relevance. Curr Rev Musculoskelet Med 2015;8(2):154–61.

6. Muraoka T, Muramatsu T, Fukunaga T, et al. Elastic properties of human Achilles tendon are correlated to muscle strength. J Appl Physiol (1985) 2005; 99(2):665–9.

7. Mueller-Wohlfahrt HW, Haensel L, Mithoefer K, et al. Terminology and classification of muscle injuries in sport: the Munich consensus statement. Br J Sports Med 2013;47(6):342–50.

8. Connell DA, Schneider-Kolsky ME, Hoving JL, et al. Longitudinal study comparing sonographic and MRI assessments of acute and healing hamstring injuries. AJR Am J Roentgenol 2004;183(4):975–84.

9. Pollock N, James SL, Lee JC, et al. British athletics muscle injury classification: a new grading system. Br J Sports Med 2014;48(18):1347–51.

10. Peetrons P. Ultrasound of muscles. Eur Radiol 2002; 12(1):35–43.

11. Valle X, Alentorn-Geli E, Tol JL, et al. Muscle Injuries in Sports: A New Evidence-Informed and Expert Consensus-Based Classification with Clinical Application. Sports Med 2017;47(7):1241–53.

12. Comin J, Malliaras P, Baquie P, et al. Return to competitive play after hamstring injuries involving disruption of the central tendon. Am J Sports Med 2013;41(1):111–5.

13. Pollock N, Patel A, Chakraverty J, et al. Time to return to full training is delayed and recurrence rate is higher in intratendinous ('c') acute hamstring injury in elite track and field athletes: clinical application of the British Athletics Muscle Injury Classification. Br J Sports Med 2016;50(5):305–10.

14. Renoux J, Brasseur JL, Wagner M, et al. Ultrasound-detected connective tissue involvement in acute muscle injuries in elite athletes and return to play: The French National Institute of Sports (INSEP) study. J Sci Med Sport 2019;22(6):641–6.

15. Yoshida K, Itoigawa Y, Maruyama Y, et al. Healing Process of Gastrocnemius Muscle Injury on Ultrasonography Using B-Mode Imaging, Power Doppler Imaging, and Shear Wave Elastography. J Ultrasound Med 2019;38(12):3239–46.

16. Hayashi D, Hamilton B, Guermazi A, et al. Traumatic injuries of thigh and calf muscles in athletes: role and clinical relevance of MR imaging and ultrasound. Insights Imaging Dec 2012;3(6):591–601.

17. Ekstrand J, Askling C, Magnusson H, et al. Return to play after thigh muscle injury in elite football players: implementation and validation of the Munich muscle injury classification. Br J Sports Med 2013;47(12):769–74.

18. Sconfienza LM, Albano D, Allen G, et al. Clinical indications for musculoskeletal ultrasound updated in 2017 by European Society of Musculoskeletal Radiology (ESSR) consensus. Eur Radiol Dec 2018; 28(12):5338–51.

19. Entrekin RR, Porter BA, Sillesen HH, et al. Real-time spatial compound imaging: application to breast, vascular, and musculoskeletal ultrasound. Semin Ultrasound CT MR 2001;22(1):50–64.

20. Woodhouse JB, McNally EG. Ultrasound of skeletal muscle injury: an update. Semin Ultrasound CT MR 2011;32(2):91–100.

21. Reeves ND, Narici MV. Behavior of human muscle fascicles during shortening and lengthening contractions in vivo. J Appl Physiol (1985) 2003;95(3): 1090–6.

22. Drakonaki EE, Sudoł-Szopińska I, Sinopidis C, et al. High resolution ultrasound for imaging complications of muscle injury: Is there an additional role for elastography? J Ultrason 2019;19(77):137–44.

23. Chang KV, Wu WT, Özçakar L. Ultrasound Imaging and Rehabilitation of Muscle Disorders: Part 1. Traumatic Injuries. Am J Phys Med Rehabil 2019;98(12): 1133–41.

24. Brasseur J-L, Renoux J. Ecographie du muscle. Echographie musculosquelettique. Montpellier, France: Sauramps Medicale; 2016. p. 294.

25. De Smet AA, Best TM. MR imaging of the distribution and location of acute hamstring injuries in athletes. AJR Am J Roentgenol 2000;174(2):393–9.

26. Boutin RD, Fritz RC, Steinbach LS. Imaging of sports-related muscle injuries. Radiol Clin North Am 2002;40(2):333–62, vii.

27. Kassarjian A, Rodrigo RM, Santisteban JM. Intramuscular degloving injuries to the rectus femoris: findings at MRI. AJR Am J Roentgenol 2014; 202(5):W475–80.

28. Balius R, Rodas G, Pedret C, et al. Soleus muscle injury: sensitivity of ultrasound patterns. Skeletal Radiol 2014;43(6):805–12.

29. Hall MM. Return to Play After Thigh Muscle Injury: Utility of Serial Ultrasound in Guiding Clinical Progression. Curr Sports Med Rep 2018;17(9):296–301.

30. Flores DV, Mejía Gómez C, Estrada-Castrillón M, et al. MR Imaging of Muscle Trauma: Anatomy, Biomechanics, Pathophysiology, and Imaging Appearance. Radiographics 2018;38(1):124–48.

31. Bianchi S, Abdelwahab IF, Mazzola CG, et al. Sonographic examination of muscle herniation. J Ultrasound Med 1995;14(5):357–60.

32. Parra JA, Fernandez MA, Encinas B, et al. Morel-Lavallée effusions in the thigh. Skeletal Radiol 1997;26(4):239–41.

33. Singh R, Rymer B, Youssef B, et al. The Morel-Lavallée lesion and its management: A review of the literature. J Orthop 2018;15(4):917–21.

34. Gilbert BC, Bui-Mansfield LT, Dejong S. MRI of a Morel-Lavallée lesion. AJR Am J Roentgenol 2004; 182(5):1347–8.

35. Mellado JM, Bencardino JT. Morel-Lavallée lesion: review with emphasis on MR imaging. Magn Reson Imaging Clin N Am 2005;13(4):775–82.

36. Mukherjee K, Perrin SM, Hughes PM. Morel-Lavallee lesion in an adolescent with ultrasound and MRI correlation. Skeletal Radiol 2007;36(Suppl 1):S43–5.

37. McLean K, Popovic S. Morel-Lavallée Lesion: AIRP Best Cases in Radiologic-Pathologic Correlation. Radiographics 2017;37(1):190–6.

38. Evans GF, Haller RG, Wyrick PS, et al. Submaximal delayed-onset muscle soreness: correlations between MR imaging findings and clinical measures. Radiology 1998;208(3):815–20.

39. Longo V, Jacobson JA, Fessell DP, et al. Ultrasound Findings of Delayed-Onset Muscle Soreness. J Ultrasound Med 2016;35(11):2517–21.

40. Edwards PH, Wright ML, Hartman JF. A practical approach for the differential diagnosis of chronic leg pain in the athlete. Am J Sports Med 2005; 33(8):1241–9.

41. van den Brand JG, Nelson T, Verleisdonk EJ, et al. The diagnostic value of intracompartmental pressure measurement, magnetic resonance imaging, and near-infrared spectroscopy in chronic exertional compartment syndrome: a prospective study in 50 patients. Am J Sports Med 2005;33(5):699–704.

42. Ringler MD, Litwiller DV, Felmlee JP, et al. MRI accurately detects chronic exertional compartment syndrome: a validation study. Skeletal Radiol 2013; 42(3):385–92.

43. Verleisdonk EJ, van Gils A, van der Werken C. The diagnostic value of MRI scans for the diagnosis of chronic exertional compartment syndrome of the lower leg. Skeletal Radiol 2001;30(6):321–5.

44. Guermazi A, Roemer FW, Robinson P, et al. Imaging of Muscle Injuries in Sports Medicine: Sports Imaging Series. Radiology 2017;285(3):1063.

45. Rajasekaran S, Beavis C, Aly AR, et al. The utility of ultrasound in detecting anterior compartment thickness changes in chronic exertional compartment syndrome: a pilot study. Clin J Sport Med 2013; 23(4):305–11.

46. Simon T, Guillodo Y, Madouas G, et al. Myositis ossificans traumatica (circumscripta) and return to sport: A retrospective series of 19 cases. Joint Bone Spine 2016;83(4):416–20.

47. Walczak BE, Johnson CN, Howe BM. Myositis Ossificans. J Am Acad Orthop Surg 2015;23(10):612–22.

48. Reurink G, Goudswaard GJ, Tol JL, et al. MRI observations at return to play of clinically recovered hamstring injuries. Br J Sports Med 2014;48(18): 1370–6.

49. Askling CM, Tengvar M, Saartok T, et al. Acute first-time hamstring strains during high-speed running: a longitudinal study including clinical and magnetic resonance imaging findings. Am J Sports Med 2007;35(2):197–206.

Peripheral Nerve Imaging
Magnetic Resonance and Ultrasound Correlation

Swati Deshmukh, MD[a,*], Kevin Sun, MD[a], Aparna Komarraju, MD[a], Adam Singer, MD[b], Jim S. Wu, MD[a]

KEYWORDS

• Peripheral nerve • Neuropathy • MRI • Ultrasound

KEY POINTS

- Peripheral nerves are susceptible to a variety of pathologic conditions including infection/inflammation, trauma, tumors, and metabolic/toxic conditions.
- Magnetic resonance (MR) imaging of peripheral nerves, or MR neurography, requires high-resolution imaging ideally performed on a 3-T magnet.
- Ultrasound imaging of peripheral nerves is ideally performed with high-resolution probes (18–24+ MHz) in the transverse and longitudinal planes.

INTRODUCTION

With advances in imaging technology, peripheral nerves can be visualized on both magnetic resonance (MR) imaging and ultrasound (US). Peripheral nerves, or nerves outside of the brain and spinal cord, are susceptible to a variety of pathologic conditions, including infection/inflammation, trauma, tumors, and metabolic/toxic conditions. Damage to peripheral nerves can result in sensory and/or motor symptoms, and if not treated, may be irreversible. Imaging complements clinical physical examination and electrodiagnostic testing and aids in the diagnosis of peripheral nerve pathologic condition, characterization of the degree of nerve injury, and assessment for end-organ damage. In some cases, imaging may play a role in preoperative planning and postoperative assessment.[1–11] Appropriate choice of imaging modality and correct imaging technique is important for ensuring optimized peripheral nerve evaluation.[12–16] This article reviews peripheral nerve imaging with attention to MR and US correlation.

PERIPHERAL NERVE ANATOMY

Peripheral nerves comprise individual axons enclosed in a layer of connective tissue termed the endoneurium. The neuronal axon is the fundamental conducting unit of a nerve and may be myelinated to allow faster conduction. Groups of axons are bundled to form fascicles and are held together by an arrangement of connective tissues termed the perineurium. Fascicles, in turn, are enclosed in a third connective tissue layer, the epineurium, that functions to protect and support the nerve. The epineurium and interfascicular connective tissues allow for mechanical adaptation of peripheral nerves. Peripheral nerves can range in size, depending on the number of fascicles within the nerve; larger nerves have more fascicles and thicker layers of connective tissue. A network of vessels coursing along and through the connective tissue layers provides vascular supply to the nerve.[2,3] The unique anatomy of peripheral nerves allows for a distinct appearance on imaging (Fig. 1). Normal fascicular architecture has a

No commercial or financial conflicts of interest.
No funding sources.
[a] Harvard Medical School, Beth Israel Deaconess Medical Center, 330 Brookline Avenue, Boston, MA 02215, USA; [b] Radiology Partners/Northside Radiology Associates
* Corresponding author.
E-mail address: sdeshmuk@bidmc.harvard.edu

Magn Reson Imaging Clin N Am 31 (2023) 181–191
https://doi.org/10.1016/j.mric.2023.01.003

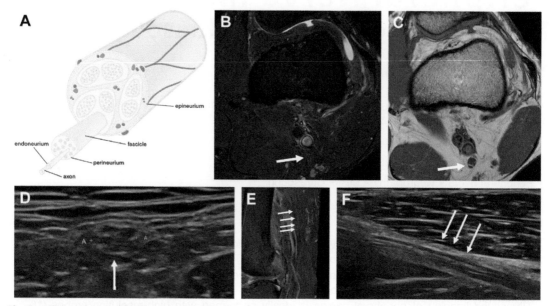

Fig. 1. MR imaging and high-resolution US of peripheral nerves. (*A*) Peripheral nerve anatomy (original artwork by Allison Wu). The fascicular architecture of peripheral nerves (*arrows*) creates a unique honeycomb appearance in the orthogonal plane on (*B, C*) axial STIR and T1-weighted MR, and (*D*) transverse US. In the parallel plane, a tubular appearance with linear tracks corresponding to fascicular bundles (*arrows*) can be identified on (*E*) sagittal STIR MR and (*F*) longitudinal US.

"honeycomb" appearance in the cross-sectional plane. In the longitudinal plane, the "tracks" of individual fascicles can be seen. In cases of nerve pathologic condition, the expected fascicular architecture may be disrupted.

PERIPHERAL NERVE PATHOLOGIC CONDITION

Peripheral neuropathy can result in various motor and/or sensory symptoms, depending on the nerve involved, and can lead to pain, weakness, and numbness. If left untreated, symptoms may be progressive and the damage irreversible. Approximately 2% to 7% of the total population in the United States is affected by peripheral neuropathy.[2] There are many potential causes of peripheral neuropathy, including congenital and hereditary disorders (ie, Charcot-Marie-Tooth disease), inflammatory/infectious conditions (poliomyelitis, leprosy, Guillian-Barre syndrome), trauma/iatrogenic nerve injury (nerve laceration, stretching, traction injury), neoplasms (schwannoma, malignant peripheral nerve sheath tumor, non-nerve-origin tumors causing mass effect on or encasement of an adjacent nerve), and metabolic/toxic conditions (diabetes mellitus, radiation, lead poisoning). Nerve injury may be focal (ie, penetrating traumatic injury) or diffuse (ie, chronic inflammatory demyelinating polyneuropathy) and can involve one or many nerves.[1,2]

Initial clinical evaluation of peripheral nerve pathologic condition entails taking a complete medical history, performing a physical examination, and obtaining general laboratory tests as indicated based on the suspected cause of neuropathy. Electrodiagnostic testing (nerve conduction studies, electromyography) may be performed to help identify the location and degree of a peripheral nerve lesion, help to identify the number of types of nerves involved, and help to formulate a differential diagnosis. Imaging plays a supplemental role in the diagnostic workup of peripheral neuropathy and can be helpful for assessing site, cause, and severity of nerve injury, extent of muscle denervation, and preoperative planning.[1,2] Prior studies have demonstrated the positive impact of MR neurography on treatment planning and surgical decision making.[2] Both MR and US imaging can aid in early detection of nerve pathologic condition, allowing for appropriate treatment and prevention of long-term disabilities (**Fig. 2**).

Recently, a multi-institutional expert consensus classification and grading system for peripheral neuropathy on MR imaging has been developed: the Neuropathy Score Reporting and Data System (NS-RADS).[2,14] NS-RADS categories for nerve lesion description on MR neurography include the folowing: NS-RADS I for nerve injuries, NS-RADS N for neoplasia, NS-RADS E

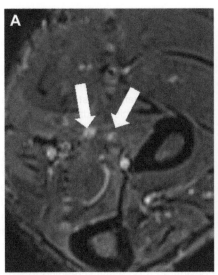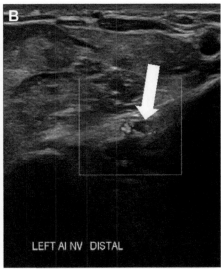

Fig. 2. MR imaging and US correlation of peripheral neuropathy. (*A*) Axial STIR MR image demonstrates signal hyperintensity of the anterior interosseous nerve and to a lesser extent the median nerve at the level of the pronator teres (*arrows*). (*B*) High-resolution US demonstrated enlargement and hypoechogenicity of the anterior interosseous nerve (*arrow*). Doppler imaging confirms adjacent vessel. Findings are compatible with neuropathy of the anterior interosseous nerve. The patient was taken to surgery where fibrous bands compressing the nerve were released. The patient's symptoms improved after surgery.

for entrapment neuropathy, NS-RADS D for diffuse nerve lesions, and NS-RADS PI for postintervention imaging. Additional categories include NS-RADS NOS (not otherwise specified) for unclear or unavailable clinical history, NS-RADS 0 for incomplete imaging, and NS-RADS U for unremarkable or normal nerve appearance. Last, NS-RADS M and M-NOS are included for classification of regional muscle findings. This consensus classification scheme allows for standardized reporting and grading of nerve injury on MR imaging.[2,14]

IMAGING TECHNIQUES
MR Imaging

MR imaging of peripheral nerves, or MR neurography, requires high-resolution imaging in order to evaluate small peripheral nerves. Ideally, MR neurography is performed on a 3-T magnet, and newer MR machines often provide optimized imaging. In some cases, however, imaging on a 1.5-T magnet may be preferred, such as in the presence of adjacent hardware in order to minimize susceptibility artifact. Of note, however, newer machines may have artifact suppression techniques that overcome the 1.5-T advantage while allowing for faster imaging and more signal. To ensure high signal-to-noise ratios and high-quality contrast imaging, multichannel flexible surface coils or joint-specific coils should be used.[2]

Standard neurography protocols include multiplanar 2-dimensional (matrix, >256; in-plane resolution, 0.2–0.8 mm) T1-weighted and T2-weighted fat-suppressed or short tau inversion recovery (STIR) sequences. T1-weighted images are important for anatomic delineation to assess peripheral nerves as well as for the evaluation of muscle size and potential fatty infiltration. T2-weighted fat-suppressed or STIR images are important for the assessment of nerve signal intensity. Slice thickness is ideally kept thin (2.5–3.5 mm with 0%–10% gap) but can be thicker (4–5 mm) as needed, such as for large coverage areas in the extremities. The field of view should include coverage of the entire area of concern of nerve injury, and if possible, associated muscles downstream from the injury site to assess for denervation changes. A plane orthogonal to the nerve's longitudinal course is necessary, which is typically the axial plane for extremities and the sagittal plane for the brachial plexus. Additional sagittal and coronal plane imaging is often obtained.[2]

Several 3-dimensional (3D) sequences are available and may be helpful for optimized nerve evaluation, particularly for smaller nerves and nerve branches. Generally, 3D STIR is best for brachial and lumbosacral plexus imaging, whereas 3D reverse fast imaging with steady-state free precession (PSIF) can be used for the extremities and pelvis (ie, pudendal nerve).[2,3,12] A postcontrast 3D STIR sampling perfection with

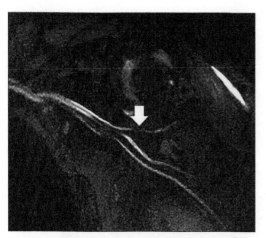

Fig. 3. 3D contrast-enhanced vascular suppression MR neurography. Coronal postcontrast SPACE STIR image in a patient presenting with persistent arm pain and weakness after a shoulder dislocation event demonstrates an area of paucity of signal within the axillary nerve (*arrow*). The patient was taken to surgery and was found to have a corresponding area of severe scarring of the axillary nerve, which ultimately required several nerve transfers to regain function.

application-optimized contrasts using different flip angle evolution (SPACE) sequence can be particularly helpful for brachial plexus imaging; contrast is used for vascular/background suppression, which aids visualization of small nerve branches (**Fig. 3**).[12] Multiplanar reconstruction of 3D images can facilitate depiction of peripheral nerves along their course.[1] Indications for intravenous contrast use in MR neurography include tumor assessment and evaluation of certain inflammatory conditions, such as acute and chronic inflammatory demyelinating polyneuropathy.[1,13] Otherwise, intravenous contrast is generally not necessary for the majority of MR neurography studies.[13] Diffusion-weighted imaging with apparent diffusion coefficient (ADC) maps is helpful for assessment of nerve tumors. Diffusion tensor imaging, although not widely used clinically, can be performed for tractography of larger peripheral nerves and fractional anisotropy measurements.[2,4]

Ultrasound

US is a noninvasive, low-cost imaging modality that is well tolerated by most patients.[3,17–19] US imaging of peripheral nerves should be performed with high-resolution probes (18–24 MHz), which can assess even small peripheral nerve branches measuring as little as 0.1 mm in size.[4] Higher-resolution probes come at the cost of reduced penetration, and in larger patients, lower-resolution (12–14 MHz) imaging may be

necessary. Ultra-high-resolution US (48+ MHz) can be used for small superficial nerves (**Fig. 4**).

Optimal patient positioning is important. Imaging should be obtained in both the transverse and the longitudinal planes and should include the entire area of concern of nerve injury as well as both proximal and distal to the primary site of injury. Sonographic evaluation of associated muscles can be performed to assess for chronic denervation changes. In some cases, dynamic US imaging may be indicated, such as to evaluate for subluxation of the ulnar nerve at the level of the cubital tunnel.[3,5,9,10] For very small peripheral nerves, doppler imaging may be helpful for differentiating nerves and vessels.[18] US can also be used for needle guidance for perineural injections and nerve biopsy.[3,19] In some cases without definitive electrodiagnostic localization, US can be considered a potential screening tool prior to MR imaging. US shear wave elastography of peripheral nerves, although not widely used clinically, is an emerging area of interest.[17]

IMAGING FINDINGS

On MR imaging, normal peripheral nerves are isointense to slightly hyperintense to muscle with preserved fascicular architecture. On US, normal peripheral nerves demonstrate isoechoic to hypoechoic fascicles surrounded by a hyperechoic epineurium.[2,18,19] Peripheral nerves are typically similar in size or smaller than the accompanying artery.[1] Both MR imaging and US can diagnose neuropathy. Abnormal nerve findings on imaging include change in size (enlarged or compressed), signal hyperintensity, or hypoechogenicity, disruption of fascicular architecture, change in course, nerve discontinuity, and mass lesion.[2,18,19] Secondary findings of nerve pathologic condition include muscle changes for motor nerves. In the early phase immediately after nerve damage ensues, innervated muscles appear normal on MR imaging. In the subacute phase, muscle edema is seen, detectable on MR imaging earlier than muscle changes on electrodiagnostic studies. In the chronic phase, denervated muscles demonstrate fatty infiltration and atrophy.[3,4] Sonographic evaluation of associated muscles may reflect hyperechogenicity and atrophy in cases of chronic muscle denervation. With US, comparison to the contralateral side may be helpful for evaluation of both nerve and muscle pathologic condition.[3,4,9,10] MR imaging and US findings of nerve pathologic condition are summarized in **Table 1**.

Nerve Injury

The severity of nerve injury on MR imaging follows clinical grading systems, including the Seddon

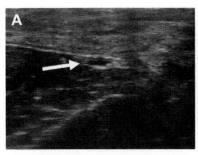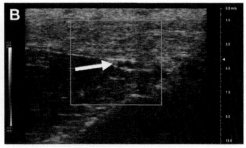

Fig. 4. Ultra-high-resolution US (Vevo Ultrasound, FUJIFILM VisualSonics. 21919 30th DR SEBothell, WA; 48 MHz). (*A*) Gray-scale and (*B*) color US images demonstrate thickening, hypoechogenicity, and fascicular enlargement of the superficial peroneal nerve (*arrow*) in a patient with chronic pain along the anterolateral lower leg, compatible with neuropathy.

and Sunderland classification schemes.[11] Grades 1 to 3 represent stretch injuries; grade 4 demonstrates a neuroma in continuity, and grade 5 reflects complete nerve discontinuity with a demonstrated nerve gap. Grade 1 injury manifests on imaging as nerve signal hyperintensity on MR imaging. Grade 2 and 3 nerve injuries can be seen on both MR imaging and US as change in signal intensity/echogenicity, nerve enlargement, and loss of normal fascicular architecture. Grade 4 injuries, or neuromas in continuity with the nerve, can be measured on both MR imaging and US. Similarly, the nerve gap in grade 5 injury can be measured on both MR imaging and US when the nerve is imaged along its longitudinal course.[2,18,19]

Nerve Tumors

In the NS-RADS classification scheme, neoplasia grading is based on suspicion of aggressiveness on MR imaging. Grades 1 to 4 reflect definitely benign, possibly benign, possibly malignant, and postoperative changes with recurrent tumor. Examples of benign nerve tumors include neural fibrolipoma, intraneural ganglion cyst, perineurioma, neurofibroma, and schwannoma. On both MR imaging and US, there should be no evidence of suspicious features, such as internal necrosis, rapid growth over time, or irregular margins, and ADC should be greater than 1.1 mm²/s on MR.[2] US can be helpful for differentiating schwannomas and neurofibromas, as a nerve eccentrically entering a mass is suggestive of schwannoma, whereas neurofibromas disrupt the normal fascicular architecture.[19] Examples of malignant nerve tumors include malignant peripheral nerve sheath tumor, lymphoma, leukemia, and metastasis. Imaging findings suspicious for malignancy include peritumoral edema, necrosis, hemorrhage, rapid growth, and heterogeneous enhancement and ADC < 1.1 mm²/s on MR imaging.[2,18,19]

Nerve Entrapment

Nerve entrapment can be categorized as mild, moderate, or severe. Entrapment can occur within an anatomic tunnel, such as the median nerve at the carpal tunnel, or secondary to an adjacent lesion, such as a ganglion cyst or hematoma. Fibrous bands, anomalous muscles, and osseous deformities can also cause nerve entrapment.[2,18] Abnormal nerve findings on imaging occur at the site of entrapment and are often short segment (2–6 cm). Imaging findings of entrapment neuropathy include nerve flattening at the entrapment site with proximal and distal nerve enlargement in higher-grade entrapment cases.[2] On US, cross-sectional area of a nerve (typically the median nerve at the carpal tunnel) can be measured to assess for nerve enlargement and compared with normative values in the literature. In cases of entrapment, nerve signal hyperintensity is seen on MR imaging and nerve hypoechogenicity on US.[2,18,19] Hypervascularity in and around the nerve and thickening of the epineurium may be seen on US.[18] Provocative dynamic maneuvers and application of sonopressure with the probe to elicit symptoms are US techniques that can be used to aid diagnosis of nerve entrapment.[19]

Diffuse Nerve Disease

Diffuse nerve disease describes long-segment nerve lesions, with nerve abnormality spanning a length greater than 6 cm. In the NS-RADS classification scheme, class D1 refers to mononeuropathies, and class D2 refers to polyneuropathies.[2] Diffuse mononeuropathies can result from infection, ischemia, traction neuropathy, idiopathic hypertrophic mononeuropathy, and lymphoma. Examples of diffuse polyneuropathies include diabetic polyneuropathy, radiation neuropathy, acute and chronic inflammatory demyelinating polyneuropathy, mononeuritis multiplex, amyloid neuropathy, lymphoproliferative diseases, and

Table 1
Nerve imaging—MR and ultrasound correlation of imaging findings

Nerve Pathologic Condition	MR Imaging Findings	US Imaging Findings
Neuropathy	Nerve enlargement Signal hyperintensity Loss of fascicular architecture	Nerve enlargement Hypoechogenicity Loss of fascicular architecture
Trauma or iatrogenic injury	Nerve discontinuity—partial or complete Perineural scarring	Nerve discontinuity—partial or complete Perineural scarring
Entrapment	Focal nerve narrowing/compression Adjacent mass lesion (ganglion cyst, lipoma, and similar)	Focal nerve narrowing/compression Adjacent mass lesion (ganglion cyst, lipoma, and similar)
Neoplasia: benign	Well-circumscribed mass in continuity with nerve, may demonstrate "tail sign" or "target sign"	Well-circumscribed mass in continuity with a nerve—schwannomas displace unaffected fascicles at the periphery, whereas neurofibromas encase fascicles of the nerve
Neoplasia: malignant	Aggressive imaging features—heterogeneous enhancement, necrosis, low ADC values, local invasiveness	Aggressive imaging features—local invasiveness, indistinct margins
Positional	Nerve compression with change of positioning (ie, arms up vs arms down for thoracic outlet syndrome)	Nerve subluxation or compression on dynamic imaging (ie, ulnar nerve at the level of the cubital tunnel with arm flexion and extension)
Secondary muscle denervation	Subacute—muscle edema Chronic—muscle fatty infiltration and atrophy	Subacute—may appear normal Chronic—muscle hyperechogenicity and atrophy

Data from Refs.[2,4,18,19]

perineural metastases. Imaging findings include nerve enlargement as well as signal hyperintensity on MR imaging and hypoechogenicity on US. Some causes may manifest in a bilateral symmetric fashion, such as diabetic polyneuropathy, whereas other causes, such as traction neuropathy or Parsonage-Turner syndrome, may be unilateral/asymmetric.[2,18,19] In infection neuropathy, such as leprosy, hypervascularity of the perineurium and endoneurium may be seen on US.[19] Hourglass constriction is a unique imaging finding that has been described in cases of Parsonage-Turner syndrome (Fig. 5).[18,20] Muscle denervation changes may be present in both class D1 and D2 cases.[2]

Postintervention

The NS-RADS postintervention category is used for patients with prior nerve surgery or intervention, when imaging is often indicated for assessment of persistent or worsening nerve damage.

Imaging may reveal near-normal appearance of the nerve, persistent nerve enlargement and signal hyperintensity/hypoechogenicity, or worsening findings of nerve enlargement and signal hyperintensity/hypoechogenicity. Perineural scarring can be seen on both MR imaging and US following intervention.[2,18,19]

MODALITY CHOICE

MR neurography and high-resolution US imaging are complementary modalities for assessment of peripheral nerve injury. Although both MR imaging and US can provide insight into localization and characterization of nerve injury, they remain specialized studies that require advanced skills and expertise for image acquisition and interpretation. Therefore, not all institutions and practices may offer both modalities for peripheral nerve imaging, or may have specific preferences on the recommended nerve imaging modality based on local expertise. Clinical collaboration and

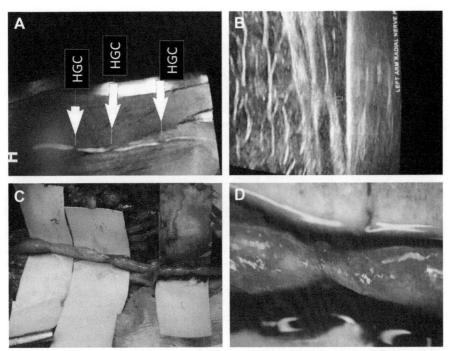

Fig. 5. Hourglass constrictions in Parsonage-Turner syndrome on MR imaging and US. (*A*) MR imaging and (*B*) high-resolution US demonstrate hourglass constrictions in the radial nerve (HCG; *arrows*) in a patient with Parsonage-Turner syndrome. The patient went to surgery where (*C, D*) intraoperative photographs confirmed the presence of constrictions. HGC, hour-glass constriction. (Intraoperative photographs courtesy of Dr Charles Daly, Medical University of South Carolina.)

consultation with radiology are encouraged to determine the best modality for nerve imaging on a case-by-case basis.

General advantages of MR imaging include a more global assessment of nerve and muscle changes, higher sensitivity for detection of subtle nerve signal changes, and the ability to assess deeper structures as well as structures traveling deep to bone (**Fig. 6**). General disadvantages of MR imaging include susceptibility artifact from

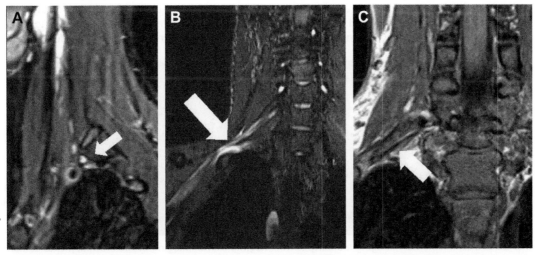

Fig. 6. MR neurography for thoracic outlet syndrome. (*A*) Sagittal and (*B*) coronal STIR MR neurography images of the brachial plexus demonstrate signal hyperintensity and enlargement of the brachial plexus at the level of a rib (*arrow*). (*C*) Coronal T1 MR image demonstrates a right cervical rib (*arrow*).

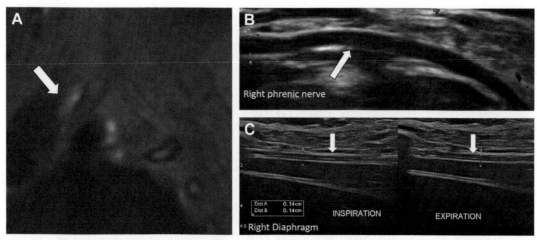

Fig. 7. MR imaging and US correlation for phrenic nerve injury. (*A*) MR neurography of the brachial plexus demonstrates an enlarged hyperintense phrenic nerve (*arrow*), compatible with neuropathy. (*B*) Longitudinal high-resolution US demonstrates an enlarged hypoechoic phrenic nerve (*arrow*), compatible with neuropathy. (*C*) Intercostal US of the diaphragm on inspiration and expiration demonstrates no change in size with respiration, compatible with diaphragm muscle dysfunction. Although both MR imaging and US provide excellent depiction of the phrenic nerve, evaluation for associated diaphragm muscle injury is best performed with US.

metal hardware, potential motion artifact in claustrophobic patients or patients otherwise limited in their ability to tolerate MR imaging, and patient factors that may be a contraindication to MR imaging. In contrast, general advantages of US include low cost, good patient tolerance, the ease with which contralateral imaging can be performed for comparison, and the ability to do dynamic imaging (**Fig. 7**). US is not affected by metal susceptibility artifact and may offer superior nerve imaging compared with MR imaging, depending on the extent of hardware and associated artifact. General disadvantages of US include limited imaging in obese patients or for deeper structures, and limited area of coverage.[2,5] Segments of nerves may not be visualized sonographically in the presence of overlying osseous

structures, such as the brachial plexus, as it courses beneath the clavicle.[3,5] Although US can be used to assess muscle changes, MR imaging offers more global and more sensitive assessment of muscle denervation.

There is limited literature directly comparing MR and US imaging of peripheral nerves. In 1 recent study of 180 nerves in 2019, the diagnostic accuracy of MR imaging performed on a 3-T magnet (using body coils owing to resource limitations) was shown to be 94% in a comparative study of imaging of peripheral neuropathy, versus 80% for US performed with a 14-Hz linear transducer.[2] In a 2017 study of 64 nerves in patients with upper-limb peripheral neuropathies, MR imaging performed with a 3-T magnet had a higher diagnostic confidence than nerve US that was performed with

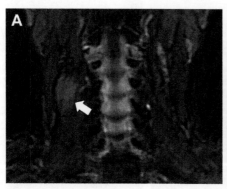
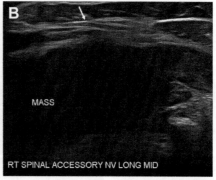

Fig. 8. US as a complementary imaging modality to MR imaging. (*A*) MR imaging of the brachial plexus demonstrates a right neck mass with suspicion for a peripheral nerve sheath tumor of the spinal accessory nerve. (*B*) High-resolution US was performed for further assessment of the spinal accessory nerve (*arrow*). The nerve is normal in size and echogenicity and is clearly separate from the mass, indicating that it is not of nerve origin.

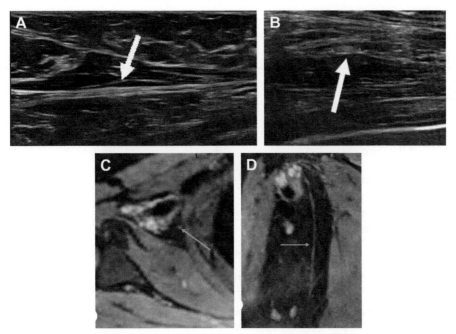

Fig. 9. High-resolution US imaging of small peripheral nerves and MR correlation. The long thoracic nerve (*arrows*) is visualized in (*A*) the longitudinal and (*B*) transverse planes with high-resolution US. The nerve is normal in size, echogenicity, and fascicular architecture. In a companion case in a different patient, an abnormal long thoracic nerve (*arrows*) is seen on (*C*) axial MR neurography image and (*D*) reformatted MR neurography image as an enlarged hyperintense structure. Although the long thoracic nerve is difficult to visualize on both US and MR neurography, an abnormal nerve may be more readily apparent owing to an enlarged size.

7- to-0-Hz frequency probe.[15] In contrast, a 2013 study of 51 nerves in 2000 found high sensitivity of US (12- or 17-Hz transducer) compared with MR imaging performed on a 1.5-T magnet without advanced neurography techniques.[16] To date, there is no comprehensive study comparing MR neurography (3 T) with high-resolution US (22 Hz+) with advanced imaging techniques and technology. Overall, diagnostic accuracy of imaging modalities likely reflects local expertise and availability of the latest imaging technology; therefore, direct consultation with the radiology practice

is suggested to determine the recommended imaging study.

In the authors' experience, MR imaging is generally preferred for larger peripheral nerves, because of the global assessment and sensitivity of nerve signal changes, whereas high-resolution US may be superior for assessment of small peripheral nerve branches (**Fig. 8**). With advances in US technology, high-resolution US with high-frequency probes can visualize small peripheral nerves that may not be well seen on MR imaging.[4] It is important to note, however, that imaging can

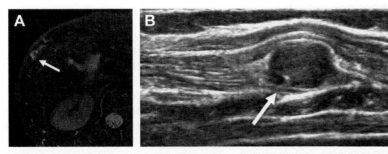

Fig. 10. MR imaging and US of chest wall lesions. (*A*) Axial STIR MR image demonstrates an STIR hyperintense heterogeneous chest wall mass (*arrow*). Image quality is degraded by respiratory artifact. (*B*) US demonstrates a well-circumscribed mass deep to the external oblique muscle and superficial to the intercostal muscle with suggestion of a tail sign, favored to represent a schwannoma (*arrow*). Follow-up US imaging to ensure stability was advised.

Table 2
Modality recommendations for imaging of peripheral nerves

Clinical Scenario	MR Neurography	High-Resolution US
Brachial plexus	3	2
Lumbosacral plexus	3	0
Extremity nerves	3	2
Small peripheral nerve/branches	2	3
Deep peripheral nerves	3	0
Metal artifact	2	3
Motion artifact/respiration artifact	2	3
Patient contraindication to MR	0	3
Suspected dynamic pathologic condition	1[a]	3
Perineural injection/biopsy	1[b]	3

Scoring is on a 3-point scale: 0, not typically performed; 1, may be performed in certain situations; 2, acceptable choice of modality; 3, preferred choice of modality.

*Suggestions are based on anecdotal experience of the authors. Nerve imaging modality availability and diagnostic accuracy reflect local expertise, and clinical consultation with radiology practices is suggested to determine the optimal imaging study.

[a] That is, MR imaging with arms down by the sides vs raised for suspected thoracic outlet syndrome.
[b] MR-guided steroid injections for pudendal neuropathy.

provide diagnostic value without necessarily visualizing small nerves through exclusion of mass or other abnormality along the expected course of a nerve and assessment of muscle changes.[4,21] Abnormal small nerves, owing to findings of enlargement and signal hyperintensity, are often more readily visualized than if they were normal (**Fig. 9**). In areas where MR imaging may be limited, such as the chest wall owing to respiratory motion artifact (**Fig. 10**) or in the presence of significant metal artifact, US may be preferred. **Table 2** outlines modality recommendations for various clinical scenarios.

SUMMARY

Recent advances in imaging technology have allowed for high-resolution diagnostic imaging of peripheral nerve pathologic condition with both MR imaging and US. Both MR neurography and high-resolution nerve US imaging are specialized studies that may not be widely offered at all radiology practices. Latest technical equipment and radiologist expertise are necessary for optimized evaluation of peripheral nerves. Although both modalities can offer excellent visualization of even small peripheral nerves with corresponding findings of nerve pathologic condition, certain clinical scenarios may lend themselves better to one modality over another. Overall, MR imaging and US are complementary modalities for peripheral nerve imaging.

CLINICS CARE POINTS

- Assessment of peripheral nerve pathologic condition on imaging should include evaluation of both primary (nerve) and secondary (muscle) injuries.
- When assessing peripheral nerves on ultrasound, high-resolution (12–24 MHz) or ultrahigh-resolution (48 MHz+) transducers are ideal.
- The Neuropathy Score Reporting and Data System is a multi-institutional expert consensus classification and grading system for peripheral neuropathy on MR imaging.

REFERENCES

1. Thawait SK, Chaudhry V, Thawait GK, et al. High-resolution MR neurography diffuse peripheral nerve lesions. AJNR Am J Neuroradiol 2011;32(8): 1365–72.
2. Chhabra A, Deshmukh SD, Lutz AM, et al. Neuropathy Score Reporting and Data System (NS-RADS): MRI Reporting Guideline of Peripheral Neuropathy Explained and Reviewed. Skeletal Radiol 2022. https://doi.org/10.1007/s00256-022-04061-1.
3. Gilcrease-Garcia BM, Deshmukh SD, Parsons MS. Anatomy, imaging, and pathologic conditions of the brachial plexus. Radiographics 2020;40(6): 1686–714.

4. Chhabra A, Ratakonda R, Zaottini F, et al. Hand and wrist neuropathies: high-resolution ultrasonography and MR neurography. Semin Musculoskelet Radiol 2021;25(2):366–78.

5. Griffith JF, Lalam RK. Top-Ten Tips for Imaging the Brachial Plexus with Ultrasound and MRI. Semin Musculoskelet Radiol 2019;23(4):405–18.

6. Agarwal A, Chandra A, Jaipal U, et al. Can imaging be the new yardstick for diagnosing peripheral neuropathy?—A comparison between high resolution ultrasound and MR neurography with an approach to diagnosis. Insights Imaging 2019;10(1):104.

7. Moller I, Miguel M, Bong DA, et al. The peripheral nerves: update on ultrasound and magnetic resonance imaging. Clin Exp Rheumatol 2018;36 Suppl 114(5):145–58.

8. Ahlawat S, Chhabra A, Blakely J. Magnetic resonance neurography of peripheral nerve tumors and tumorlike conditions. Neuroimaging Clin N Am 2014;24(1):171–92.

9. Brown JM, Yablon CM, Morag Y, et al. US of the peripheral nerves of the upper extremity: a landmark approach. Radiographics 2016;36(2):452–63.

10. Yablon CM, Hammer MR, Morag Y, et al. US of the peripheral nerves of the lower extremity: a landmark approach. Radiographics 2016;36(2):464–78.

11. Chhabra A, Ahlawat S, Belzberg A, et al. Peripheral nerve injury grading simplified on MR neurography: as referenced to Seddon and Sunderland classifications. Indian J Radiol Imaging 2014;24(3):217–24.

12. Deshmukh S, Tegtmeyer K, Kovour M, et al. Diagnostic contribution of contrast-enhanced 3D MR imaging of peripheral nerve pathology. Skeletal Radiol 2021;50(12):2509–18.

13. Harrell AD, Johnson D, Samet J, et al. With or without? A retrospective analysis of intravenous contrast utility in magnetic resonance neurography. Skeletal Radiol 2020;49(4):577–84.

14. Chhabra A, Deshmukh SD, Lutz AM, et al. Neuropathy Score Reporting and Data System: A Reporting Guideline for MRI of Peripheral Neuropathy With a Multicenter Validation Study. AJR Am J Roentgenol 2022;1–11. https://doi.org/10.2214/AJR.22.27422.

15. Aggarwal A, Srivastava DN, Jana M, et al. Comparison of different sequences of magnetic resonance imaging and ultrasonography with nerve conduction studies in peripheral neuropathies. World Neurosurg 2017;108:185–200.

16. Zaidman CM, Seelig MJ, Baker JC, et al. Detection of peripheral nerve pathology: comparison of ultrasound and MRI. Neurology 2013;80(18):1634–40.

17. Wee TC, Simon NG. Ultrasound elastography for the evaluation of peripheral nerves: a systematic review. Muscle Nerve 2019;60(5):501–12.

18. Kalia V, Jacobson JA. Imaging of peripheral nerves of the upper extremity. Radiol Clin North Am 2019; 57(5):1063–71.

19. Ali ZS, Pisapia JM, Ma TS, et al. Ultrasonographic evaluation of peripheral nerves. World Neurosurg 2016;85:333–9.

20. Krishnan KR, Wolfe SW, Feinberg JH, et al. Imaging and treatment of phrenic nerve hourglass-like constrictions in neuralgic amyotrophy. Muscle Nerve 2020;62(5):E81–2.

21. Deshmukh S, Fayad LM, Ahlawat S. MR neurography (MRN) of the long thoracic nerve: retrospective review of clinical findings and imaging results at our institution over 4 years. Skeletal Radiol 2017;46(11): 1531–40.

Sarcoma Imaging Surveillance
MR Imaging–Ultrasound (US) Correlation

Alberto Bazzocchi, MD, PhD[a],*, Giuseppe Guglielmi, MD[b,c],
Maria Pilar Aparisi Gómez, MBChB, FRANZCR[d,e]

KEYWORDS

• Soft tissue sarcomas • Tumor • US • MR imaging

KEY POINTS

• MR imaging remains the usual imaging method for recurrence surveillance, and the use of dynamic contrast enhancement and diffusion-weighted imaging has improved its efficiency on the diagnosis, reducing false positives.
• The use of ultrasound for surveillance of local recurrence of soft tissue sarcomas has some clear advantages. It has been proven to efficiently identify the majority of patients who do not have a recurrence. It is being progressively considered as an alternative to MR imaging as first-line assessment in different guidelines.
• Comparative studies on the performance of both techniques are still scarce. Ultrasound may be comparable in accuracy to MR imaging and could be used as surveillance in expert hands, but multi-institutional prospective trials to increase power and reproducibility are still needed.

INTRODUCTION

Soft tissue sarcomas (STS) are a rare and complex heterogeneous group of solid tumors with mesenchymal origin. Their rarity means they benefit from a multidisciplinary approach to management and adherence to recommendations and guidelines.

There are many histologic subtypes, with some common clinical and pathological characteristics, but also specific features impacting management.

The prognosis depends on multiple factors. Local recurrence of soft tissue tumors has been reported to be as high as 23.4%. The histologic type and lack of wide resection have been detected as factors impacting local recurrence. Patients with recurrence have a poorer prognosis. On this basis, surveillance of patients with STS is extremely important. MR imaging and ultrasound play an important role in the evaluation of local recurrence.

The purpose of this review is to analyze the particularities MR imaging and ultrasound bring to the surveillance of STS, and how they correlate and potentially complement each other. The recommendations for use in different guidelines are also reviewed.

Soft Tissue Sarcomas, Epidemiology and Risk of Relapse

STS are a heterogeneous group of solid tumors which have a mesenchymal origin and are rare. Their estimated incidence is 4 to 5 cases/1,00,000 inhabitants/year in Europe.[1]

In the United States, updated estimations suggest 13,190 people will be diagnosed with STS in 2022, with approximately 5,130 deaths (Siegel).

Risk factors for the development of an STS are previous radiation to the site,[2] use of certain

[a] Diagnostic and Interventional Radiology, IRCCS Istituto Ortopedico Rizzoli, Via G. C. Pupilli 1, Bologna 40136, Italy; [b] Department of Radiology, Hospital San Giovanni Rotondo, Italy; [c] Department of Radiology, University of Foggia, Viale Luigi Pinto 1, Foggia 71100, Italy; [d] Department of Radiology, Auckland City Hospital, 2 Park Road, Grafton, Auckland 1023, New Zealand; [e] Department of Radiology, IMSKE, Calle Suiza, 11, Valencia 46024, Spain
* Corresponding author.
E-mail address: abazzo@inwind.it

Magn Reson Imaging Clin N Am 31 (2023) 193–214
https://doi.org/10.1016/j.mric.2023.01.004

chemicals (eg, herbicides), and genetic syndromes (eg, neurofibromatosis).[3]

They can appear anywhere in the body, but most are found in the extremities (43%), followed by the trunk (10%), visceral (19%), retroperitoneum (15%), and head and neck (9%).[3,4] The location of the tumor is an important variable influencing treatment and outcome.

They are more common in middle-aged or older adults, but can also affect children and young adults. Indeed, as a proportion of pediatric malignancies, they comprise 7 to 10% of childhood cancers, and are an important cause of death in the 14 to 29 age group.[5,6]

The management of STS should always be channeled through a multidisciplinary team. STS are rare and complex, and this is one of the reasons following guidelines/recommendations is so important. Voss and colleagues[7] analyzed data from 15,957 patients with STS from the National Cancer database and concluded adherence to the National Comprehensive Cancer Network (NCCN) guidelines was associated with improved outcomes regarding survival.

There are more than 50 histologic subtypes of STS; they share clinical and pathological characteristics, but also have some specific features impacting management. STS most commonly metastasize to the lungs. If occurring intraabdominally, liver and peritoneum metastasis occur.[3] Approximately 50% of STS patients with intermediate or high-grade tumors develop metastatic disease.[8] The overall survival is approximately 55% at 5 years.[9–11]

Traditionally, the most common type of STS in adults was considered the malignant fibrous histiocytoma, which, in the past, was named fibrosarcoma and is currently labeled (2013 WHO classification) pleomorphic undifferentiated sarcoma. These are considered to represent 25 to 40% of adult STS.[12] Pleomorphic undifferentiated sarcoma has a predilection for extremities (50% lower, 20% upper).[13] It represents the most frequent STS appearing after radiotherapy.

The second most common type are liposarcomas.[12] Liposarcomas typically present between 40 and 60 years of age. They appear in the limbs (75%), and more frequently in the thigh.

There are five different histological types, with increasing aggressiveness (well-differentiated, myxoid, round-cell, pleomorphic, mixed). The most common is the well-differentiated one (50%).[14] The higher the grade, the more likely to recur.[15]

Rhabdomyosarcoma is the most common STS in children and adolescents (19% of sarcomas), and less common in adults.[3] Desmoid tumors or aggressive fibromatosis are a special soft tissue tumor subtype that demonstrate local infiltration rather than distant metastasis.

The prognosis after treatment may be estimated by the analysis of the type of tumor, grade, depth, size at diagnosis, as well as age of the patient.[16] In some environments, there are calculators available.[17]

Local recurrence of soft tissue tumors has been seen to range from 4.1% to 23.4% in large studies.[18–20] The histologic type and lack of wide resection have been detected as factors impacting local recurrence.[20–23] The tumor location is associated with local recurrence, with tumors deep to the superficial fascia and tumors located in the trunk or upper extremities at a higher risk.[22] Other studies on high-grade tumors have related the increasing size to poor survival.[24,25]

A few years ago, a retrospective study from an American institution detected that local recurrence predicted an increased likelihood of distal metastasis and worse overall survival,[18] in agreement with a previous retrospective study[20] that demonstrated that local recurrence and positive margins correlated with worse survival. Results from a large Italian cohort of patients (997)[19] suggested that long-term survival was only impacted by local control of the tumor, and that relapse was related to surgical margins, radiation therapy, and histology type. Interestingly, a recent study reported that non-resection of the core biopsy tract was not found to increase local recurrence (8.5%) in a group of patients who were also being treated with radiation and chemotherapy as adjuvant therapies.[26]

A study in the past decade[27] found that recurrent tumors tended to be located deeper and were higher in grade than primary lesions, and that patients with recurrence had a poor prognosis. In their series, amputation did not prevent death in comparison with limb salvage surgery.

The size of the recurrence has been linked with survival[28] and with morbidity.[29] Based on gathered evidence, surveillance for local recurrence is important.

High-risk extremity STS usually relapses within 2 to 3 years, mainly to the lungs, although there are some subtypes (epithelioid, clear cell, synovial sarcoma, or rhabdomyosarcoma) that metastasize to lymph nodes, and typically, retroperitoneal sarcoma relapses locally and extends to the liver or peritoneum.[4]

Most recurrences will happen in the first 5 years following diagnosis, but late relapses may occur, described in retroperitoneal or very large tumors.[30] There are subtypes, such as alveolar sarcoma, clear cell sarcoma, or extraskeletal

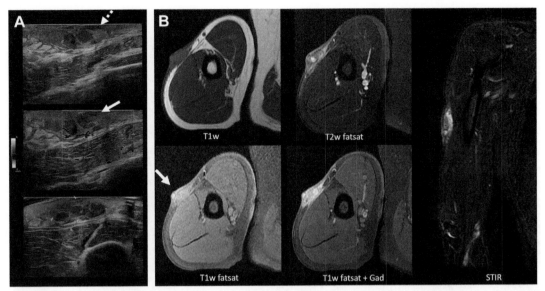

Fig. 1. Myxofibrosarcoma recurrence. (*A*). Typical ultrasound appearances of myxofibrosarcoma recurrence. Lobulated hypoechoic lesions surrounded by iso/hyperechoic tissue (*dotted arrow*). Moderate vascularization on Doppler interrogation (*bold arrow*). Mass effect, displacing and infiltrating surrounding tissue. Ultrasound approach allows the radiologist to palpate and clinically examine the postoperative area and the lesions. (*B*). MR imaging appearance of the same lesion; a single but inhomogeneous lesion is confirmed (*bold arrow*), with clearer infiltration of the superficial aponeurosis.

chondrosarcoma that may relapse even after 10 years, and therefore, longer follow-up is advised.[4]

Clinical Findings: Initial Diagnosis and Staging

Clinically, STS present as soft tissue lumps. History and physical examination are paramount in the initial assessment. In general, any lump which is increasing in size, has a size of more than 5 cm, or is painful should be considered malignant unless otherwise proven.[31] Increasing size is the most suspicious indicator.

The vast majority of soft tissue lumps are benign. Benign lesions such as superficial lipomas and ganglia are by far the most common soft tissue masses and can be readily identified and excluded on ultrasound in a few minutes, thereby reducing the need for more complex investigations and biopsies.

Ultrasonographic assessment of soft tissue masses is an ideal triaging tool in many countries. There are many reasons ultrasound lends itself to this purpose. Compared to MR imaging, ultrasound is cheap, has a high resolution, is readily available in most health care settings, has no contraindications, is well tolerated, and is safe. Ultrasound allows dynamic assessment of the lesions to assess features such as consistency, compressibility, mobility, relationship to structures such as tendons, muscles, and joints, and also

offers the possibility of Doppler interrogation (color, power, spectral) (**Fig. 1**). The use of new techniques such as elastography and contrast is promising.[12]

The American College of Radiology Appropriateness Criteria[32] consider ultrasound as "usually appropriate" for the initial assessment of superficial or palpable soft tissue masses. MR imaging (without contrast) is deemed "may be appropriate", MR imaging with contrast is considered "usually not appropriate". If the mass is deep, or located in a region difficult to assess with radiographs, or the clinical assessment is not specific, ultrasound is still considered as "may be appropriate" as an initial tool before MR imaging or MR imaging with and without contrast, where a note is made of the existence of panel disagreement.

In the United Kingdom, the National Institute for Health and Care Excellence (NICE) implemented some guidelines aimed at primary care for the early diagnosis of STS.[33] Any patient with a soft tissue mass that is growing or has more than 5 cm, independently of the presence of pain, should be referred for an urgent ultrasound, or if there is a high suspicion of malignancy (and ultrasound may introduce delay) directly referred, following suspected cancer priority pathways, to a sarcoma center.

If ultrasound does not confidently confirm benignity, a sarcoma center referral should be warranted. Any lesions previously considered

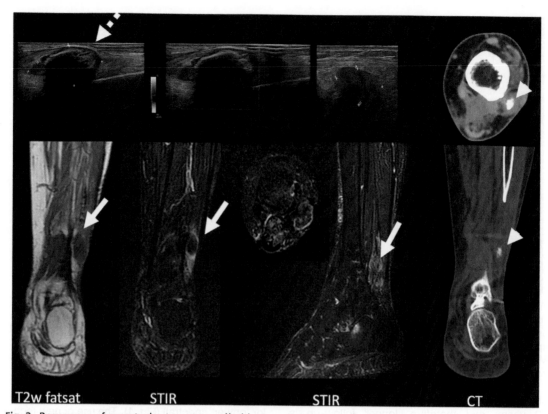

Fig. 2. Recurrence of parosteal osteosarcoma (*bold arrows* in MR, *arrowhead* in CT, *dotted arrow* in ultrasound). Despite recurrence can be detected on the superficial planes by ultrasound, imaging follow-up is typically performed with MR imaging and CT.

benign that increase in size or develop other suspicious features should be referred for further investigation in a sarcoma center (**Fig. 2**).

Any retroperitoneal or intraabdominal mass with imaging appearances suggestive of a STS should be referred to a sarcoma center as well, before biopsy or surgical treatment is considered.[33]

After the introduction of the NICE guidelines, an improvement in survival was seen in patients with STS, especially those with high-grade tumors, mainly given to the fact more patients were referred at an earlier stage.[34]

If the soft tissue mass is deemed suspicious, a detailed imaging evaluation of the tumor and a carefully planned biopsy (core needle or incisional biopsy) are performed.

The general recommendation (joint guidelines from the European Society for Medical Oncology (ESMO), European Reference Network for Rare Adult Solid Cancers (EURACAN), and European Reference Network for Genetic Tumour Risk Syndromes (GENTURIS), NCCN) is to perform cross-sectional imaging, able to provide details of tumor size and volume and spatial relations to nearby anatomical structures.

Both groups recommend MR imaging (the NCCN panel recommends MR imaging with contrast), adding Computed tomography (CT) with or without contrast. CT is useful in calcified lesions, and to rule out myositis ossificans. In pleuropulmonary sarcomas and retroperitoneal sarcomas, the performance is the same as MR imaging.[35] Radiographs are useful to rule out an underlying bone tumor, erosions at risk of fracture, and calcifications. Specific studies such as CT angiograms are indicated in selected circumstances.

The European group (ESMO–EURACAN–GENTURIS) specifically states that ultrasound may be considered as first-line imaging, but if there is suspicion of STS, it should be followed by CT or MR imaging.[35] It is recommended this is performed by an experienced, specialized operator.

Once a careful imaging assessment of the tumor is performed, the histological diagnosis should be achieved through biopsy. Ideally, material for analysis should be obtained by core biopsy using 14 to 16 G needles. Ultrasound is extremely useful as an imaging guiding tool, and is the method of choice for superficial lesions (**Fig. 3**). Closed biopsies do not require general anesthesia or hospital stay

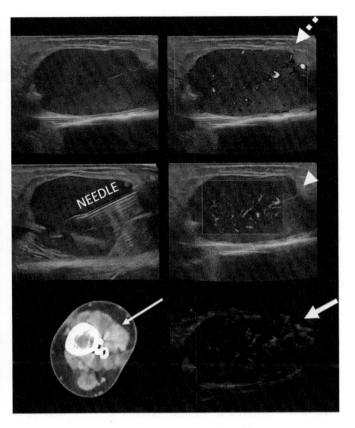

Fig. 3. Recurrence of osteosarcoma. Bone tumors can locally recur in soft tissues. Ultrasound can be used for assessing possible soft tissue recurrence, and in this case, can easily show the relapse. Additional methods of characterization are vascular assessment–color-Doppler (*dotted arrow*), microvascular imaging (MVI) (*arrowhead*), and B-flow imaging mode (*bold short arrow*). Ultrasound and contrast-enhanced CT (lesion signaled by *thin long arrow*) are often preferred, as metal implants may cause artifacts precluding the detection of small nodules, especially in MR imaging, and because of the possible calcified pattern of recurrence. Ultrasound is the favored imaging method to guide the biopsy of suspected soft tissue tumor recurrence ("*NEEDLE*" labeled in the left central image).

and have the same excellent diagnostic performance, compared to open biopsies.[36] The needle needs to be targeted to regions where the tumor appears active. Doppler assessment or contrast enhancement is useful to reveal these regions.[37,38] Fusion imaging can also help with biopsy planning.

Open biopsies may be another option in selected cases. Excisional biopsies may be the most logical option for small superficial lesions (less than 3 cm).[11]

Biopsies may underestimate the tumor malignancy grade, so when preoperative treatment is an option, imaging is useful, in addition to pathology, in providing information regarding malignancy grade.

The presence of metastatic disease at diagnosis may change how treatment of the primary lesion is approached, and overall management planned. Different sarcoma types have different patterns of spread, and as such, imaging should be individualized based on the subtype of sarcoma.

The general recommendation for staging is to perform imaging of the chest (CT without contrast preferred). In a small number of cases, radiographs may suffice, for example, frail elderly patients or very small, low-grade lesions.[11] Atypical lipomatous tumors of the extremities have a very low risk of metastatic spread, so chest radiographs may be adequate for staging.[11]

In cases of angiosarcoma, leiomyosarcoma, myxoid/round-cell liposarcoma, or epithelioid sarcoma and sarcoma in which definitive pathology before surgical treatment is not available, abdominopelvic CT should be warranted. Whole-body MR imaging is feasible for detecting bone and soft tissue metastasis in myxoid liposarcoma.[35,39] Some groups suggest this should be considered in lower extremity sarcomas, depending on grade.[11,40]

Some specific types require additional imaging for staging. In cases of myxoid/round-cell liposarcoma, there is an increased risk for metastasis to the spine, so a whole spine MR imaging is recommended. In the case of alveolar sarcoma (especially in cases of stage IV, or lung metastases present),[41] clear cell sarcoma and angiosarcoma, central nervous system metastases may occur, so brain MR imaging (or CT if this is contraindicated) is recommended.[11,42] Regional MR imaging or CT is recommended to detect potential nodal involvement in synovial sarcoma, clear cell sarcoma, or epithelioid sarcoma.[11]

According to the latest NCCN guidelines, Positron Emission Tomography (PET CT) may be useful in staging, grading, assessment of prognosis, and monitorization of chemotherapy.[3,43–45] The maximum standardized uptake value of F18-deoxyglucose (FDG) has been correlated with grade and prognosis, seen to represent an independent predictor of survival and disease progression.[46,47] The ESMO–EURACAN–GENTURIS group includes FDG-PET CT as a useful imaging tool to adequately estimate malignancy grade in association with biopsy results.

According to the British Sarcoma Group (BSG) guidelines, FDG-PET CT may be reserved as a problem-solving tool, for example, for the characterization of equivocal CT findings such as affected lymph nodes in relevant sarcoma types.[11,48]

Based on the initial workup, with imaging and histology, correct staging can be carried out, assigning patients to stages I, II, III, unresectable disease, stage IV (metastatic disease), and recurrent disease.

SURVEILLANCE, CURRENT GUIDELINES, AND PRACTICE

Given early detection of local or metastatic recurrence might be potentially curable, surveillance is important. The paucity of data is general for follow-up protocols in STS patients. Very limited data of effective strategies have been published.[49–53] The risk of relapse does not disappear, even after 5 years, so long-term follow-up is indicated.[54] After 10 years, the likelihood decreases so follow-up can be individualized.

Early detection of local relapse or metastasis may improve prognosis, so this is an urgent field for research. Recommendations for surveillance have been issued by different groups. Ultimately, the plan should be adequately discussed with the patient and the reasons and limitations addressed.

The role of imaging is still an item of debate. Results from a prospective randomized single-center noninferiority trial comparing standard follow-up with greater intensity follow-up (in terms of frequency of visits and mode of imaging, radiographs, or CT) in patients with extremity sarcomas failed to demonstrate the difference in outcome.[55] In a recent update of their results they concluded radiographs at 6-monthly intervals and patient examination of the site of surgery will detect most recurrences without negative effects on the eventual outcome.[56] Their cohort included 500 patients with sarcoma and found that 90% of local recurrences were clinically detected.

Rothermundt and colleagues[53] analyzed data on 174 consecutive patients with a STS of the limb undergoing follow-up (local imaging performed with MR imaging), and concluded that in the case of local recurrence, relapse is almost always detected by patients or physicians, and that routine scanning is of doubtful benefit. Local recurrences were detected clinically in 30/31 patients. The MR imaging identified only one local recurrence.

A recent retrospective study[57] analyzed surveillance imaging in a large group of patients with intermediate/high localized extremity or trunk STS, treated with radical surgery and radiotherapy. Their results showed that although surveillance chest imaging may be very useful for the detection of metastasis, local primary site imaging may only be useful for patients at high risk of local recurrence.

However, a subsequent, more recent study by Park and colleagues[58] including 325 patients with STS with a local recurrence rate of 11%, surveilled with MR imaging found that a rate of 60% of local recurrences was not detected clinically, especially those in the thigh or buttock, those of small size or without mass formation. They also noted patients with MR imaging-detected that local recurrence tended to have better post-local recurrence survival, without reaching statistical significance.

From a slightly different point of view, a recent study by Kraus and colleagues[59] retrospectively examined the efficacy and cost-benefit of MR imaging for detecting the recurrence of STS in extremities and trunk. The authors collected data on patient demographics, tumor characteristics, treatment, and follow-up, and correlated imaging with clinical course, sensitivity, specificity, and predictive values. The study concluded that MR imaging is more cost-effective than clinical examination, but recommended both modalities be performed together to detect the maximum number of recurrences.

All expert guidelines acknowledge the use of clinical evaluation, and most of them include imaging in combination.

Higher grade and larger tumors have a higher risk of dissemination, and in this regard, more intensive follow-up recommendations, especially in the first 3 years.

Based on NCCN recommendations, stage I tumors should be followed with anamnesis/physical examination every 3 to 6 months for 2 to 3 years and then annually. Chest imaging with radiographs or CT (preferred) is recommended every 6 to 12 months. Postoperative baseline and regular imaging of the primary tumor site is recommended based on the estimated risk of locoregional

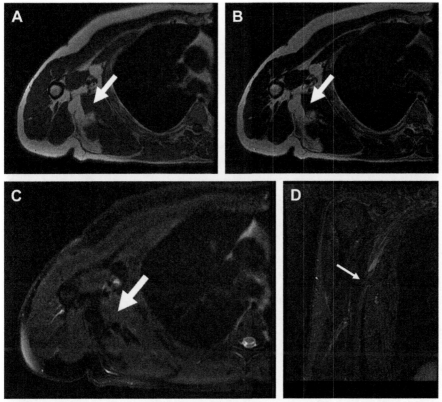

Fig. 4. Recurrence of atypical lipomatous tumor (right posterior axillary region). MR axial T1w (*A*), T2w (*B*), and T2 fat-sat (*C*) imaging showing a mass (*thick arrow*) which shows shape and signal intensity typical of fat, with complete suppression in STIR (coronal view, *D, thin arrow*). Administration of contrast medium was not necessary in this case.

recurrence. The recommendation is to use MR imaging (± contrast) and/or contrast CT. Ultrasound (performed by an experienced, specialized operator) may be considered for the detection of local recurrence in patients with small, superficial lesions. In situations in which the area is adequately assessed by physical examination, imaging may not be necessary.[60]

The European group (ESMO–EURACAN–GEN-TURIS) recommends that patients with low-grade tumors are followed every 6 months for the first 5 years, and then annually for at least 10 years. CT is recommended for chest surveillance and MR imaging for locoregional surveillance.

For stages II, III, and IV, the NCCN recommends anamnesis/physical examination every 2 to 6 months for 2 to 3 years and then annually, then every 6 months for the following 2 to 3 years (up to 5 years), and then annually. Postoperative baseline and regular imaging of the primary tumor site is recommended based on the estimated risk of locoregional recurrence (MR imaging and/or CT). Ultrasound (performed by an experienced, specialized operator) may be considered for the detection

of local recurrence in patients with small, superficial lesions.

The European group (ESMO–EURACAN–GEN-TURIS) guidelines are similar, and recommend that patients with intermediate/high-grade tumors are followed every 3 to 4 months for the first 2 to 3 years, and then every 6 months to 5 years, and then, annually. CT is recommended for chest surveillance and MR imaging for locoregional surveillance.

The BSG[48] and the Sociedad Española de Oncología Médica [4] mostly adhere to these guidelines. It is important to mention that these groups specifically consider the use of the ultrasound for the detection of local recurrence.

It is important to mention that a further value of follow-up is to monitor for adverse, late effects of treatment.[61]

MR IMAGING AND ULTRASOUND: EXCLUSIVE OR COMPLEMENTARY?

All groups, led by NCCN, list MR imaging (± contrast) and/or contrast CT as preferred tools

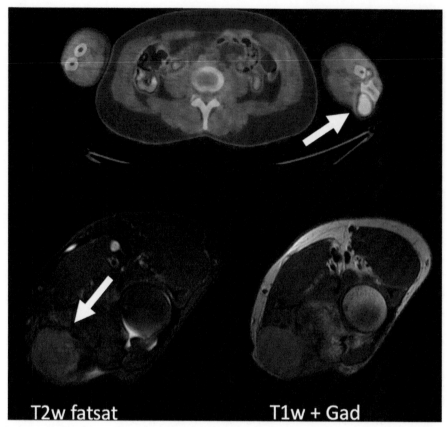

Fig. 5. Recurrence of rhabdomyosarcoma (left forearm). Follow-up of certain tumors may benefit from PET CT, as they can show avid FDG uptake, as in the case presented here (*image on the top–arrow*). MR imaging also shows and comprehensively characterizes and delineates the recurrence (*images on the bottom–arrow*).

in their recommendations for locoregional surveillance.

In the latest edition of the appropriateness criteria of the American College of Radiology regarding surveillance of local recurrence in patients with malignant or aggressive primary soft tissue tumors in the limbs or trunk, MR imaging of the area of interest, is considered as "usually appropriate". Both options, with or without contrast, are considered equivalent alternatives (**Fig. 4**).

Ultrasound, CT with intravenous (IV) contrast, as well as whole-body FDG-PET CT or MR imaging are considered "may be appropriate" tools (**Fig. 5**). Interestingly, and as a novelty, in the latest edition, the concept of "disagreement" among members of the panel was introduced, regarding the use of ultrasound. The panel considered that there are still limited data comparing the utility of ultrasound relative to other established methods.

CT without contrast and radiographs are considered "usually not appropriate".

Recently, the suggestion has been made to perform imaging if there is clinical suspicion of local recurrence, leaving imaging surveillance to sites than cannot be accessed clinically.[60]

The Role of MR Imaging on the Surveillance of Soft Tissue Sarcomas

In recent years, several studies on the utility of MR imaging for the assessment of local recurrence in STS have been published. Comparative studies are still scarce, and likely because of its characteristics, MR imaging has been adopted as the usual imaging method (**Fig. 6**).

A study by Park and colleagues[58] on a group of 325 patients with STS surveilled with MR imaging found that 60% of local recurrences were not detected clinically, especially those in the thigh or buttock, small in size or without mass formation (**Fig. 7**). As an aside, but without statistical significance, they noted patients with MR imaging-detected local recurrence tended to have better post-local recurrence survival.

One of the downsides of MR imaging appears to be the high frequency of false positive results.[62] Labarre and colleagues[63] reported MR imaging

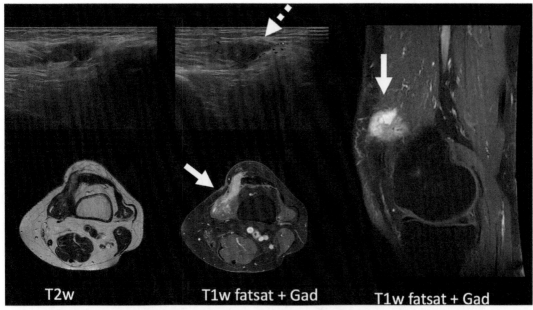

Fig. 6. Low-grade myxofibrosarcoma recurrence. Recurrence of soft tissue tumor often shows similar features to the original tumor. In this case of recurrence, on MR imaging, the typical «tail» of myxofibrosarcoma is identified in the axial plane but not cranio-caudally *(bold arrows)*. Post surgical change can modify the imaging features of the tumors. Despite big improvements in Doppler technology, ultrasound can still miss important features of vascularization *(dotted arrow)*.

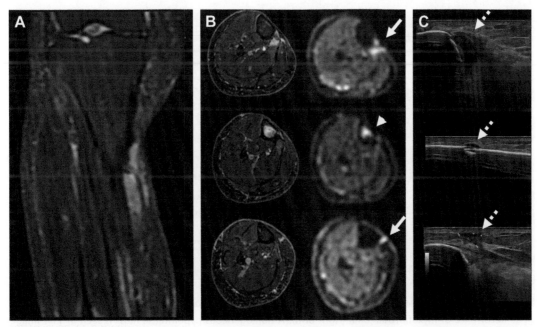

Fig. 7. Low-grade myxofibrosarcoma recurrence in the leg ((*A*), Sagittal STIR; (*B*), Axial T2 fat-sat and DWI; (*C*), Ultrasound). Recurrence of myxofibrosarcoma often shows multiple nodules, and it can involve the bone. DWI despite having relatively low spatial resolution can detect very small foci of recurrence (*white arrows*), as well as bone involvement (*arrowhead*, *B*). The extremely high spatial resolution of ultrasound allows for a confident identification of the nodules, and invasion of bone surfaces (*dotted arrows*, *C*).

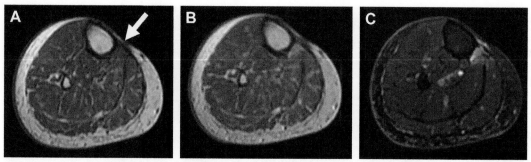

Fig. 8. Low-grade myxofibrosarcoma recurrence in the right leg. Same case as in **Fig. 7** ((*A*), Ax T1w; (*B*), T1w + Gad; (*C*), T2w fat-sat). It is important to note that high-field (≥ 1.5 T) MR imaging equipment should be favored for follow-up imaging and that contrast medium may be very helpful in detecting and discriminating the recurrence, which may be unconspicuous on non contrast imaging (*white arrow in T1w sequence*).

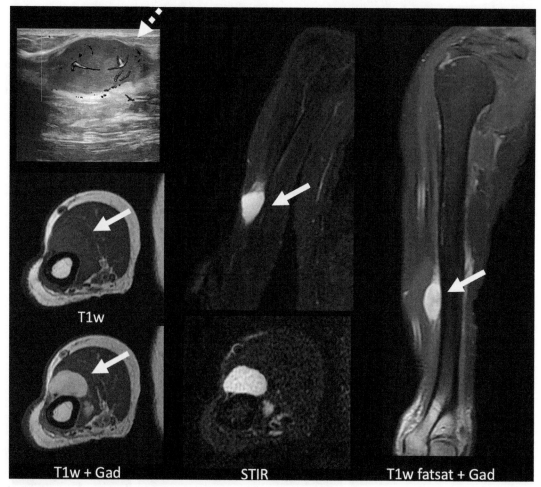

Fig. 9. Recurrence of myxofibrosarcoma (right arm). A homogeneous hypointense mass is seen in T1w images, with homogeneous diffuse contrast enhancement. Note how the appearances of the vascular pattern are different between post-Gd MR images and color-Doppler ultrasound (*dotted arrow on ultrasound image*). Post-contrast MR accurately detects the typical «tail» at the poles of the lesion. In general, fat suppressed in pre- and post-contrast MR imaging is desirable, when possible and when artifacts can be avoided. The lesion is in contact with the humerus, however, this is not involved.

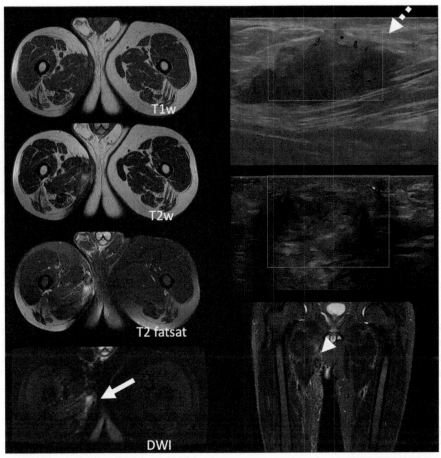

Fig. 10. Recurrence of extraskeletal osteosarcoma (right thigh). In the context of postsurgical changes (*arrow-head on coronal image*), DWI assists to identify the relapse (*bold arrow*). Ultrasound can also detect the firm solid nodule (*right top, dotted arrow;* note the paucity of Doppler signal), though MR sequences were more useful in assessing the involvement of the superficial aponeurosis.

to have a positive predictive value of only 42%, which reinforces the suggestion of some groups to base surveillance on clinical assessment. However, the study by Park and colleagues,[58] with a significantly larger group (325 patients, recurrence rate 11%) than the one from Labarre and colleagues[63] (124 patients, recurrence rate 8.9%) reported a positive predictive value of 93%.

Contrast allows better differentiation of benign and malignant lesions[64] (**Fig. 8**).

Several recent studies[65,66] reported that the use of contrast improves reader confidence for inexperienced but also experienced readers, and the accuracy of inexperienced readers (from 65% to 72%).[66]

A recent retrospective study[67] on the diagnostic efficacy of contrast for the detection of recurrent STS compared with non-contrast sequences concluded contrast improved diagnostic performance in the detection of recurrence. If fat-sat

T2-weighted images were added, sensitivity increased slightly. Specificity was not significantly different (**Fig. 9**).

Beyond the conventional use of contrast and morphologic assessment, the use of functional sequences such as dynamic contrast-enhanced MR imaging (DCE-MR imaging) and quantitative diffusion-weighted imaging (DWI) with apparent diffusion coefficient mapping was proven useful in the evaluation of response to neoadjuvant therapy in STS, and to increase the sensitivity for detection.[68]

As a general rule, tumor tissue enhances fast during the first pass of contrast, whereas reactive, fibrotic tissue enhances at a slower rate, later.[69] Solid tumors have an increased number of cells and intact cell membranes, which typically translates into restricted diffusion (low apparent diffusion coefficient - ADC - values), while successful treatment results in cell membrane rupture and

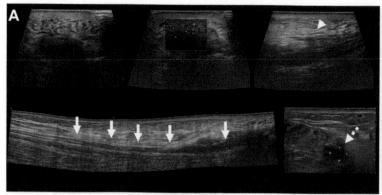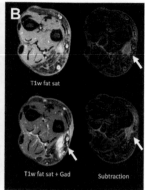

Fig. 11. Recurrence of pleomorphic sarcoma after surgery and radiation therapy (forearm/wrist). For follow-up in superficial regions, such as extremities, high-frequency ultrasound is very useful. In complex cases, after different treatments and scarring, it may be very difficult to discern recurrence from fibrosis with ultrasound–despite the possibility of using very high-frequency probes (such as a linear probe 6–24 Mhz–images shown in *A*). Scars, edema *(arrowhead)*, and postsurgical change (see the ulnar nerve alteration from proximal to distal in the panoramic view at the bottom–*A*) may mimic recurrence (a nodule of recurrence is identified though–*dotted arrow*). MR imaging with contrast enhancement *(B)* is fundamental to provide a comprehensive and safe detection of possible multiple nodules. Subtraction imaging (pre-post Gad) emphasizes this *(arrow)*.

reduction in number, with increased diffusion of water molecules (high ADC values). There is some overlap though because not all malignant tumors present more cellularity than the benign and the benign may have an extracellular matrix similar to the malignant.[70]

The addition of DCE-MR imaging was reported to offer a specificity of more than 95% for distinguishing recurrent sarcoma from postsurgical changes (fibrosis/scarring).[71]

Hirschmann and colleagues[72] highlight the value of DCE-MR imaging in combination with knowledge of surgical margins for the detection of local recurrence and differentiation from postsurgical changes. The authors reported that differentiation of local recurrence from post-treatment changes was the highest combining conventional MR imaging, DCE-MR imaging, and knowledge of surgical margins (Area under curve - AUC 0.779), followed by DCE-MR imaging (AUC 0.706) and conventional MR imaging (AUC 0.648), concluding that the use of DCE-MR imaging and knowledge of surgical margins substantially increase the ability of MR imaging to detect recurrences when these are not clinically evident.

Ongoing research supports the use of DCE-MR imaging with their results. A prospective study by Erber and colleagues[73] analyzed the use of the quantitative DCE-MR imaging parameters relative plasma flow (rPF) and relative mean transit time, using ADC mapping to quantify diffusion restriction, in comparison to morphological assessment, showing that rPF had a distinct higher specificity and true positive predictive value than morphological assessment.

Del Grande and colleagues,[71] in their study comparing the accuracy of conventional MR imaging with the use of functional sequences, also analyzed the performance of quantitative DWI with apparent diffusion coefficient mapping to detect recurrences. Their group included 37 patients (6 histologically proven recurrences). Sensitivity and specificity were 100% and 97%, respectively, with the addition of DCE-MR imaging and 60% and 97% with the addition of DWI and ADC mapping. The average ADC of recurrence (1.08 mm2/s $\pm$ 0.19) was significantly different from those with postoperative fibrosis/scarring (0.9 mm2/s $\pm$ 0.00) ($P = .03$) and hematomas (2.34 mm2/s $\pm$ 0.72) ($P = .03$).

Multiple other recent studies[74–76] have proven that ADC values obtained from DWI have high sensitivity and specificity in differentiating recurring STS from postsurgical changes (**Fig. 10**).

The study by Moustafa and colleagues[75] included 12 patients with aggressive fibromatosis, and showed that lesions with favorable response to chemotherapy or radiotherapy (8/12 patients) demonstrated significantly lower ADC values than those showing disease progression.

ElDaly and colleagues[76] showed that the joint use of contrast and quantitative DWI with ADC mapping offers added value in the detection of recurrence. They achieved 100% sensitivity and 90.48% specificity with a cut-off average ADC value of $\leq 1.3 \times 10^{-3}$ mm2/s, for nonmyxoid tumors. Their results showed limited value of DWI with ADC mapping in assessing myxoid tumor recurrences.

Myxoid tumors have higher diffusion coefficients than nonmyxoid tumors, because of their contents of increased mucin, decreased collagen, and increased amount of water.[77]

Baseline imaging after treatment is extremely important.[78] Radiation therapy can induce vascularization, which results in increased perfusion[79] (**Fig. 11**). Granulation tissue can initially demonstrate contrast uptake, which may make MR imaging assessment equivocal. After 2 to 6 months, only a slow contrast uptake should be detectable.[78] Postsurgical baseline examinations should be delayed to 6 to 8 weeks so that these immediate postsurgical changes are not confounding. Follow-up imaging is necessary because the perfusion of a reactive mass decreases, whereas, in the case of residual tumor or recurrence, there is growth and increase in perfusion.[80]

The Role of Ultrasound on the Surveillance of Soft Tissue Sarcomas. How Does It Compare to MR Imaging?

Ultrasound can be used to detect the recurrence of STS. Most studies comparing the effectiveness of ultrasound compared with MR imaging are outdated[81–83] because both techniques have undergone significant advances.

Choi and colleagues,[81] in the early nineties, in a comparative study that included 21 patients, reported a 100% sensitivity and 79% specificity for ultrasound, compared to 83% and 93%, respectively, for MR imaging (no statistical difference). Ultrasound was indeterminate in two cases, performed 2 and 4 months after surgery. Ultrasound was used to guide fine-needle aspiration biopsy of impalpable lesions. The authors concluded that ultrasound and MR imaging were equally useful for the detection of local recurrence, but ultrasound may be more difficult to interpret than MR imaging in the early postoperative period and MR imaging should be used if ultrasound is inconclusive.

Two years later, a study on 26 patients by Pino and colleagues,[82] reported a sensitivity of 87% for ultrasound, compared to 69.6% for CT. They reported the accuracy of diagnosis for the US on lesions as small as 5 mm.

Arya and colleagues[83] used ultrasound to follow-up on 50 patients after sarcoma surgery. Ultrasound detected 26 recurrences, 18 non-recurrences, benign disease in 4 cases, and 2 indeterminate lesions. In the 26 patients with suspected recurrence, histology confirmed 24 (one false negative and one patient not operated on). Out of the 18 considered non-recurrence, 13 were operated, all negative. Ultrasound fine-needle aspiration was

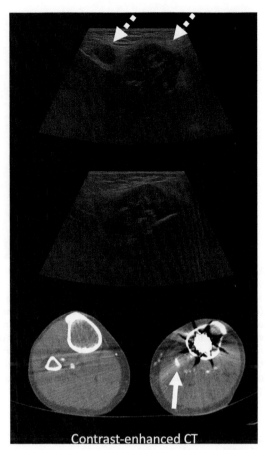
Fig. 12. Recurrence of dedifferentiated chondrosarcoma. Bone tumors can locally recur in soft tissues. Ultrasound can be used for assessing possible soft tissue recurrence, and in this case, can show multiple nodules (*dotted arrows*). Ultrasound and contrast-enhanced CT are often preferred when metal implants may cause artifacts preventing the detection of small nodules on MR imaging, and because of the possible calcified pattern of recurrences (*bold arrow*).

positive in 14 out of 17 patients (88%). The authors reported sensitivity for the ultrasound of 92.3% and a specificity of 94.4%.

Ultrasound also has the advantage of cost efficiency, calculated to be approximately 75% cheaper than MR imaging.[84]

Aside from the described advantages for primary diagnosis, in the particular setting of postsurgical status, ultrasound has the added benefit of not being subject to artifact from hardware (**Fig. 12**). Ultrasound is extremely helpful to assess relatively early postsurgical complications (fluid collections, for example), and potentially guide drainage (and obviously, biopsy).

It is also very useful in the assessment of superficial sarcoma recurrences, including those of very

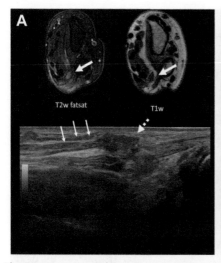
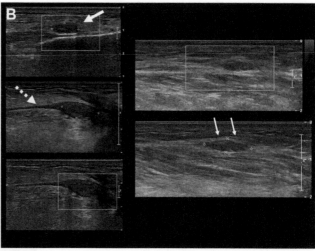

Fig. 13. Neuroma and stump neuromas are classic findings and pitfalls in sarcoma surveillance. Whether caused by voluntary resection of nerves or incidental resection or damage, neuromas are common after surgery for STS. In (*A*) a hyperintense lesion in T2w images, and hypointense T1w, is seen on the course of the ulnar nerve on the wrist (*white thick arrow*). It was known that the surgery had to sacrifice the ulnar nerve, resulting on the existence of a nerve stump. A stump neuroma may be detected and characterized by ultrasound (stump neuroma pointed with *dotted arrow*), showing continuity with the ulnar nerve, which shows normal echotexture proximally (*thin arrows*). In (*B*), two different neuromas are presented (*thick arrow* on the right and *thin arrows* on the left, respectively). It is important to be familiar with the specific district anatomy, and to carefully check for continuity with nerve structures (*dotted arrows*) also when the affected nerves are thin. Note the complete absence of Doppler signal.

small size, due to its superb spatial resolution[85,86] (**Fig. 13**).

The presence of a solid lesion in the context of postsurgical assessment should be assumed to represent a recurrence and managed as such (**Fig. 14**).

In the cases in which the existence of scar tissue may pose a challenge for diagnosis, the use of Doppler can help in the differentiation of fibrous tissue from tumor recurrence[87] (**Fig. 15**). However, the absence of vascularity does not rule out malignancy in these cases, given scarring may interfere with the proliferation of vessels.[88]

In general, lesions that are not completely cystic or suggestive of hematoma or seroma should be considered suspicious. Recurrences may have solid but also cystic components, or contain necrosis, especially if the patient has received radiotherapy.

A recent retrospective study on 68 patients by Tagliafico and colleagues[84] consolidates ultrasound as a highly sensitive and specific test. The authors concluded that the diagnostic accuracy of ultrasound was high and that ultrasound can efficiently identify the majority of patients who do not have a recurrence (positive likelihood ratio of 14.9 and negative predictive value of 0.96).

On this basis, they suggest that ultrasound can be considered as a first-line tool for post-

treatment follow-up, together with clinical examination.

The false negatives they encountered (2) were attributed to the location (deep) and appearance of the lesions. There were three false positives. Accuracy concerning tumor grading was not assessed, but this has been seen to not correlate well even on MR imaging[89] (**Figs. 16–18**).

There is a lack of studies on the specific application of contrast-enhanced ultrasound (CEUS) and elastography on the surveillance of the recurrence of STS.

There are only limited published data on the role of elastography and CEUS in the evaluation of musculoskeletal soft tissue masses.[90–99]

The malignant soft tissue lesions show variable elasticity according to tissue characteristics and cellular differentiation.[90,91,95,96] It has been reported that real-time shear-wave elastography may be useful for malignancy prediction, in combination with conventional ultrasound techniques.[100]

De Marchi and colleagues[97] evaluated CEUS and MR imaging accuracy in comparison to histology in differentiating malignant from nonmalignant superficial soft tissue masses and demonstrated that CEUS showed a sensitivity higher than MR imaging, whereas positive predictive value (PPV) and

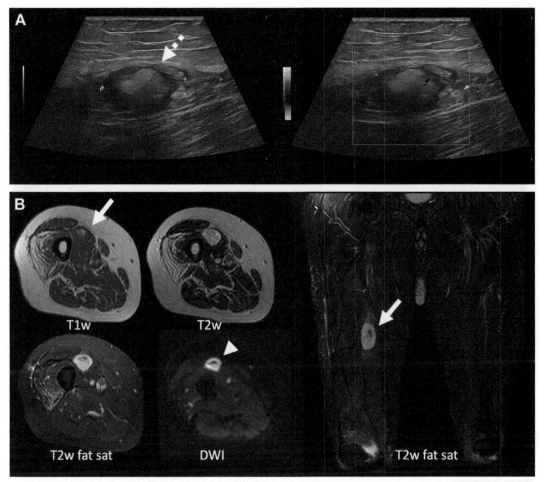

Fig. 14. Recurrence of a well-differentiated liposarcoma (right thigh). In (*A*), the recurrence is clearly depicted and well-characterized by ultrasound, with an echogenic central component (*dotted arrow*). MR imaging (*B*) shows the lesion in T1w imaging (*arrow* on the *left*), T2w, and T2w fat-sat axial and coronal (*right*) and DWI (*bottom right*). Note a locule of fat, with low diffusivity in the center of it (*arrowhead*).

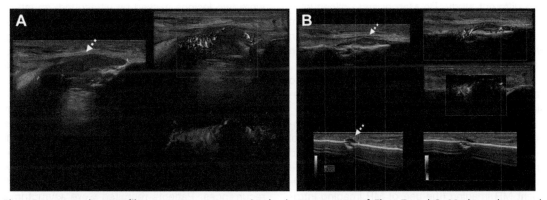

Fig. 15. Low-grade myxofibrosarcoma recurrence in the leg–same case of **Figs. 7** and **8.** Modern ultrasound equipment greatly improves vascular pattern evaluation of lesions. In (*A*), recurrence is presented as a hypoechoic mass (*dotted arrow*) on B-mode on the left, with detailed vascular characterization with color-Doppler (*up*) and B-flow imaging mode (*bottom*) on the right. In (*B*), other foci of recurrence involving the tibia are present. Appearances on B-mode are shown on the left of the image (*dotted arrow*), power-Doppler assessment demonstrates vascularity (*up* and *bottom*). Microvascular imaging (MIV) is shown in the *box in the middle image*.

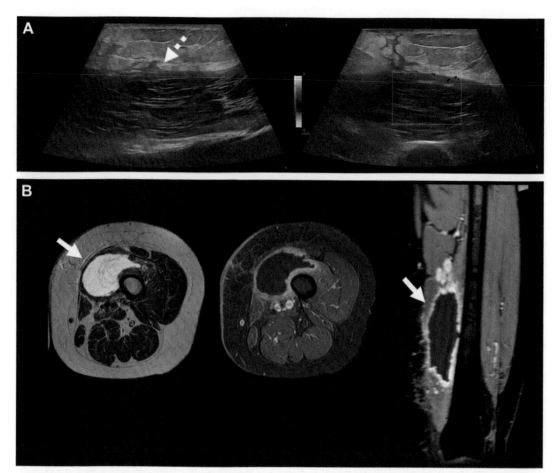

Fig. 16. Post-surgery findings after resection of Evans tumor (left thigh). Ultrasound showed a rather big and mixed multiloculated mass in the surgical bed (*dotted arrow*), without a significant Doppler signal (*A*). MR imaging (T2w, T1w fat-sat with Gad and multiplanar reconstruction) (*B*) shows this as a postsurgical collection (seroma)–*bold arrow*. The radiologist experience is very important. Follow-up exams should be performed in sarcoma-dedicated centers.

negative predictive value (NPV) were comparable. In a different study, De Marchi and colleagues[98] reported intense inhomogeneous enhancement with avascular areas and rapid vascularization time could be useful in discriminating benign from malignant soft tissue tumors.

CEUS has been reported as an accurate way to safely target representative areas of soft tissue lesions for biopsy.[99]

In a recent study, Singer and colleagues[101] proposed a novel scanning and reporting protocol (novel lexicon), and using it, compared ultrasound and MR imaging accuracy and agreement. The outcome was defined by histology or by subsequent MR imaging (the use of MR imaging introducing a bias for reference standard). They analyzed 68 scans in 55 patients. Their results showed the overall accuracy was the same for ultrasound and MR imaging (92.6%). Ultrasound was less sensitive (75.0%) than MR imaging

(91.7%) but more specific (97.6% vs 92.9%). There were two lesions missed by ultrasound, an intraosseous one and a millimetric skin nodule. The agreement between ultrasound and MR imaging with outcome was strong (k = 0.787 and 0.801, respectively). Their data suggest their ultrasound method is comparable in accuracy to MR imaging, and could be used as surveillance, but multi-institutional prospective trials to increase power and reproducibility are still needed.

The magnetic resonance imaging or ultrasound in soft tissue tumors (MUSTT) trial[102] is a prospective monocentric study designed to independently compare these two methods for the detection of recurrences. Patients recruited were asymptomatic, non-metastatic and were followed up with ultrasound and MR imaging every 4 months for the first 5 years and 24 months for negative ultrasound and MR imaging findings after 5 years (clinical assessment, chest CT, and relevant assessment

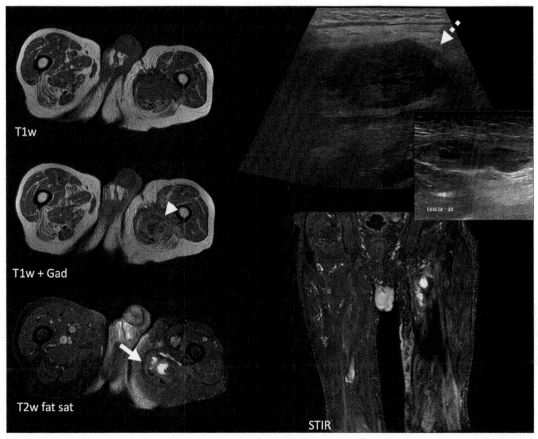

Fig. 17. Pleomorphic sarcoma recurrence (left thigh). As its pattern is very heterogenous, pleomorphic sarcoma looks like a multicystic complex lesion (*arrow*), and may even mimic a collection. Note the inhomogeneous contrast enhancement (*arrowhead*). Ultrasound also depicts the heterogeneity, with hypo-anechoic central areas (*dotted arrow*), suggesting necrosis, found in high-grade sarcomas.

to exclude metastatic disease were performed as per current protocols). Outcome measures were compared using Receiver Operating Characteristic (ROC) curve analysis and the X^2 test, on a per-follow-up event basis (232 events).

The analysis showed an AUC of 0.909 for ultrasound (95% confidence interval 0.832–0.981) and an AUC of 0.966 (0.939–0.989) for MR imaging, with prob $> X^2 = 0$.

The authors concluded each test had satisfactory accuracy, with MR imaging slightly superior but with no statistical significance (if X^2 statistics was used considering the number of events included in the analysis). They noted, however, that ultrasound had some false negative and positive results.

Ultrasound resulted in being highly specific for the detection of recurrences, with the false positives due to presence of scarring and granulation tissue mimicking a mass. The false negatives were deep lesions and lesions containing fat.

The results of these two recent studies are overall coincidental, none of them showing the superiority of ultrasound over MR imaging.

MR imaging may also present false negatives[89] and is not able to characterize every lesion, even if advanced techniques are used.[71,103] Local recurrences may be missed on inadequate protocols.

A recent study found that the systematic use of MR imaging was not effective for the detection of local recurrences in the cases in which these were asymptomatic.[63]

The main limitation of ultrasound is the inability to deep penetration and difficult access to some anatomical locations in some cases. A possible disadvantage is that it is operator-dependent, but it is important to note that these patients should always be managed in the context of a tumor center, by experienced operators.

As a sub-study from the MUSTT trial, Tagliafico and colleagues[104] performed a radiomics analysis on 1.5T images from 33 follow-up events, with a total of 198 data sets per patient of both

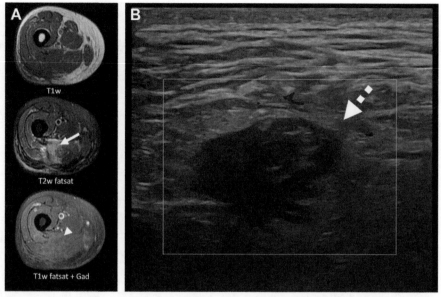

Fig. 18. Undetermined nodule after sarcoma resection. On follow-up MR imaging (*A*) a nodule was detected, which was hyperintense on T2w (*bold arrow*), hypointense on T1w, and hypoechoic on ultrasound (*dotted arrow* in *B*). This nodule was in the course of the sciatic nerve, apparently in continuity with it. This does not show enhancement after Gadolinium injection (*arrowhead*). It is essential for the radiologist to receive information on the surgical procedure performed.

pathological and normal tissue analyzed. Four radiomics features were significantly correlated to tumor size ($P < 0.02$) and four radiomics features were correlated with grading ($P < 0.05$). The ROC analysis showed an AUC for T1w images of 0.71 (95% CI 0.55–0.87) and 0.96 for post-Gadolinium T1w imaging (95% CI 0.87–1.00). Their results show radiomics features on MR imaging allow to differentiate normal from the pathological tissue. The potential application of radiomics is currently a clear advantage favoring the use of MR imaging in the assessment of STS recurrence.

SUMMARY

MR imaging and ultrasound have different advantages in the assessment of soft tissue sarcoma recurrence.

Ultrasound is cost-efficient, lacks interference from hardware, and has a high spatial resolution for superficial lesions. It also presents the advantage of providing guidance for biopsy. It has been proven to efficiently identify the majority of patients who do not have a recurrence. Despite this, it cannot be used in certain deep anatomical locations, is still operator-dependent, and may pose difficulties to interpretation in the early postoperative period. Its use is being progressively considered in different guidelines. There is a lack of evidence on the use of novel ultrasound

techniques, like CEUS and elastography, for the specific assessment of local tumor recurrence.

MR imaging remains the usual imaging method for recurrence surveillance, and the use of DCE-MR imaging and DWI has improved its efficiency in the diagnosis, reducing false positives in the cases of postsurgical fibrosis.

Comparative studies on the performance of both techniques are still scarce. Recent studies are overall coincidental, none of them showing the superiority of ultrasound over MR imaging. Ultrasound may be comparable in accuracy to MR imaging, and could be used as surveillance, but multi-institutional prospective trials to increase power and reproducibility are still needed.

The potential application of radiomics could favor the use of MR imaging in the assessment of STS recurrence.

CLINICS CARE POINTS

- Ultrasound as a surveillance tool of local recurrence of soft tissue sarcomas has been proven to have high negative predictive value, besides from having a number of other advantages. Different guidelines present it as an alternative to MR imaging as first-line assessment.

- MR imaging is still the preferred method for recurrence surveillance. The use of advanced techniques (such as dynamic contrast enhancement and diffusion-weighted imaging) has improved its efficiency on the diagnosis, reducing false positives.
- Comparative studies on the performance of US and MR imaging are scarce. US may be comparable in accuracy to MR imaging in expert hands, but multi-institutional prospective trials to increase power and reproducibility are still needed.

DISCLOSURE

The authors have no funding information to disclose.

REFERENCES

1. Gatta G, Capocaccia R, Botta L, et al. Burden and centralised treatment in Europe of rare tumours: results of RARECAREnet-a population-based study. Lancet Oncol 2017;18(8):1022–39.

2. Penel N, Grosjean J, Robin YM, et al. Frequency of certain established risk factors in soft tissue sarcomas in adults: a prospective descriptive study of 658 cases. Sarcoma 2008;2008:459386.

3. von Mehren M, Kane JM, Bui MM, et al. NCCN guidelines insights: soft tissue sarcoma, version 1.2021. J Natl Compr Canc Netw 2020;18(12):1604–12.

4. de Juan Ferré A, Álvarez Álvarez R, Casado Herráez A, et al. SEOM Clinical Guideline of management of soft-tissue sarcoma (2020). Clin Transl Oncol 2021;23(5):922–30.

5. Albritton K, Bleyer WA. The management of cancer in the older adolescent. Eur J Cancer 2003;39(18):2584–99.

6. Geraci M, Birch JM, Alston RD, et al. Cancer mortality in 13 to 29-year-olds in England and Wales, 1981-2005. Br J Cancer 2007;97(11):1588–94.

7. Voss RK, Chiang YJ, Torres KE, et al. Adherence to National Comprehensive Cancer Network Guidelines is Associated with Improved Survival for Patients with Stage 2A and Stages 2B and 3 Extremity and Superficial Trunk Soft Tissue Sarcoma. Ann Surg Oncol 2017;24(11):3271–8.

8. Coindre JM, Terrier P, Guillou L, et al. Predictive value of grade for metastasis development in the main histologic types of adult soft tissue sarcomas: a study of 1240 patients from the French Federation of Cancer Centers Sarcoma Group. Cancer 2001;91(10):1914–26.

9. NCIN Bone and soft tissue sarcomas. UK incidence and survival. 1996–2010. 2nd edn; 2013. p. 1–17. Available at: http://www.ncin.org.uk/cancer_type_and_topic_specific_work/cancer_type_specific_work/sarcomas/.

10. Kotilingam D, Lev DC, Lazar AJF, et al. Staging soft tissue sarcoma: evolution and change. CA Cancer J Clin 2006;56(5):282–91 [quiz: 314-315].

11. Dangoor A, Seddon B, Gerrand C, et al. UK guidelines for the management of soft tissue sarcomas. Clin Sarcoma Res 2016;6:20.

12. Aparisi Gómez MP, Errani C, Lalam R, et al. The role of ultrasound in the diagnosis of soft tissue tumors. Semin Musculoskelet Radiol 2020;24(2):135–55.

13. Kumar V, Abbas AK, Fausto N, et al. In: *Robbins and cotran pathologic basis of disease*. 7th edition. Amsterdam, The Netherlands: Elsevier Saunders; 2005.

14. Murphey MD, Arcara LK, Fanburg-Smith J. From the archives of the AFIP: imaging of musculoskeletal liposarcoma with radiologic-pathologic correlation. Radiographics 2005;25(5):1371–95.

15. Gaskin CM, Helms CA. Lipomas, lipoma variants, and well-differentiated liposarcomas (atypical lipomas): results of MRI evaluations of 126 consecutive fatty masses. AJR Am J Roentgenol 2004;182(3):733–9.

16. Grobmyer SR, Brennan MF. Predictive variables detailing the recurrence rate of soft tissue sarcomas. Curr Opin Oncol 2003;15(4):319–26.

17. Memorial Sloan Kettering Cancer Centre. Prediction tools, Available at: https://www.mskcc.org/cancer-care/types/soft-tissue-sarcoma/prediction-tools. Accessed July 11, 2022.

18. Sabolch A, Feng M, Griffith K, et al. Risk factors for local recurrence and metastasis in soft tissue sarcomas of the extremity. Am J Clin Oncol 2012;35(2):151–7.

19. Gronchi A, Lo Vullo S, Colombo C, et al. Extremity soft tissue sarcoma in a series of patients treated at a single institution: local control directly impacts survival. Ann Surg 2010;251(3):506–11.

20. Novais EN, Demiralp B, Alderete J, et al. Do surgical margin and local recurrence influence survival in soft tissue sarcomas? Clin Orthop Relat Res 2010;468(11):3003–11.

21. Salas S, Stoeckle E, Collin F, et al. Superficial soft tissue sarcomas (S-STS): a study of 367 patients from the French Sarcoma Group (FSG) database. Eur J Cancer 2009;45(12):2091–102.

22. Sugiura H, Nishida Y, Nakashima H, et al. Surgical procedures and prognostic factors for local recurrence of soft tissue sarcomas. J Orthop Sci 2014;19(1):141–9.

23. Alamanda VK, Crosby SN, Archer KR, et al. Predictors and clinical significance of local recurrence in extremity soft tissue sarcoma. Acta Oncol 2013;52(4):793–802.

24. Nakamura T, Grimer RJ, Carter SR, et al. Outcome of soft-tissue sarcoma patients who were alive and event-free more than five years after initial treatment. Bone Joint Lett J 2013;95-B(8):1139–43.

25. Kolovich GG, Wooldridge AN, Christy JM, et al. A retrospective statistical analysis of high-grade soft tissue sarcomas. Med Oncol 2012;29(2):1335–44.

26. Binitie O, Tejiram S, Conway S, et al. Adult soft tissue sarcoma local recurrence after adjuvant treatment without resection of core needle biopsy tract. Clin Orthop Relat Res 2013;471(3):891–8.

27. Abatzoglou S, Turcotte RE, Adoubali A, et al. Local recurrence after initial multidisciplinary management of soft tissue sarcoma: is there a way out? Clin Orthop Relat Res 2010;468(11):3012–8.

28. Stojadinovic A, Leung DHY, Allen P, et al. Primary adult soft tissue sarcoma: time-dependent influence of prognostic variables. J Clin Oncol 2002; 20(21):4344–52.

29. Cipriano CA, Jang E, Tyler W. Sarcoma Surveillance: A Review of Current Evidence and Guidelines. J Am Acad Orthop Surg 2020;28(4):145–56.

30. Toulmonde M, Le Cesne A, Mendiboure J, et al. Long-term recurrence of soft tissue sarcomas: prognostic factors and implications for prolonged follow-up. Cancer 2014;120(19):3003–6.

31. Johnson CJ, Pynsent PB, Grimer RJ. Clinical features of soft tissue sarcomas. Ann R Coll Surg Engl 2001;83(3):203–5.

32. ACR Appropriateness Criteria® follow-up of malignant or aggressive musculoskeletal tumors, Available at: https://acsearch.acr.org/docs/69428/Narrative/. Accessed July 20, 2022.

33. Suspected cancer: recognition and referral NICE Guidance NG12 June 2015, Section 1.11, Available at: http://www.nice.org.uk/guidance/ng12. Accessed July 20, 2022.

34. Fujiwara T, Grimer RJ, Evans S, et al. Impact of NICE guidelines on the survival of patients with soft-tissue sarcomas. Bone Joint Lett J 2021;103-B(3):569–77.

35. Gronchi A, Miah AB, Dei Tos AP, et al. Soft tissue and visceral sarcomas: ESMO-EURACAN-GENTURIS Clinical Practice Guidelines for diagnosis, treatment and follow-up. Ann Oncol 2021; 32(11):1348–65.

36. Pohlig F, Kirchhoff C, Lenze U, et al. Percutaneous core needle biopsy versus open biopsy in diagnostics of bone and soft tissue sarcoma: a retrospective study. Eur J Med Res 2012;17:29.

37. Peer S, Freuis T, Loizides A, et al. Ultrasound guided core needle biopsy of soft tissue tumors; a fool proof technique? Med Ultrason 2011;13(3):187–94.

38. De Marchi A, Brach del Prever EM, Linari A, et al. Accuracy of core-needle biopsy after contrast-enhanced ultrasound in soft-tissue tumours. Eur Radiol 2010;20(11):2740–8.

39. Seo SW, Kwon JW, Jang SW, et al. Feasibility of whole-body MRI for detecting metastatic myxoid liposarcoma: a case series. Orthopedics 2011; 34(11):e748–54.

40. King DM, Hackbarth DA, Kilian CM, et al. Soft-tissue sarcoma metastases identified on abdomen and pelvis CT imaging. Clin Orthop Relat Res 2009;467(11):2838–44.

41. Portera CA, Ho V, Patel SR, et al. Alveolar soft part sarcoma: clinical course and patterns of metastasis in 70 patients treated at a single institution. Cancer 2001;91(3):585–91.

42. ESMO/European Sarcoma Network Working Group. Soft tissue and visceral sarcomas: ESMO Clinical Practice Guidelines for diagnosis, treatment and follow-up. Ann Oncol 2014;25(Suppl 3):iii102–12.

43. Kubo T, Furuta T, Johan MP, et al. Prognostic significance of (18)F-FDG PET at diagnosis in patients with soft tissue sarcoma and bone sarcoma; systematic review and meta-analysis. Eur J Cancer 2016;58:104–11.

44. Lim HJ, Johnny Ong CA, Tan JWS, et al. Utility of positron emission tomography/computed tomography (PET/CT) imaging in the evaluation of sarcomas: a systematic review. Crit Rev Oncol Hematol 2019;143:1–13.

45. Schuetze SM. Utility of positron emission tomography in sarcomas. Curr Opin Oncol 2006;18(4):369–73.

46. Eary JF, O'Sullivan F, Powitan Y, et al. Sarcoma tumor FDG uptake measured by PET and patient outcome: a retrospective analysis. Eur J Nucl Med Mol Imaging 2002;29(9):1149–54.

47. Folpe AL, Lyles RH, Sprouse JT, et al. (F-18) fluorodeoxyglucose positron emission tomography as a predictor of pathologic grade and other prognostic variables in bone and soft tissue sarcoma. Clin Cancer Res 2000;6(4):1279–87.

48. On behalf of the British Sarcoma Group, Gerrand C, Athanasou N, Brennan B, et al. UK guidelines for the management of bone sarcomas. Clin Sarcoma Res 2016;6(1):7.

49. Whooley BP, Mooney MM, Gibbs JF, et al. Effective follow-up strategies in soft tissue sarcoma. Semin Surg Oncol 1999;17(1):83–7.

50. Whooley BP, Gibbs JF, Mooney MM, et al. Primary extremity sarcoma: what is the appropriate follow-up? Ann Surg Oncol 2000;7(1):9–14.

51. Kane JM. Surveillance strategies for patients following surgical resection of soft tissue sarcomas. Curr Opin Oncol 2004;16(4):328–32.

52. Patel SR, Zagars GK, Pisters PWT. The follow-up of adult soft-tissue sarcomas. Semin Oncol 2003; 30(3):413–6.

53. Rothermundt C, Whelan JS, Dileo P, et al. What is the role of routine follow-up for localised limb soft tissue sarcomas? A retrospective analysis of 174 patients. Br J Cancer 2014;110(10):2420–6.

54. Lewis JJ, Leung D, Casper ES, et al. Multifactorial analysis of long-term follow-up (more than 5 years) of primary extremity sarcoma. Arch Surg 1999; 134(2):190–4.

55. Puri A, Gulia A, Hawaldar R, et al. Does intensity of surveillance affect survival after surgery for sarcomas? Results of a randomized noninferiority trial. Clin Orthop Relat Res 2014;472(5):1568–75.

56. Puri A, Ranganathan P, Gulia A, et al. Does a less intensive surveillance protocol affect the survival of patients after treatment of a sarcoma of the limb? updated results of the randomized TOSS study. Bone Joint Lett J 2018;100-B(2):262–8.

57. Patel SA, Royce TJ, Barysauskas CM, et al. Surveillance Imaging Patterns and Outcomes Following Radiation Therapy and Radical Resection for Localized Extremity and Trunk Soft Tissue Sarcoma. Ann Surg Oncol 2017;24(6):1588–95.

58. Park JW, Yoo HJ, Kim HS, et al. MRI surveillance for local recurrence in extremity soft tissue sarcoma. Eur J Surg Oncol 2019;45(2):268–74.

59. Kraus D, Oettinger F, Kiefer J, et al. Efficacy and cost-benefit analysis of magnetic resonance imaging in the follow-up of soft tissue sarcomas of the extremities and trunk. J Oncol 2021;2021:5580431.

60. Cheney MD, Giraud C, Goldberg SI, et al. MRI surveillance following treatment of extremity soft tissue sarcoma. J Surg Oncol 2014;109(6):593–6.

61. Aparisi Gómez MP, Aparisi F, Morganti AG, et al. Effects of radiation therapy and chemotherapy on the musculoskeletal system. Semin Musculoskelet Radiol 2022;26(3):338–53.

62. Richardson K, Potter M, Damron TA. Image intensive soft tissue sarcoma surveillance uncovers pathology earlier than patient complaints but with frequent initially indeterminate lesions. J Surg Oncol 2016;113(7):818–22.

63. Labarre D, Aziza R, Filleron T, et al. Detection of local recurrences of limb soft tissue sarcomas: is magnetic resonance imaging (MRI) relevant? Eur J Radiol 2009;72(1):50–3.

64. Kransdorf MJ, Murphey MD. The use of gadolinium in the MR evaluation of soft tissue tumors. Semin Ultrasound CT MR 1997;18(4):251–68.

65. Chou SHS, Hippe DS, Lee AY, et al. Gadolinium contrast enhancement improves confidence in diagnosing recurrent soft tissue sarcoma by MRI. Acad Radiol 2017;24(5):615–22.

66. Diana Afonso P, Kosinski AS, Spritzer CE. Following unenhanced MRI assessment for local recurrence after surgical resection of mesenchymal soft tissue tumors, do additional gadolinium-enhanced images change reader confidence or diagnosis? Eur J Radiol 2013;82(5): 806–13.

67. Amini B, Murphy WA, Haygood TM, et al. Gadolinium-based contrast agents improve detection of recurrent soft-tissue sarcoma at MRI. Radiol Imaging Cancer 2020;2(2):e190046.

68. Soldatos T, Ahlawat S, Montgomery E, et al. Multiparametric assessment of treatment response in high-grade soft-tissue sarcomas with anatomic and functional MR imaging sequences. Radiology 2016;278(3):831–40.

69. Verstraete KL, De Deene Y, Roels H, et al. Benign and malignant musculoskeletal lesions: dynamic contrast-enhanced MR imaging–parametric "first-pass" images depict tissue vascularization and perfusion. Radiology 1994;192(3):835–43.

70. Rimondi E, Benassi MS, Bazzocchi A, et al. Translational research in diagnosis and management of soft tissue tumours. Cancer Imag 2016;16(1):13.

71. Del Grande F, Subhawong T, Weber K, et al. Detection of soft-tissue sarcoma recurrence: added value of functional MR imaging techniques at 3.0 T. Radiology 2014;271(2):499–511.

72. Hirschmann A, van Praag VM, Haas RL, et al. Can we use MRI to detect clinically silent recurrent soft-tissue sarcoma? Eur Radiol 2020;30(9):4724–33.

73. Erber BM, Reidler P, Goller SS, et al. Impact of dynamic contrast enhanced and diffusion-weighted MR imaging on detection of early local recurrence of soft tissue sarcoma. J Magn Reson Imaging 2022. https://doi.org/10.1002/jmri.28236.

74. Aktas E, Arikan SM, Ardıç F, et al. The importance of diffusion apparent diffusion coefficient values in the evaluation of soft tissue sarcomas after treatment. Pol J Radiol 2021;86:e291–7.

75. Moustafa AFI, Eldaly MM, Zeitoun R, et al. Is MRI diffusion-weighted imaging a reliable tool for the diagnosis and post-therapeutic follow-up of extremity soft tissue neoplasms? Indian J Radiol Imaging 2019;29(4):378–85.

76. ElDaly MM, Moustafa AFI, Abdel-Meguid SMS, et al. Can MRI diffusion-weighted imaging identify postoperative residual/recurrent soft-tissue sarcomas? Indian J Radiol Imaging 2018;28(1):70–7.

77. Maeda M, Matsumine A, Kato H, et al. Soft-tissue tumors evaluated by line-scan diffusion-weighted imaging: influence of myxoid matrix on the apparent diffusion coefficient. J Magn Reson Imaging 2007;25(6):1199–204.

78. Noebauer-Huhmann IM, Chaudhary SR, Papakonstantinou O, et al. Soft tissue sarcoma follow-up imaging: strategies to distinguish post-treatment changes from recurrence. Semin Musculoskelet Radiol 2020;24(06):627–44.

79. Verstraete KL, Lang P. Bone and soft tissue tumors: the role of contrast agents for MR imaging. Eur J Radiol 2000;34(3):229–46.

80. Costa FM, Martins PH, Canella C, et al. Multiparametric MR imaging of soft tissue tumors and pseudotumors. Magn Reson Imaging Clin N Am 2018; 26(4):543–58.

81. Choi H, Varma DG, Fornage BD, et al. Soft-tissue sarcoma: MR imaging vs sonography for detection of local recurrence after surgery. AJR Am J Roentgenol 1991;157(2):353–8.

82. Pino G, Conzi GF, Murolo C, et al. Sonographic evaluation of local recurrences of soft tissue sarcomas. J Ultrasound Med 1993;12(1):23–6.

83. Arya S, Nagarkatti DG, Dudhat SB, et al. Soft tissue sarcomas: ultrasonographic evaluation of local recurrences. Clin Radiol 2000;55(3):193–7.

84. Tagliafico A, Truini M, Spina B, et al. Follow-up of recurrences of limb soft tissue sarcomas in patients with localized disease: performance of ultrasound. Eur Radiol 2015;25(9):2764–70.

85. Morel M, Taïeb S, Penel N, et al. Imaging of the most frequent superficial soft-tissue sarcomas. Skeletal Radiol 2011;40(3):271–84.

86. Hung EHY, Griffith JF, Ng AWH, et al. Ultrasound of musculoskeletal soft-tissue tumors superficial to the investing fascia. AJR Am J Roentgenol 2014; 202(6):W532–40.

87. Vanel D, et al. Post treatment assessment of soft tissue tumors. In: DeSchepper AM, Vanhoenacker F, Gielen J, et al, editors. *Imaging of soft tissue tumors*. 3rd edition. Berlin: Springer Verlag; 2006. p. 375–81.

88. Belli P, Costantini M, Mirk P, et al. Role of color Doppler sonography in the assessment of musculoskeletal soft tissue masses. J Ultrasound Med 2000;19(12):823–30.

89. Zhao F, Ahlawat S, Farahani SJ, et al. Can MR imaging be used to predict tumor grade in soft-tissue sarcoma? Radiology 2014;272(1):192–201.

90. Magarelli N, Carducci C, Bucalo C, et al. Sonoelastography for qualitative and quantitative evaluation of superficial soft tissue lesions: a feasibility study. Eur Radiol 2014;24(3):566–73.

91. Park HJ, Lee SY, Lee SM, et al. Strain elastography features of epidermoid tumours in superficial soft tissue: differences from other benign soft-tissue tumours and malignant tumours. Br J Radiol 2015; 88(1050):20140797.

92. Drakonaki EE, Allen GM, Wilson DJ. Ultrasound elastography for musculoskeletal applications. Br J Radiol 2012;85(1019):1435–45.

93. Taljanovic MS, Gimber LH, Becker GW, et al. Shear-Wave Elastography: Basic Physics and Musculoskeletal Applications. Radiographics 2017;37(3):855–70.

94. Lee YH, Song HT, Suh JS. Use of strain ratio in evaluating superficial soft tissue tumors on ultrasonic elastography. J Med Ultrason (2001) 2014; 41(3):319–23.

95. Pass B, Johnson M, Hensor EMA, et al. Sonoelastography of musculoskeletal soft tissue masses: a pilot study of quantitative evaluation. J Ultrasound Med 2016;35(10):2209–16.

96. Pass B, Jafari M, Rowbotham E, et al. Do quantitative and qualitative shear wave elastography have a role in evaluating musculoskeletal soft tissue masses? Eur Radiol 2017;27(2):723–31.

97. De Marchi A, Pozza S, Charrier L, et al. Small Subcutaneous Soft Tissue Tumors (<5 cm) Can Be Sarcomas and Contrast-Enhanced Ultrasound (CEUS) Is Useful to Identify Potentially Malignant Masses. Int J Environ Res Public Health 2020;17(23):E8868.

98. De Marchi A, Prever EBD, Cavallo F, et al. Perfusion pattern and time of vascularisation with CEUS increase accuracy in differentiating between benign and malignant tumours in 216 musculoskeletal soft tissue masses. Eur J Radiol 2015;84(1): 142–50.

99. Daniels SP, Mankowski Gettle L, Blankenbaker DG, et al. Contrast-enhanced ultrasound-guided musculoskeletal biopsies: our experience and technique. Skeletal Radiol 2021;50(4):673–81.

100. Li A, Peng XJ, Ma Q, et al. Diagnostic performance of conventional ultrasound and quantitative and qualitative real-time shear wave elastography in musculoskeletal soft tissue tumors. J Orthop Surg Res 2020;15(1):103.

101. Singer G, Cichocki M, Schalamon J, et al. A study of metatarsal fractures in children. J Bone Joint Surg Am 2008;90(4):772–6.

102. Bignotti B, Rossi F, Signori A, et al. Magnetic Resonance Imaging or Ultrasound in Localized Intermediate- or High-Risk Soft Tissue Tumors of the Extremities (MUSTT): Final Results of a Prospective Comparative Trial. Diagnostics 2022;12(2):411.

103. Sen J, Agarwal S, Singh S, et al. Benign vs malignant soft tissue neoplasms: limitations of magnetic resonance imaging. Indian J Cancer 2010;47(3): 280–6.

104. Tagliafico AS, Bignotti B, Rossi F, et al. Local recurrence of soft tissue sarcoma: a radiomic analysis. Radiol Oncol 2019;53(3):300–6.

Pain After Hip Arthroplasty
MR Imaging/Ultrasound Correlation

Meghan E. Sahr, MD*, Theodore T. Miller, MD

KEYWORDS

- Total hip arthroplasty • MRI • Multispectral imaging • Ultrasound

KEY POINTS

- MR imaging assessment requires technical modifications to reduce metal artifact, such as multi-spectral imaging, optimization of image quality, and a high-performance 1.5-T system.
- Ultrasound (US) is particularly helpful for periarticular soft tissue, tendon, and nerve evaluation at high-spatial resolution without interference of metal artifact.
- US permits real-time dynamic evaluation and is useful for procedure guidance.
- Causes of synovitis after hip arthroplasty include polymeric wear, adverse reaction to metal debris, infection, mechanical irritation, and recurrence of inflammatory or crystal deposition arthropathy. Synovial appearance can suggest the causitive etiology, particularly on MR imaging.
- Bone complications are diagnosed primarily with MR imaging.

INTRODUCTION

Total hip arthroplasty (THA) is a successful surgical procedure for the treatment of incapacitating arthritis, performed on more than 600,000 patients in the United States annually[1]. Despite its success, postoperative pain is a common complaint, affecting up to 25% of patients at 1 year.[2,3] MR imaging and ultrasound (US) have complementary roles for the assessment of the painful hip replacement. MR imaging provides a comprehensive evaluation, demonstrating abnormalities such as synovitis, periarticular fluid collections, bone abnormalities such as periprosthetic fracture and osteolysis, some types of prosthesis failure, tendon and muscle tears, and neurovascular impingement. US can also evaluate synovitis, periarticular fluid collections, and pathologic condition of the overlying muscles and tendons. It has unique capabilities for dynamic assessment of soft tissue impingement and to guide aspiration and injection procedures. The relative indications for each modality for the evaluations of hip arthroplasty complications are compared in **Table 1**. Many of these complications necessitate revision, performed on more than 50,000 patients per year in the United States, at a risk of 1% to 2% per year.[4–6] Lumbar radiculopathy or medical diseases may cause pain referred to the hip, which is outside the scope of this review.

DISCUSSION
Imaging Technique

MR imaging conventional pulse sequences must be optimized to reduce susceptibility artifact generated from the prosthesis. Differences in susceptibility between the prosthesis and surrounding tissues result in altered precessional frequencies and accelerated dephasing, causing image distortion owing to spatial misregistration in the frequency-encoding and slice selecting directions, as well as inhomogeneous fat suppression. This can be mitigated by both minimizing metal artifact and optimizing image quality (**Table 2**).[7] Of note, use of these techniques requires a high-performance

Department of Radiology and Imaging, Hospital for Special Surgery, 535 East 70th Street, New York, NY 10021, USA
* Corresponding author.
E-mail address: sahrm@hss.edu

Magn Reson Imaging Clin N Am 31 (2023) 215–238
https://doi.org/10.1016/j.mric.2023.01.005

Table 1
Comparison of MR imaging and ultrasound evaluation of hip arthroplasty complications

	MR Imaging	US
Synovitis	+++	++
Periarticular fluid collection	+++	+++
Bone (fracture, osteolysis)	+++	−
Tendon tears/muscle quality	+++	++
Neurovascular impingement	+++	++
Prosthesis component failure	+	+
Dynamic evaluation	−	+++
Procedure guidance	−	+++

1.5-T system capable of high-gradient amplitude and radiofrequency power, available from all major vendors.

Proprietary 3-dimensional (3D) MR imaging pulse sequences to reduce metal artifact have been developed that further reduce susceptibility artifact around metal. These include MAVRIC (Multiacquisition Variable-Resonance Image Combination; GE), SEMAC (slice-encoding metal artifact correction; Siemens), O-MAR (Orthopedic Metal Artifact Reduction; Philips), and HiMAR (Hitachi Metal Artifact Reduction; Hitachi).[8] These techniques decrease the volume of susceptibility artifact adjacent to the prosthesis at the cost of decreased signal-to-noise (SNR) and longer acquisition times.[9] More recently, a hybrid sequence combining SEMAC and MAVRIC called Multi-Acquisition with Variable Resonance Image Combination SeLective (MAVRIC SL) has been developed that mitigates aliasing artifact seen on MAVRIC and reduces metal artifacts even at higher field strengths.[10] Isotropic MAVRIC SL further improves SNR, conspicuity of lesions, visualization of synovium and periprosthetic bone, and decreases blurring compared with a nonisotropic acquisition.[11]

US is particularly advantageous for the evaluation of the periarticular soft tissues after hip replacement owing to its high-spatial resolution and lack of metal artifact. The examination is targeted to the clinical concern, as is done for diagnostic evaluation about the native hip. A high-frequency linear transducer (9–15 mHz) is preferred. Although preoperative MR imaging is being investigated to predict postoperative range of motion and potential sites of bone, prosthesis, and soft tissue impingement,[12] only US permits dynamic examination and direct visualization of such processes postoperatively.

Hip Arthroplasty Types and Techniques

THA prostheses can be grouped based on the combination of bearing surfaces used. A metal femoral head on a polyethylene acetabular liner (metal-on-polyethylene, MoP), a ceramic head on polyethylene, a ceramic head on a ceramic liner, and a metal head on a metal acetabular component without a liner (metal-on-metal, MoM) are commonly encountered designs (**Fig. 1**). Of note, all THA designs include an interface between the separately fabricated but attached prosthetic femoral head and stem, called the trunnion, resulting in a component of modularity and customization in every THA design. Resurfacing hip arthroplasty (HRA) spares the native femoral neck, using a noncemented acetabular component and a large prosthetic head with a short stem. It is often performed in younger patients requiring hip replacement so that bone stock is better preserved for potential revisions.

There are multiple surgical approaches in use, each one associated with specific soft tissue complications caused either directly by the surgical incision or by stretching from excessive traction. If the surgery was recently performed, the tract will normally contain a small amount of fluid, and the adjacent soft tissues will be edematous and mildly hyperemic. After healing, it can be identified on MR imaging as a hypointense line with subtle

Table 2
Strategies to minimize metal artifact on MR imaging

Minimization of Metal Artifacts	Optimization of Image Quality
Lower field strength (1.5 T, not 3 T)	Use intermediate TE fluid-sensitive sequences
FSE sequences (avoid gradient-echo)	Large matrix in frequency-encoding direction
High receiver (readout) bandwidth	High number of excitations (increase SNR)
Thin sections	Inversion recovery fat suppression (avoid frequency-selective fat suppression)

Adapted with permission from Fritz et al.[7]

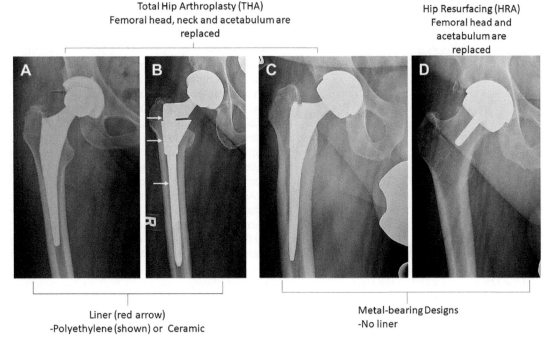

Total Hip Arthroplasty (THA)
Femoral head, neck and acetabulum are
replaced

Hip Resurfacing (HRA)
Femoral head and
acetabulum are
replaced

Liner (red arrow)
-Polyethylene (shown) or Ceramic

Metal-bearing Designs
-No liner

Fig. 1. Arthroplasty design. Anteroposterior (AP) radiographs of a THA using metal femoral and acetabular components and a radiolucent polyethylene liner (*red arrow*) (MoP; *A, B*). Interfacing stem components (*yellow arrows*) in panel B indicate a modular design. MoM THA (*C*) and HRA (*D*) using metal components and no liner (HRA; *D*). Note the preservation of the femoral neck in resurfacing (*D*). Close apposition of the femoral head and acetabular component is diagnostic of the MoM, linerless design (*C, D*). Image / Video reused with permissions from Complete Anatomy (www.3d4medical.com), copyright 3D4Medical LTD, 2021.

distortion of tissue planes and usually a few foci of susceptibility artifact. On US, only subtle tissue distortion will be detectable, although the surgical scar is usually readily visualized on direct inspection while scanning. Identification of the surgical approach should cue a search for its commonly associated complications (**Fig. 2, Table 3**).

INTRAARTICULAR COMPLICATIONS
Effusion and Synovitis

Normally, the postarthroplasty hip synovium should be thin with or without a small amount of intraarticular fluid (**Figs. 3** and **4**).[13] The capsule is incised during surgery and is thereafter referred to as the pseudocapsule. If intraarticular fluid accumulates, it often decompresses into the greater trochanteric bursa, particularly if a posterior, transgluteal approach was used, or the iliopsoas or subiliac bursa if an anterior approach was used.[14,15] As in the native hip, the US appearance of synovitis is of hypoechoic synovial thickening with or without hyperemia and/or an anechoic effusion.[16] Nonspecific synovitis is diagnosed when the synovium is thickened with accumulation of intraarticular fluid that is uniformly high signal on MR imaging or anechoic on US, thought to be

caused by mechanical irritation by the components, which can be asymptomatic (**Figs. 5** and **6**).[17] MR imaging with metal artifact reduction techniques is highly sensitive for detection of synovitis, and its appearance is suggestive of the causative cause (**Box 1**).

Polymeric liner wear generates intraarticular particles that can induce synovitis, often accompanied by osteolysis and loosening. Although highly cross-linked polyethylene has a lower wear rate than the ultrahigh-molecular-weight polyethylene used in the past, polymeric wear

---

Box 1
Causes of synovitis after hip arthroplasty

- Mechanical irritation
- Infection
- Polyethylene wear
- Adverse reaction to metal debris (metallosis and ALVAL)
- Recurrent inflammatory arthropathy/crystal deposition/tumor
- Hemarthrosis

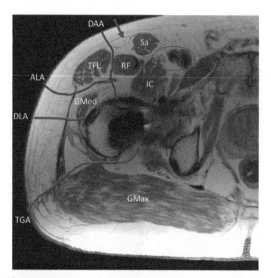

Fig. 2. Hip surgical approaches. Axial intermediate-weighted MRimage of a THA at the level of the proximal femur shows the expected locations of various surgical tracts in use to perform the procedure (*blue lines*). ALA, anterolateral approach; DAA, direct anterior approach; DLA, direct lateral approach; Gmed, gluteus medius muscle; Gmax, Gluteus maximus muscle; lateral femoral cutaneous nerve (*red arrow*), femoral neurovascular bundle (*red oval*); IC, iliocapsularis muscle; RF, rectus femoris muscle; Sa, sartorius muscle; TGA, posterior/transgluteal approach; TFL, tensor fascia lata.

continues to be a leading cause of postoperative synovitis, particularly for the MoP design.[18] Polyethylene wear-induced synovitis is characterized on MR imaging by distention of the pseudocapsule

by thick, low- to intermediate-signal intensity synovial proliferation and debris with variable amounts of fluid, which may extend into the overlying bursae (**Fig. 7**).[13,19,20] Because of this signal profile, synovitis may be difficult to detect on fat-suppressed sequences and is most conspicuous on fast spin-echo (FSE) sequences with intermediate tissue weighting. On US, synovitis appears bulky with heterogeneous echogenicity. Occasionally, characteristic intrasynovial punctate hyperechoic dots are observed, producing a "starry sky" appearance, although this is more commonly seen at the knee.

Adverse local tissue reaction (ALTR) refers to an inflammatory reaction incited by metal wear debris, corrosion products, and metal ions shed by the prosthesis. They are classically associated with metal-bearing (MoM and HRA) designs, but can be generated even with MoP and metal-on-ceramic designs owing to fretting by abnormal contact between the femoral component and cup, as well as at the metal interfaces of modular designs such as at the trunnion (see **Fig. 1**).[21–23] Metallosis is a nonhypersensitivity subcategory of ALTR associated with high wear rates and shedding of metallic particles (**Fig. 8**). It causes a characteristic synovitis on MR imaging, appearing as low-signal-intensity synovial debris, which is either confluent or coats the synovial surface, often with susceptibility, and associated hypointense periprosthetic osteolysis (**Figs. 9** and **10**). The periarticular soft tissues are usually preserved; however, low-signal foci and susceptibility may also be seen in the periprosthetic soft tissues

Table 3
Hip surgical approaches and complications

Approach	Tract	Complication
Posterior (transgluteal)	Divides gluteus maximus, short external rotators, and posterior capsule	Dislocation (posterior), more common without capsular repair[13] Sciatic nerve palsy, especially the common peroneal branch
Anterolateral approach (Watson-Jones)	Extend between tensor fascia lata and gluteus medius, often detaches abductors	Abductor weakness and tears Superior gluteal nerve injury
Direct lateral	Splits gluteus medius and vastus lateralis	Abductor weakness and tears Superior gluteal nerve injury
Direct anterior (Smith-Peterson)	Between rectus femoris and tensor fascia lata Only internervous and intermuscular approach	Lateral femoral cutaneous nerve and femoral neurovascular injury Short external rotator injury Postoperative hematomas Dislocation (anterior) Femoral perforation and periprosthetic fracture Wound dehiscence

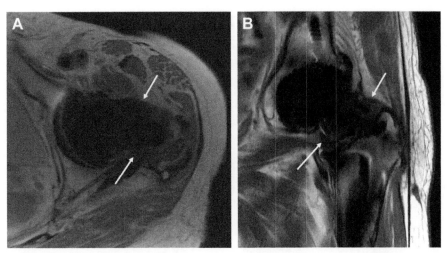

Fig. 3. Normal MR imaging appearance of a THA in an 85-year-old female patient on straight axial (*A*) and coronal (*B*) proton density (PD) -weighted FSE sequences without dedicated metal artifact reduction. The joint pseudocapsule is scar thickened (*arrows*), and a trace amount of intraarticular fluid is also common (not shown).

and regional lymph nodes. The US appearance is of a nonspecific synovitis, as the metal particles are sonographically occult (see **Fig. 9C**).

Metal hypersensitivity, or aseptic lymphocytic vasculitis-associated lesion (ALVAL), is a term that describes a type IV hypersensitivity ALTR to metal ions, generally associated with lower wear rates and smaller particles than metallosis.[23,24] ALVAL is most associated with MoM (43% at revision) and modular designs and may be asymptomatic with an indolent course.[18,25,26] When severe, ALVAL can cause painful, aggressive soft tissue destruction, including necrosis; therefore, early diagnosis and revision are essential to limit tissue damage. The severity of ALVAL is determined histologically, scored for synovial integrity, components of the inflammatory infiltrate, and degree of tissue organization, with a high score of 10.

Severity does not correlate well with preoperative serum metal ion levels[27]; therefore, imaging has a pivotal diagnostic role. MR imaging features predictive of a moderate to severe histologic ALVAL (score ≥5) are synovial thickness ≥7 mm and a solid and cystic synovial appearance. Pseudocapsular dehiscence, a mixed pattern of synovitis with extracapsular decompression of synovium and periarticular soft tissue edema are most predictive of tissue damage found at revision (**Fig. 11**).[28] A poor zone of demarcation between the periarticular muscles and pseudocapsule indicates necrosis (**Fig. 12**).[28] Extracapsular soft tissue masses, or "pseudotumors," that do not communicate with the joint associated with ALVAL can be graded on severity with several classification systems; they are most likely to be symptomatic when solid and anterior in location (**Fig. 13**).[23,29,30] US is also

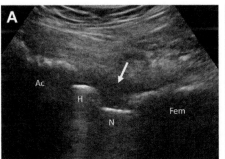
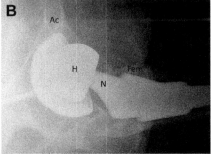

Fig. 4. Normal US appearance of THA (*A*) correlated with a frog-lateral radiograph of the same hip (*B*). Reverberation artifact is generated by the prosthetic femoral head (H) and neck (N); the bony acetabulum (Ac) and femur (Fem) have an echogenic cortex with deeper acoustic shadowing. There is expected mild capsular/synovial thickening (*arrow*) at the anterior aspect of the joint, without anechoic fluid distention of the anterior recess, imaged supine.

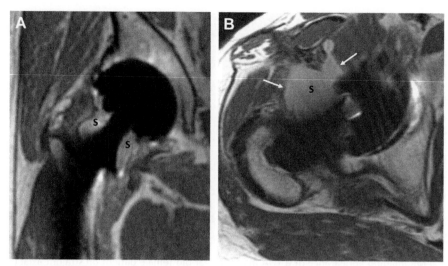

Fig. 5. MR imaging appearance of nonspecific synovitis (S) in a 62-year-old woman after recent hip dislocation after THA using the anterior approach. Coronal MAVRIC PD-weighted (A) and axial conventional 2-dimensional (2D) PD (B) images of the right hip show homogeneous, hyperintense distension of the pseudocapsule with anterior disruption (arrows).

able to demonstrate high-volume synovitis with hypoechoic synovial thickening and any cystic components, pseudocapsular dehiscence, periarticular collections, and extraarticular soft tissue masses suggestive of ALVAL (see **Fig. 11C**).

Infection must be excluded in the setting of painful hip arthroplasty. Incidence is 1.63% within the first 2 years, decreasing to 0.59% between years 2 and 10.[31] Definitive diagnosis requires arthrocentesis with synovial fluid and histologic synovial analysis, the latter routinely obtained at the time of explantation or staged revision surgery;

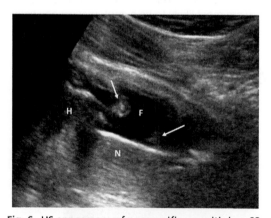

Fig. 6. US appearance of nonspecific synovitis in a 68-year-old man 3 years after total hip replacement. An anterior image of the hip shows reverberation artifact from the head (H) and stem/neck (N) of the prosthesis and anechoic intraarticular fluid (F) with small foci of synovial hypertrophy (arrows).

however, imaging can be predictive. On MR imaging, features of infection include synovitis and effusion, edematous enhancing synovium, pericapsular soft tissues, and bone, sinus tracts, bone destruction, and lymphadenopathy (**Fig. 14**). The synovitis of infection often has a hyperintense, lamellated appearance, which can increase diagnostic confidence when present.[32,33] Absence of osteomyelitis features does not exclude septic arthritis. On US, the synovium is thickened and markedly hyperemic, although the lamellated appearance is not apparent. Sinus tracts are depicted as a hypoechoic tract extending from the joint or a periarticular collection to the skin surface, often with surrounding soft tissue hyperemia (**Fig. 15**). Periarticular fluid collections contain fluid of various echotextures that can be targeted for aspiration, differentiated from soft tissue by lack of color flow, compressibility, and swirling mobile debris.

Hemarthrosis may also complicate hip arthroplasty with causes including pseudoaneurysm or bleeding directly from the geniculate vessels or the synovium. Patients with coagulopathy or taking anticoagulant medications are at increased risk. On both MR imaging and US, hemarthrosis may have a variable appearance depending on age, but is often complex, consisting of clotted components that are heterogenous in signal and echotexture, as well as fluid-fluid levels (**Fig. 16**). Evaluation with MRA can often diagnose pseudoaneurysm or hyperemic synovium as the cause and identify feeding vessels as potential targets for embolization.[34]

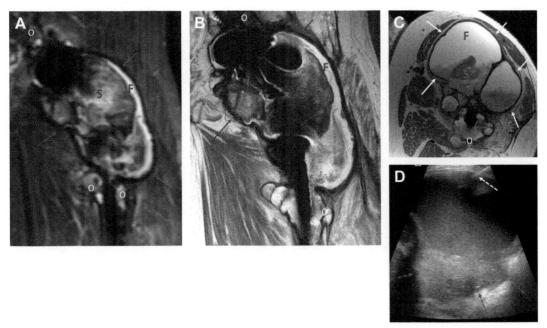

Fig. 7. Severe case of polymeric wear-induced synovitis in a 66-year-old man with a painful revision proximal femoral replacing THA. MR imaging coronal MAVRIC inversion recovery (A), coronal (B), and axial (C) PD FSE images of the left hip show exuberant synovial expansion (*red arrows*) with bulky intermediate-low solid (S) and fluid signal (F) components decompressing into the extracapsular soft tissues (*yellow arrows*). Foci of periprosthetic osteolysis (O) with similar heterogeneous signal characteristics in the acetabulum and femur are also present. Transverse US image taken during aspiration (D) at the level of the anterior proximal thigh corresponding to figure component (C) illustrates the hypoechoic fluid component and bulky solid components containing echogenic dots: the "starry sky" appearance suggestive of polymeric wear (*dashed red arrows*). Aspiration needle (*dashed white arrow*).

US-guided procedures serve a major role in the diagnosis of the cause of intraarticular complications. Hip aspiration is part of the standard workup to rule out infection in the setting of postoperative pain (**Fig. 17**). In the authors' experience, there is almost always some fluid in the hip after arthroplasty. Either a longitudinal approach, parallel to the neck, or transverse approach, perpendicular to the neck can be used. If no native fluid is encountered initially, the needle is redirected off the side of the neck to access the fluid. The femur can also be internally/externally rotated and flexed/extended while aspirating, which can sometimes move dependent fluid to the needle. Alternatively, if no intraarticular fluid is identified during preprocedural scanning of the anterior

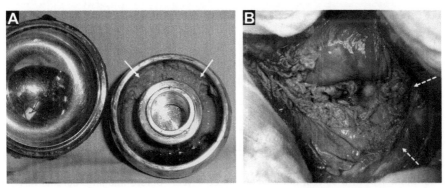

Fig. 8. Metallosis. Excised hip arthroplasty components (A) and hip synovium through an open incision (B) demonstrate green-gray staining of adherent debris (*solid arrows*) and synovium (*dashed arrows*) by metal particles.

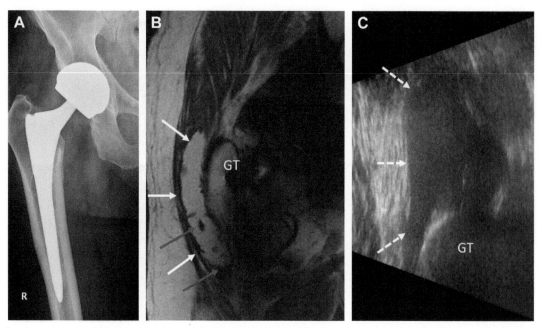

Fig. 9. A 68-year-old man with a painful right MoM THA placed 10 years before imaging using a posterior approach is shown with a contemporaneously obtained AP radiograph (*A*), coronal MAVRIC FSE MR imaging image (*B*), and lateral US image rotated to simulate the coronal MR imaging slice (*C*). There are characteristic features of metallosis, including relatively homogeneous synovial expansion decompressing into the greater trochanteric bursa (*white arrows*) with low-signal synovial staining (*red arrows, B*). Corresponding US image (*C*) shows nonspecific fluid distension of the greater trochanteric bursa (*dashed arrows*). GT, greater trochanter.

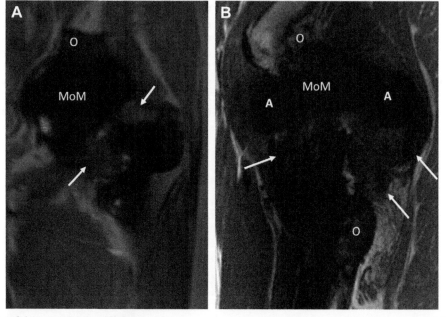

Fig. 10. Painful MoM THA in a 55-year-old woman placed 7 years before imaging. Coronal MAVRIC (*A*) and sagittal conventional 2D (*B*) FSE PD-weighted MR images show susceptibility artifact associated with the prosthesis (MoM), including large side lobes adjacent to the head on the 2D FSE sequence (*A*). Low-signal intensity, thickened synovium (*arrows*), and low-signal osteolysis (O) are characteristic of metallosis.

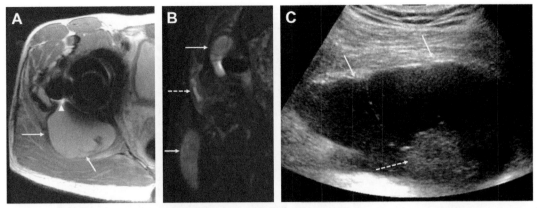

Fig. 11. ALVAL in a 56-year-old man with a history of right THA 2 years before imaging. Axial PD (*A*) and coronal STIR (*B*) MR images show an ALTR characterized by posterior pseudocapsular dehiscence (*arrowhead*) with fluid distention (*long white arrows*) and synovial thickening in the greater trochanteric bursa (*dashed white arrows*). The collection extends further distally along the superficial fascia of the lateral thigh (*yellow arrow*). US image of the lateral hip (*C*) in the same patient also shows fluid distention and synovial thickening of the greater trochanteric bursa.

hip, the patient can be turned onto their side to assess for the presence of greater trochanter bursal fluid, which may have accumulated through a dehiscent posterior joint capsule (see **Figs. 11** and **14**). An advantage of US over fluoroscopically guided aspirations is that the joint and periprosthetic collections can be separately targeted for sampling, without contaminating the joint if only a superficial infection is suspected. Occasionally, synovial biopsy is desired for the preoperative diagnosis of bulky synovitis or if there is a question of an alternative cause, such as tumor (**Fig. 18**).

Liner Displacement or Fracture

The most common type of hip arthroplasty design includes a polyethylene liner within the acetabular cup, articulating with the metal femoral head.

Occasionally, this liner may displace, sometimes preceded by liner fracture. On MR imaging, this appears as a C-shaped or circular signal void in the vicinity of the prosthesis (**Fig. 19**). Eccentric seating of the femoral head in the cup, diagnostic of wear on radiographs, is usually not detectable on MR imaging owing to metal artifact. On US, liner displacement is only detectable if it is sufficiently displaced and superficial for detection, appearing as a smooth contoured, shadowing structure in the periarticular soft tissues.

BONE COMPLICATIONS

MR imaging readily demonstrates bone abnormalities following hip replacement, such as osteolysis, periprosthetic fracture, stress reaction, and

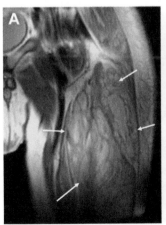
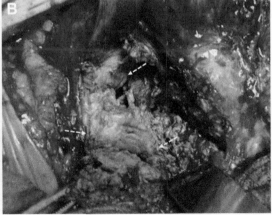

Fig. 12. ALVAL in a 51-year-old man with a MoM THA. MR imaging coronal MAVRIC PD-weighted image (*A*) shows extracapsular decompression of synovitis with destruction of the quadriceps muscle group indicative of myonecrosis (*solid arrows*). (*B*) Tissue necrosis (*dashed arrows*) was confirmed at revision.

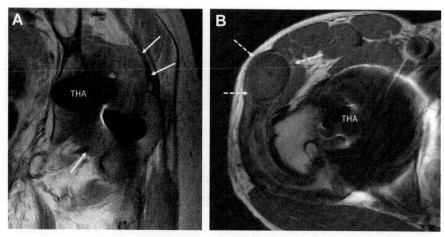

Fig. 13. Extracapsular soft tissue mass in a patient with ALVAL. Coronal (*A*) and axial (*B*) MR images of the right hip in a patient after THA demonstrate marked synovial thickening (*solid arrows*) and development of a periarticular soft tissue mass (*dashed arrows*), or "pseudotumor."

heterotopic ossification (HO). US is unable to penetrate bone or the prosthesis and currently has a limited role for evaluation of these complications.

After hip arthroplasty, implant fixation is achieved by bone ingrowth onto the prosthesis, creating a sharp interface between the marrow and prosthetic signal void on MR imaging. A fibrous membrane may form at the prosthesis-bone or cement-bone interface, characterized by linear signal hyperintensity measuring 1 to 2 mm in thickness and a surrounding hypointense rim (**Fig. 20**). This may be asymptomatic and may exist in the setting of adequate implant fixation.[35] When this high-signal interface reaches greater than 2 mm in thickness, it is termed bone resorption or osteolysis, which is caused by either

mechanical stress or an inflammatory response to wear debris or corrosion products shed from the prosthesis over time. There will be accompanying synovitis. Osteolysis owing to polymeric wear appears geographic, periprosthetic intermediate-high signal replacing bone (**Fig. 21**), whereas osteolysis associated with ALTR tends to be lower in signal (see **Fig. 10**); MR imaging is the most accurate means of diagnosis.[35–37] Circumferential osteolysis at the prosthesis-bone or cement-bone interface is suggestive of loosening, or lost implant fixation.[15] Migration or fracture of implant components, cement mantle fractures (if cement was used), is diagnostic of loosening (**Fig. 22**).[38]

Periprosthetic fractures may occur during placement or later in the postoperative period.

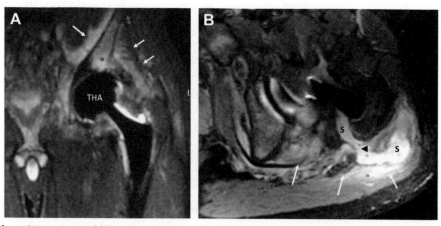

Fig. 14. Infected THA. Coronal (*A*) and axial (*B*) STIR images demonstrate synovitis (S) with pseudocapsular dehiscence (*arrowhead*). Periprosthetic bone marrow edema pattern (*red asterisks*, BME) and periarticular soft tissue edema (*arrows*) are particularly worrisome for infection.

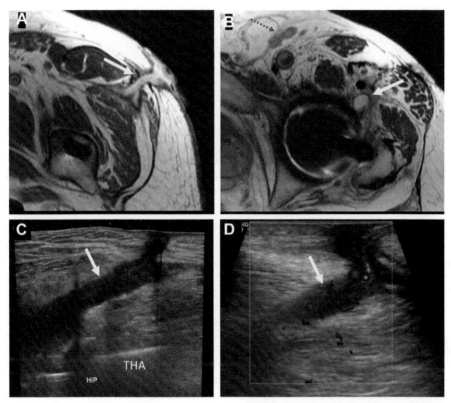

Fig. 15. Infected THA in an 84-year-old man. Axial MR imaging PD-weighted images (*A, B*) of the left hip show a sinus tract (*yellow arrows*) extending from the hip joint to the skin surface and inguinal lymphadenopathy (*red dashed arrow*). US grayscale (*C*) and power doppler images (*D*) obtained 3 weeks later show persistence of the sinus tract, filled with hypoechoic and hyperemic granulation tissue. Joint aspiration was performed, and cultures were positive for enterococcus faecalis.

Fractures are more common adjacent to the femoral component and appear as they would elsewhere, that is, a low-signal-intensity line surrounded by bone marrow edema pattern, sometimes with adjacent periosteal reaction (**Fig. 23**). Predisposing factors for later fractures include loss of bone owing to osteolysis or bone resorption, deterioration of bone quality owing to

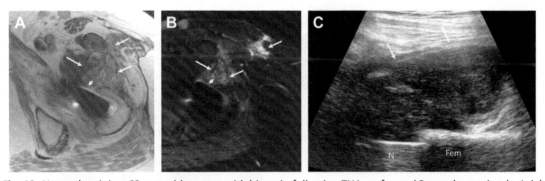

Fig. 16. Hemarthrosis in a 68-year-old woman with hip pain following THA performed 3 months previously. Axial PD (*A*) and STIR (*B*) MR images at the level of the inferior hip joint shows an intraarticular hematoma characterized by hyperintense fluid and intermediate signal clots (*long white arrows*). Note the deficient iliofemoral ligament (*short white arrows*) and soft tissue edema along the anterior approach incisional tract (*yellow arrows*). US image of the anterior hip parallel to the prosthetic femoral neck (N) in the same patient (*C*) 6 months later shows persistent heterogenous echotexture hemarthrosis (*long white arrows*). Aspiration yielded a small amount of fluid and clots.

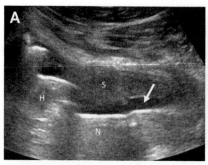
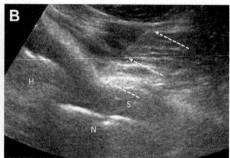

Fig. 17. US-guided hip aspiration. US images of the anterior hip after THA before (*A*) and during (*B*) US-guided arthrocentesis show bulky, mildly hypoechoic synovial thickening (S) and a small effusion (*solid arrow*), which was successfully sampled. Needle (*dashed arrow*).

osteoporosis, and component malpositioning; therefore, these concomitant findings should be sought when a periprosthetic fracture is visualized.[7] Stress reactions are characterized on MR imaging as marrow and endosteal signal hyperintensity, cortical and periosteal thickening and

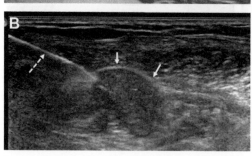

Fig. 18. Percutaneous soft tissue biopsy. Axial MR PD image of the right hip (*A*) shows decompression of synovitis (S) through a dehiscent posterior pseudocapsule into the GT and synovial thickening (*solid arrows*). US-guided biopsy was requested, and the more accessible, superficial bursal synovium was targeted (*B*). Biopsy needle (*dashed arrow*).

hyperintensity without a fracture line, and overlying soft tissue edema.[7] Metal artifact reduction is essential to detect these findings.

Medullary reaming and compaction used to prepare the femur for the prosthetic stem produce postoperative marrow signal hyperintensity adjacent to the prosthesis that can last for months, are usually most prominent at the tip of the stem, and should not be mistaken for a stress reaction. The absence of associated soft tissue edema and periosteal reaction are helpful discriminators, as is stability or a gradual decrease in signal over time.

Heterotopic ossification (HO) refers to the formation of bone in an abnormal, extraskeletal location. Reported rates after THA range from 2% to 90%, variable depending on patient risk factors, surgical approach, and postoperative prophylaxis.[39] Symptoms of HO include pain, impingement on adjacent structures, and significantly limited hip motion. Once formed, lesions require surgical resection. HO progresses through various stages of maturation, classified on MR imaging as grades 1 to 4, with 4 as the most mature, described by Ledermann and colleagues.[40] On MR imaging, this progression begins as tissue signal hyperintensity and enhancement at stage 1, which gradually decreases and is replaced by increasing fat and cortical bone, and finally by mature bone with a low-signal-intensity cortex and fatty marrow, which suppresses on STIR sequences at stage 4 (**Figs. 24** and **25**). This is not to be confused with the Brooker classification, which attempts to classify HO by its clinical importance and also has 4 categories, with class 4 disease representing hip ankylosis.[41] The recognizable appearance of mature HO is seen at about 8 weeks after surgery, although in the acute phase, extensive soft tissue edema may raise concern for infection. HO is detectable on US through all stages; acute lesions have been described as heterogeneously hyperechoic and

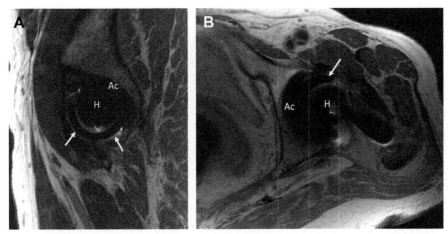

Fig. 19. Polyethylene liner displacement. Sagittal (*A*) and axial (*B*) PD MR images of an MoP THA show inferior displacement and rotation of the low-signal polyethylene liner (*arrows*) from between the prosthetic femoral head (H) and acetabular component(Ac).

hyperemic. With maturation, the hypervascularity resolves and shadowing ectopic internal foci of echogenic bone form at days 10 to 14.[42] Acute lesions have also been described as hypoechoic, although this may have been confounded with denervation edema in a series of patients with spinal cord injury.[43]

PERIARTICULAR SOFT TISSUE COMPLICATIONS
Tendon Injury

Hip abductor tendon tears and dysfunction are common postoperatively. Deterioration of these components of the soft tissue envelope is a clinically important cause of lateral hip pain and predisposes to dislocation of the prosthesis. Causes include injury or release during intraoperative joint access using the transgluteal, direct lateral, or anterolateral approaches, impingement by arthroplasty components and heterotopic bone, disruption by an encroaching ALTR, progression of preexisting tendinopathy and degenerative tears, and trauma. Tendinopathy and tears are diagnosed on both MR imaging and US as they are for patients with native hips. Tendinopathy appears as hyperintense (MR imaging) or hypoechoic (US) thickened tendons. When acute, tears appear

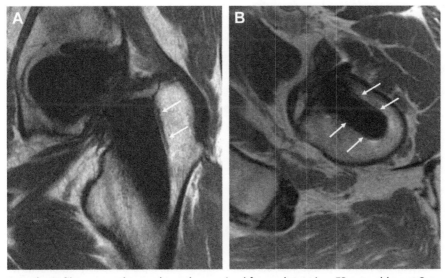

Fig. 20. Periprosthetic fibrous membrane about the proximal femoral stem in a 53-year-old man. Coronal (*A*) and axial (*B*) PD MR images show a low-signal fibrous interface adjacent to the stem that measures less than 2 mm in thickness (*arrows*).

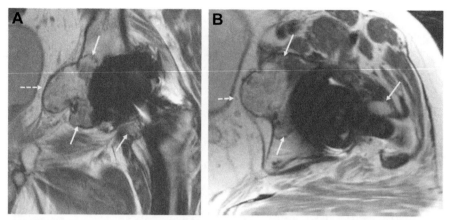

Fig. 21. Expansile polyethylene wear-induced osteolysis in a patient with a painful THA placed 15 years prior. Coronal (*A*) and axial (*B*) MR images of the hip show geographic, bulky intermediate signal osteolysis adjacent to the acetabular component (*white solid arrows*), which remodels the medial acetabular wall (*dashed arrows*). Accompanying synovitis is mild (*yellow arrows*).

as partial- or full-thickness defects, with fluid in the tear gap and/or greater trochanteric bursa and associated muscle edema. Chronic attritional tears are depicted as generalized tendon attenuation, often with fatty muscle atrophy, without visible tendon slip retraction (**Figs. 26 and 27**). Chronically torn abductor tendons may also become scar adherent to the greater trochanter or to adjacent structures, such as the iliotibial band or pseudocapsule, and are functionally insufficient, demonstrated to better advantage on MR imaging.

Iliopsoas impingement is a known cause of postoperative anterior hip and groin pain, seen in up to 4.3% of patients.[7,44] Causes include acetabular component oversizing or malposition, retained cement, long or aberrant screws, or a large prosthetic femoral head. MR imaging findings include iliopsoas tendinosis and tears that may be partial or complete, iliopsoas, and subiliacus bursal fluid (**Fig. 28**). Atrophy of the muscle is an indirect sign of iliopsoas dysfunction, characterized by loss of muscle mass and fatty infiltration. MR imaging may also demonstrate anterior prominence

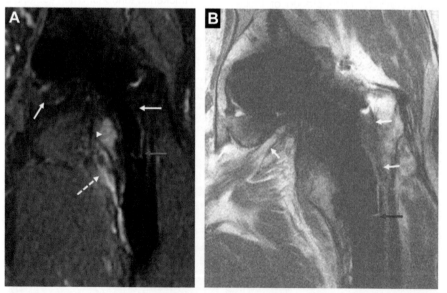

Fig. 22. Femoral stem hip fracture in a 63-year-old man with a revision hip arthroplasty. Coronal MAVRIC (*A*) and coronal PD (*B*) MR images of the right hip show periprosthetic osteolysis (*white arrows*) and a fluid signal intensity cleft (*red arrows*) through the stem, diagnostic of fracture. There is a severe stress response medial to the prosthesis with bone (*white arrowhead*) and soft tissue (*dashed arrow*) edema pattern.

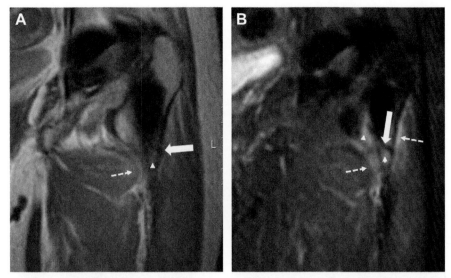

Fig. 23. Periprosthetic fracture after MoM THA. Coronal PD (*A*) and MAVRIC IR (*B*) sequences depict the low-signal fracture line (*solid white arrows*), surrounding bone marrow (*arrowheads*) and periosteal edema (*dashed arrows*).

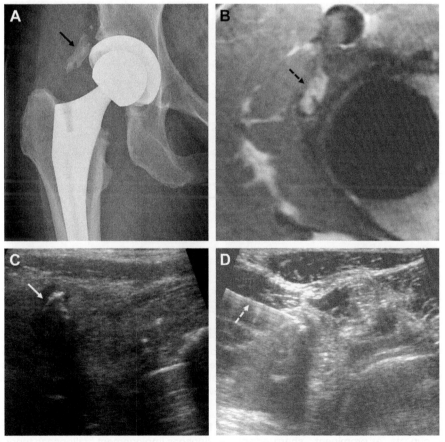

Fig. 24. HO in a 53-year-old woman with groin pain after hip replacement. AP radiographs (*A*) demonstrate a small focus of heterotopic bone formation lateral to the acetabular component (*black arrow*). Axial PD MR image (*B*) shows a mature focus of bone containing fatty marrow within the reflected head of rectus femoris (*dashed arrow*). On US, this appears as echogenic, shadowing cortical bone (*C; white arrow*). The HO was targeted for ultrasound-guided injection with anesthetic and steroid (*D*) with immediate postprocedural pain relief. Needle, dashed white arrow.

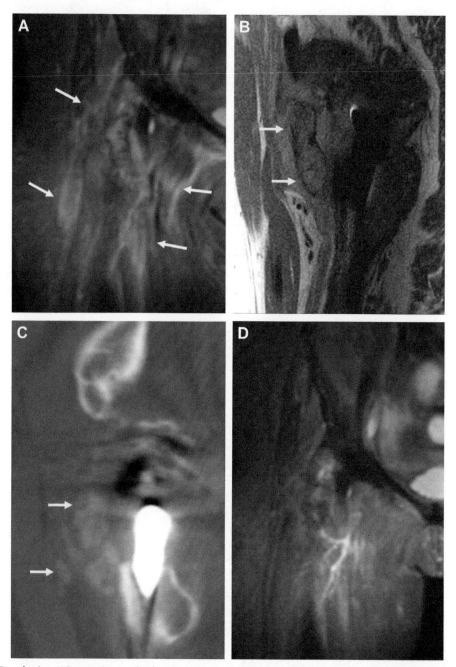

Fig. 25. Developing HO anterior to the hip in a 78-year-old man who underwent THA 6 weeks prior. Coronal MAVRIC STIR (*A*), sagittal PD (*B*), and sagittal CT (*C*) images of the affected hip show marked soft tissue edema (*white arrows*) and organizing HO (*yellow arrows*). Coronal MAVRIC STIR image from an MR imaging performed 6 months (*D*) later shows the soft tissue edema has improved.

of the acetabular component. US shows the acetabular cup as a prominent, sharp-edged structure generating reverberation artifact extending into the deep field adjacent to shadowing acetabular bone. Sonographic visibility of the acetabular cup and iliopsoas tendinopathy is highly sensitive, and cup contact with the iliopsoas tendon and iliopsoas bursitis is highly specific for iliopsoas impingement.[45] Iliopsoas tendon attrition or tears as well as echogenic muscle fatty atrophy may be seen on US, with the added benefit of dynamic evaluation and direct visualization of the site of impingement, correlated with symptoms (**Fig. 29**). US can also be used to guide therapeutic

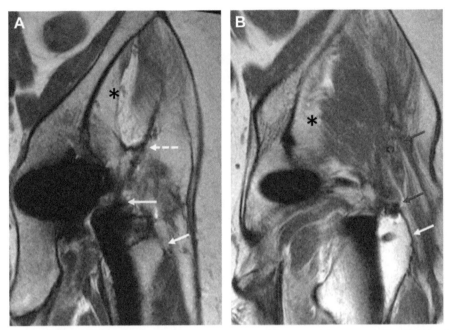

Fig. 26. Chronic, retracted gluteus minimus and medius tears in a 68-year-old woman with a history of abductor repair and THA performed 4 years prior. Coronal PD MR images (*A, B*) show exposure of the greater trochanter (*white arrows*) and retraction of the tendons, which have scarred to each other (*white dashed arrow*) and the pseudocapsule (*yellow arrow*). Note the gluteal muscle atrophy (*asterisk*) and foci of susceptibility (*red arrows*) associated with anchors and suture material used for the repair, some of which are also proximally retracted.

injection of steroid and anesthetic into the iliopsoas bursa (**Fig. 30**).[46,47]

BURSITIS AND EXTRACAPSULAR FLUID COLLECTIONS
Hematoma

Hematomas may develop in the periarticular soft tissues, as well as in the retroperitoneum and thigh in the early postoperative period (within 2 weeks of surgery). Reported incidence is 0.6% of primary and 2.2% of revision THA.[48] They are most common after the anterior approach both owing to the greater risk of vascular injury and

because there is no overlying fascia to contain bleeding as there is for the other approaches. Postoperative hematomas may be intramuscular, intrafascial, or subcutaneous in location. Symptoms include pain, limited range of motion, and paresthesias, dysesthesias, and ischemia owing to neurovascular compression. They also increase the risk for HO and prosthetic joint infection.[49]

MR imaging reliably detects periprosthetic fluid collections (**Fig. 31**). On MR imaging, intramuscular hematomas are initially isointense on T1- and hyperintense on T2-weighted images, developing at T1 hyperintense rim owing to oxidation

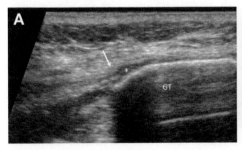
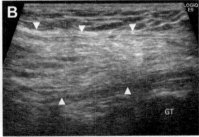

Fig. 27. Chronic partial gluteus medius insertional tear. Sagittal US images of the lateral hip in an 81-year-old woman (*A, B*) demonstrate longitudinal stripping of the tendon undersurface (*white arrow*), undermined by hypoechoic fluid (*asterisk*), comprising 50% of its thickness. The muscle is echogenic and thin (*arrowheads*), indicative of atrophy.

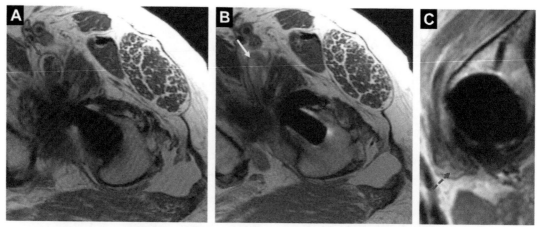

Fig. 28. Iliopsoas tendon partial tear in a 78-year-old man with a painful THA placed 5 months prior. Iliopsoas high-grade partial tear with retraction on MR imaging axial PD (*A* slightly superior to *B*) and sagittal MAVRIC PD (*C*) sequences. There is severe iliopsoas tendinosis (*A*; *red arrow*) and partial absence of the tendon slightly more inferiorly (*B*), replaced by bursal fluid (*yellow arrow*). The torn and retracted fibers are better seen on the sagittal image (*C*; *red dashed arrows*).

of hemoglobin to methemoglobin after 24 to 48 hours. A T2 hypointense rim develops after 7 days owing to hemosiderin deposition.[50,51] Signal loss on gradient echo sequences is seen in hematomas of all ages. Of course, if there is persistent bleeding, blood products of different ages will produce a more heterogenous appearance. MR imaging well depicts soft tissue disruption as a cause of the hematoma, as well as the location of any nerve compression.

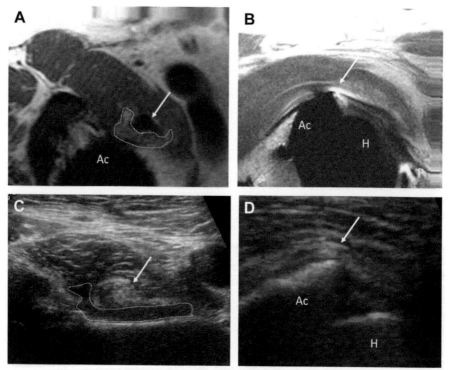

Fig. 29. A 63-year-old man with groin pain after hip replacement. Axial and rotated sagittal intermediate-weighted MR imaging sequences (*A, B*) and corresponding US images (*C, D*) of the iliopsoas tendon (*arrows*) at the level of the hip joint show impingement of the Ac on the tendon and iliopsoas bursitis (*dashed line*) characterized by hyperintense/hypoechoic bursal thickening. The patient's symptoms resolved after therapeutic US-guided injection of the iliopsoas bursa.

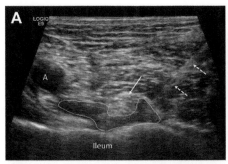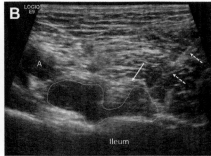

Fig. 30. US-guided iliopsoas bursa injection. US images with the transducer anterior and transverse to the iliopsoas tendon (*arrow*) at the level of the pelvic brim before (*A*) and during (*B*) the injection show the needle in plane to the transducer (*dashed arrows*). Preinjection, there is hypoechoic bursal thickening (*yellow outline*). During injection, the bursa distends with fluid (*blue outline*). A, femoral artery.

US accurately diagnoses and quantifies postoperative fluid collections, up to 53% of which are undetectable with physical examination.[49] On US, hematomas have variable echotextures and may appear complex, echogenic, heterogenous of hypoechoic, regardless of age, although complex hematomas are more likely to be more recent. Large or symptomatic hematomas are often aspirated to treat symptoms and to prevent a superimposed infection from developing. As these are usually superficially located, US is used to guide aspiration procedures (see **Fig. 31**). Although hematomas that are anechoic or intraarticular are more easily aspirated, most are at least partially aspirable, regardless of age or echotexture.[52,53]

Bursal Fluid Collections

Fluid commonly accumulates in the greater trochanteric bursa, particularly if a posterior approach was used, owing to pseudocapsular repair dehiscence, or if repair was not performed.

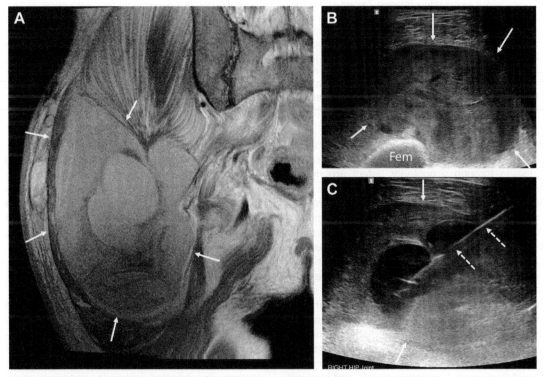

Fig. 31. Hematoma in a 59-year-old man after THA. Coronal PD (*A*) and transverse US (*B*, *C*) images demonstrate a large hematoma with fluid and solid components distending the greater trochanteric bursa (*arrows*). Aspiration was performed with an 11-gauge trocar (*dashed arrows*), yielding 530 mL dark red fluid and clots, with improvement in symptoms.

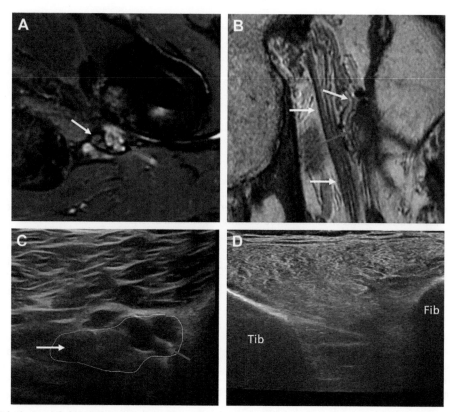

Fig. 32. Sciatic nerve injury imaged 2 years after posterior approach THA in a 61-year-old man with onset of foot drop immediately after surgery. Axial STIR (*A*) and high-resolution coronal PD (*B*) MR images show fascicular enlargement and hyperintensity of the sciatic nerve common peroneal component (*red arrow*), contrasted with the normal appearance of the tibial component (*white arrow*). This is caused by suture tethering to the capsule, indicated by kinking of the nerve adjacent to susceptibility generated by the suture (*yellow arrow*). US image transverse (*C*) to the affected sciatic nerve (*yellow outline*) shows fascicular enlargement of the common peroneal component (*red arrow*) contrasted with the normal tibial component (*white arrow*). Transverse US image of the anterior calf (*D*) shows echogenic fatty denervation atrophy of the anterior compartment muscles. Fib, fibula; Tib, tibia.

This may be asymptomatic and characterized on both US and MR imaging as joint fluid decompressing through a posterior defect around the greater trochanter to distend the bursa (see **Figs. 9, 11, 14,** and **18**). If this is recognized before performing US-guided arthrocentesis, accessing the more superficial greater trochanteric bursa is equivalent to joint aspiration, which makes the procedure both technically easier and better tolerated by the patient. Patients may also develop symptoms of greater trochanteric bursitis in the setting of hip abductor tendinopathy or tear, or if the arthroplasty positioning disadvantageously altered the mechanics of the abductors. Findings on both modalities include bursal fluid, hyperintense on MR imaging and hypoechoic on US, bursal thickening, hyperemia on US, and contrast enhancement (if given) on MR imaging. US can be used to guide therapeutic intrabursal injections with steroid.

Fluid collections may also be seen in the iliopsoas and subiliacus bursae, usually in the setting of anterior pseudocapsular dehiscence with expansion of synovitis from the hip joint. This may be due to use of an anterior approach or excess fluid production, a harbinger of ALTR or infection. Bursitis associated with iliopsoas impingement was described earlier.

NERVE INJURY

Nerve injury complicates 0.17% to 7.6% of hip arthroplasties, most commonly in revisions, in patients with developmental dysplasia, if limb lengthening is performed, and when placing a cementless prosthesis.[54] Mechanisms are compression, traction, ischemia, and transection. The sciatic nerve is most commonly injured after THA, particularly the common peroneal branch, which is vulnerable to traction owing to its relative

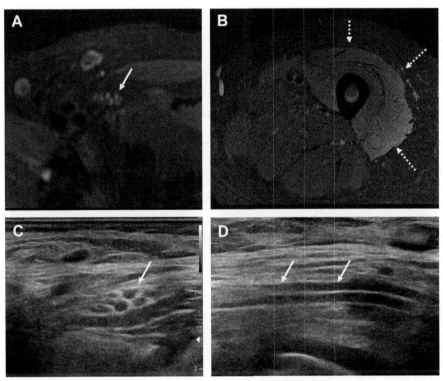

Fig. 33. Femoral nerve traction injury after lateral approach THA in a 59-year-old woman. Axial T2 fat-saturated images at the left of the hip (*A*) and proximal thigh (*B*) show an enlarged and hyperintense femoral nerve (*solid arrow*) and denervation edema in the quadriceps muscle group (*dashed arrows*). The fascicles are contiguous. Transverse (*C*) and longitudinal (*D*) US images of the femoral nerve in the same patient show fascicular enlargement.

fixation between the greater sciatic notch and the fibular head (**Fig. 32**).[55] Superior gluteal, lateral femoral cutaneous, femoral, and obturator nerve injuries have been reported.

MR imaging that is optimized to image peripheral nerves is called MR neurography (MRN). Usually performed on a 3-T system, protocol optimization must still be performed to reduce susceptibility artifact in the presence of metal, as detailed by Sneag and colleagues.[56] US also readily diagnoses peripheral nerve injury about the hip. The nerve is scanned in short and long axis along its entire accessible length using the highest frequency transducer possible. US often provides the highest-resolution imaging of superficial nerves; however, deep nerves, such as the obturator nerve, can only be seen on MR imaging. Both MR imaging and US can also detect causes of nerve compression or impingement, including arthroplasty components, synovial expansion, fluid collections, HO, or scar encasement.

On MR imaging and US, an intact nerve has a caliber similar to its accompanying artery (if present), has an internal architecture of roughly equally sized hyperintense/hypoechoic fascicles, and is surrounded by intact fat planes.[57] Intrinsic

MR imaging signal should be similar or slightly brighter than normal skeletal muscle, without enhancement.[55] In the mildest type of nerve injury, termed neuropraxia, injury to the myelin sheath around the axon results in transient functional loss, characterized by abnormal intraneural signal hyperintensity on MR imaging, and mild enlargement on both modalities (**Fig. 33**). If axons are damaged, termed axonotmesis, MRN and US show the findings of neuropraxia as well as effacement, enlargement, or disruption of nerve fascicles (see **Fig. 32**). The most severe type of nerve injury, neurotmesis, involves complete nerve transection and functional loss. Acutely, MRN shows nerve discontinuity with a gap filled with hyperintense fluid and granulation tissue, replaced by less-intense, enhancing fibrous tissue in the chronic setting. The ends usually retract and form stump neuromas within days, consisting of tangles of attempted axonal regeneration and fibrosis.[58] If the peripheral nerve axons are disrupted but the epineurium remains intact, MRN and US depict a neuroma in continuity with focal nerve enlargement with partial or complete effacement of the normal fascicles. Progression of intraneural signal hyperintensity distally is indicative of Wallerian degeneration.[59] Both transection and neuroma-in-continuity are high-grade injuries with a low potential for spontaneous recovery and are important to diagnose so that surgical repair or grafting can be performed.

Denervation edema pattern, or increased signal in muscles supplied by the injured nerve 24 to 48 hours after injury, is seen on MR imaging only (see **Fig. 33**). If the nerve regenerates or surgical repair is successful, these signal abnormalities will regress.[60] Otherwise, the muscles atrophy and infiltrate with fat over months to years, resulting in permanent functional loss, seen with both MR imaging and US (see **Fig. 32**D).

SUMMARY

MR imaging and US have essential and complementary roles in the imaging evaluation of painful hip arthroplasty. MR imaging with metal artifact reduction techniques, including 3D multispectral sequences, is the most accurate imaging test to evaluate for periprosthetic bone and soft tissue complications. US can evaluate the periprosthetic soft tissues without the interference of metal artifact, permits dynamic evaluation, and is used to guide diagnostic and therapeutic interventions.

CLINICS CARE POINTS

- MR imaging and ultrasound have complementary roles for the evaluation of hip arthroplasty complications.

- Determination of the type of arthroplasty performed and the surgical approach that was used should cue a targeted search for commonly associated complications.

- MR imaging is the best imaging modality to diagnose and characterize synovitis, periprosthetic fracture and osteolysis, tendon tears, and muscle injury and for nerve impingement about the hip.

- Ultrasound is an effective modality for the evaluation of synovitis, periarticular fluid collections, tendon tears, muscle atrophy, and for nerve injury, particularly in areas obscured by metal artifact on MR imaging.

- Ultrasound permits dynamic evaluation and can be used for procedure guidance.

- Although adverse local tissue reaction is most commonly associated with the metal-on-metal design, it can be caused by any hip arthroplasty design with metal interfaces.

- Early-stage heterotopic ossification causes marked soft tissue edema on MR imaging and can be discriminated from infection by the appearance of ectopic bone 10 to 14 days after surgery on follow-up imaging.

- Nerve injuries can be caused by tissue retraction or transection and should be sought in every case by evaluating nerve integrity and the appearance of the muscles it innervates.

DISCLOSURE

The authors have nothing to disclose.

REFERENCES

1. Arshi A, Leong NL, Wang C, et al. Outpatient Total Hip Arthroplasty in the United States: A Population-based Comparative Analysis of Complication Rates. J Am Acad Orthop Surg 2019;27(2):61–7.
2. Kavanagh BF, Dewitz MA, Ilstrup DM, et al. Charnley total hip arthroplasty with cement. Fifteen-year results. J Bone Joint Surg Am 1989;71(10):1496–503.
3. Harris WH, Barrack RL. Developments in diagnosis of the painful total hip replacement. Orthop Rev 1993;22(4):439–47.
4. Gwam CU, Mistry JB, Mohamed NS, et al. Current Epidemiology of Revision Total Hip Arthroplasty in the United States: National Inpatient Sample 2009 to 2013. J Arthroplasty 2017;32(7):2088–92.
5. Kurtz S, Mowat F, Ong K, et al. Prevalence of primary and revision total hip and knee arthroplasty in the United States from 1990 through 2002. J Bone Joint Surg Am 2005;87(7):1487–97.
6. Katz JN, Wright EA, Wright J, et al. Twelve-year risk of revision after primary total hip replacement in the U.S. Medicare population. J Bone Joint Surg Am 2012;94(20):1825–32.
7. Fritz J, Lurie B, Miller TT, et al. MR imaging of hip arthroplasty implants. Radiographics 2014;34(4):E106–32.
8. Sahr M, Tan ET, Sneag DB. 3D MRI of the Spine. Semin Musculoskelet Radiol 2021;25(3):433–40.
9. Talbot BS, Weinberg EP. MR Imaging with Metal-suppression Sequences for Evaluation of Total Joint Arthroplasty. Radiographics 2016;36(1):209–25.
10. Gutierrez LB, Do BH, Gold GE, et al. MR imaging near metallic implants using MAVRIC SL: initial clinical experience at 3T. Acad Radiol 2015;22(3):370–9.
11. Zochowski KC, Miranda MA, Cheung J, et al. MRI of Hip Arthroplasties: Comparison of Isotropic Multiacquisition Variable-Resonance Image Combination Selective (MAVRIC SL) Acquisitions With a Conventional MAVRIC SL Acquisition. AJR Am J Roentgenol 2019;213(6):W277–86.

12. Kebbach MSC, Meyenburg C, Kluess D, et al. A MRI-Based Patient-Specific Computational Framework for the Calculation of Range of Motion of Total Hip Replacements. Appl Sci 2021;11(6): 2852.

13. Potter HG, Nestor BJ, Sofka CM, et al. Magnetic resonance imaging after total hip arthroplasty: evaluation of periprosthetic soft tissue. J Bone Joint Surg Am 2004;86(9):1947–54.

14. Pellicci PM, Bostrom M, Poss R. Posterior approach to total hip replacement using enhanced posterior soft tissue repair. Clin Orthop Relat Res 1998;355: 224–8.

15. Hayter CL, Koff MF, Potter HG. Magnetic resonance imaging of the postoperative hip. J Magn Reson Imaging 2012;35(5):1013–25.

16. Walther M, Harms H, Krenn V, et al. Synovial tissue of the hip at power Doppler US: correlation between vascularity and power Doppler US signal. Radiology 2002;225(1):225–31.

17. Murakami AM, Hash TW, Hepinstall MS, et al. MRI evaluation of rotational alignment and synovitis in patients with pain after total knee replacement. J Bone Joint Surg Br 2012;94(9):1209–15.

18. Koff MF, Esposito C, Shah P, et al. MRI of THA Correlates With Implant Wear and Tissue Reactions: A Cross-sectional Study. Clin Orthop Relat Res 2019; 477(1):159–74.

19. Malchau H, Karrholm J, Wang YX, et al. Accuracy of migration analysis in hip arthroplasty. Digitized and conventional radiography, compared to radiostereometry in 51 patients. Acta Orthop Scand 1995; 66(5):418–24.

20. Fritz J, Lurie B, Miller TT. Imaging of hip arthroplasty. Semin Musculoskelet Radiol 2013;17(3):316–27.

21. Campbell J, Rajaee S, Brien E, et al. Inflammatory pseudotumor after ceramic-on-ceramic total hip arthroplasty. Arthroplast Today 2017;3(2):83–7.

22. Nodzo SR, Esposito CI, Potter HG, et al. MRI, Retrieval Analysis, and Histologic Evaluation of Adverse Local Tissue Reaction in Metal-on-Polyethylene Total Hip Arthroplasty. J Arthroplasty 2017;32(5):1647–53.

23. Campbell P, Ebramzadeh E, Nelson S, et al. Histological features of pseudotumor-like tissues from metal-on-metal hips. Clin Orthop Relat Res 2010; 468(9):2321–7.

24. Schmalzried TP. Metal-metal bearing surfaces in hip arthroplasty. Orthopedics 2009;32(9). https://doi.org/10.3928/01477447-20090728-06.

25. Ebreo D, Bell PJ, Arshad H, et al. Serial magnetic resonance imaging of metal-on-metal total hip replacements. Follow-up of a cohort of 28 mm Ultima TPS THRs. Bone Joint J 2013;95-B(8):1035–9.

26. Koff MF, Gao MA, Neri JP, et al. Adverse Local Tissue Reactions are Common in Asymptomatic Individuals After Hip Resurfacing Arthroplasty: Interim Report from a Prospective Longitudinal Study. Clin Orthop Relat Res 2021;479(12):2633–50.

27. Liow MH, Urish KL, Preffer FI, et al. Metal Ion Levels Are Not Correlated With Histopathology of Adverse Local Tissue Reactions in Taper Corrosion of Total Hip Arthroplasty. J Arthroplasty 2016;31(8): 1797–802.

28. Nawabi DH, Gold S, Lyman S, et al. MRI predicts ALVAL and tissue damage in metal-on-metal hip arthroplasty. Clin Orthop Relat Res 2014;472(2): 471–81.

29. van der Weegen W, Brakel K, Horn RJ, et al. Asymptomatic pseudotumours after metal-on-metal hip resurfacing show little change within one year. Bone Joint Lett J 2013;95-B(12):1626–31.

30. Smeekes C, Schouten BJM, Nix M, et al. Pseudotumor in metal-on-metal hip arthroplasty: a comparison study of three grading systems with MRI. Skeletal Radiol 2018;47(8):1099–109.

31. Ong KL, Kurtz SM, Lau E, et al. Prosthetic joint infection risk after total hip arthroplasty in the Medicare population. J Arthroplasty 2009;24(6 Suppl):105–9.

32. Li AE, Johnson CC, Sneag DB, et al. Frondlike Synovitis on MRI and Correlation With Polyethylene Surface Damage of Total Knee Arthroplasty. AJR Am J Roentgenol 2017;209(4):W231–7.

33. Plodkowski AJ, Hayter CL, Miller TT, et al. Lamellated hyperintense synovitis: potential MR imaging sign of an infected knee arthroplasty. Radiology 2013;266(1):256–60.

34. Koff MF, Burge AJ, Potter HG. Clinical magnetic resonance imaging of arthroplasty at 1.5 T. J Orthop Res 2020;38(7):1455–64.

35. Nam D, Salih R, Nahhas CR, et al. Is a modular dual mobility acetabulum a viable option for the young, active total hip arthroplasty patient? Bone Joint J 2019;101-B(4):365–71.

36. Cooper HJ, Ranawat AS, Potter HG, et al. Early reactive synovitis and osteolysis after total hip arthroplasty. Clin Orthop Relat Res 2010;468(12):3278–85.

37. Walde TA, Weiland DE, Leung SB, et al. Comparison of CT, MRI, and radiographs in assessing pelvic osteolysis: a cadaveric study. Clin Orthop Relat Res 2005;437:138–44.

38. Harris WH, McGann WA. Loosening of the femoral component after use of the medullary-plug cementing technique. Follow-up note with a minimum five-year follow-up. J Bone Joint Surg Am 1986;68(7): 1064–6.

39. Cohn RM, Schwarzkopf R, Jaffe F. Heterotopic ossification after total hip arthroplasty. Am J Orthop (Belle Mead NJ) 2011;40(11):E232–5.

40. Ledermann HP, Schweitzer ME, Morrison WB. Pelvic heterotopic ossification: MR imaging characteristics. Radiology 2002;222(1):189–95.

41. Hug KT, Alton TB, Gee AO. Classifications in brief: Brooker classification of heterotopic ossification

after total hip arthroplasty. Clin Orthop Relat Res 2015;473(6):2154–7.

42. Bodley R, Jamous A, Short D. Ultrasound in the early diagnosis of heterotopic ossification in patients with spinal injuries. Paraplegia 1993;31(8):500–6.

43. Rosteius T, Suero EM, Grasmucke D, et al. The sensitivity of ultrasound screening examination in detecting heterotopic ossification following spinal cord injury. Spinal Cord 2017;55(1):71–3.

44. Bricteux S, Beguin L, Fessy MH. [Iliopsoas impingement in 12 patients with a total hip arthroplasty]. Rev Chir Orthop Reparatrice Appar Mot 2001;87(8): 820–5. Le conflit ilio-psoas - prothese dans les arthroplasties totales de hanche douloureuses.

45. Guillin R, Bertaud V, Garetier M, et al. Ultrasound in Total Hip Replacement: Value of Anterior Acetabular Cup Visibility and Contact With the Iliopsoas Tendon. J Ultrasound Med 2018;37(6):1439–46.

46. Adler RS, Buly R, Ambrose R, et al. Diagnostic and therapeutic use of sonography-guided iliopsoas peritendinous injections. AJR Am J Roentgenol 2005;185(4):940–3.

47. Nunley RM, Wilson JM, Gilula L, et al. Iliopsoas bursa injections can be beneficial for pain after total hip arthroplasty. Clin Orthop Relat Res 2010;468(2): 519–26.

48. Nichols CI, Vose JG. Clinical Outcomes and Costs Within 90 Days of Primary or Revision Total Joint Arthroplasty. J Arthroplasty 2016;31(7):1400–6. e3.

49. Smith D, Berdis G, Singh V, et al. Postoperative Fluid Collections in Total Joint Arthroplasty: A Narrative Review. Orthop Res Rev 2022;14:43–57.

50. Unger EC, Glazer HS, Lee JK, et al. MRI of extracranial hematomas: preliminary observations. AJR Am J Roentgenol 1986;146(2):403–7.

51. Lee YS, Kwon ST, Kim JO, et al. Serial MR imaging of intramuscular hematoma: experimental study in a rat model with the pathologic correlation. Korean J Radiol 2011;12(1):66–77.

52. Dave RB, Stevens KJ, Shivaram GM, et al. Ultrasound-guided musculoskeletal interventions in American football: 18 years of experience. AJR Am J Roentgenol 2014;203(6):W674–83.

53. Yoon ES, Lin B, Miller TT. Ultrasound of Musculoskeletal Hematomas: Relationship of Sonographic Appearance to Age and Ease of Aspiration. AJR Am J Roentgenol 2021;216(1):125–30.

54. Hasija R, Kelly JJ, Shah NV, et al. Nerve injuries associated with total hip arthroplasty. J Clin Orthop Trauma 2018;9(1):81–6.

55. Wolf M, Baumer P, Pedro M, et al. Sciatic nerve injury related to hip replacement surgery: imaging detection by MR neurography despite susceptibility artifacts. PLoS One 2014;9(2):e89154.

56. Sneag DB, Zochowski KC, Tan ET. MR Neurography of Peripheral Nerve Injury in the Presence of Orthopedic Hardware: Technical Considerations. Radiology 2021;300(2):246–59.

57. Chhabra A, Andreisek G, Soldatos T, et al. MR neurography: past, present, and future. AJR Am J Roentgenol 2011;197(3):583–91.

58. Wijntjes J, Borchert A, van Alfen N. Nerve Ultrasound in Traumatic and Iatrogenic Peripheral Nerve Injury. Diagnostics 2020;11(1). https://doi.org/10.3390/diagnostics11010030.

59. Koltzenburg M, Bendszus M. Imaging of peripheral nerve lesions. Curr Opin Neurol 2004;17(5):621–6.

60. Wessig C, Koltzenburg M, Reiners K, et al. Muscle magnetic resonance imaging of denervation and reinnervation: correlation with electrophysiology and histology. Exp Neurol 2004;185(2):254–61.

Spectrum of Hand Arthritis

Doppler Ultrasound, Diffusion-Weighted MR Imaging, and Perfusion MR Imaging Evaluation

Parham Pezeshk, MD[a], Theodoros Soldatos, MD[b], Fatemeh Ezzati, MD[c],
Nidhi Bhatnagar, MD[d], Avneesh Chhabra, MD, MBA[a,e,f,*]

KEYWORDS

• Hand and wrist arthritis • Inflammatory arthropathy • Rheumatoid arthritis • US • MRI

KEY POINTS

- Early diagnosis of inflammatory arthritis can be challenging owing to temporal dissemination of the symptoms; imaging plays an important role in early detection as well as in monitoring of the treatment response.
- Radiography and ultrasound are commonly used imaging modalities to evaluate arthritis; however, they have limitations compared with MR imaging.
- Advanced MR imaging techniques, such as 3-dimensional isotropic imaging, diffusion-weighted imaging, and dynamic-enhanced imaging, can provide invaluable information with regard to activity and extent of the disease.

INTRODUCTION

Hand arthritis includes degenerative and inflammatory disorders, which involve the joints of the wrist, hand, and fingers. The heterogeneous nature of these diseases and their presentations often makes the final diagnosis challenging to render and treat.[1] Early detection of inflammatory changes is important to prevent and arrest progressive bone destruction and structural changes. Although conventional radiography is still considered the first choice for the initial imaging assessment of hand arthritis,[2] Doppler ultrasonography (US) and advanced MR imaging techniques, including diffusion-weighted (DW) and perfusion imaging, are increasingly being used for the early detection and follow-up of peripheral joint inflammatory activity.[3–5]

Doppler US is sensitive in detecting increased blood flow in and around the peripheral joints as a sign of inflammation. Inherent advantages of US include widespread availability, low cost, quick scanning time, high patient acceptance, and the ability to perform dynamic real-time imaging with contralateral comparison in the same setting.[6] The method is limited by its operator skill and patient dependency with imaging limited owing to patient size, noncompliance, and regional injury/ prior surgical changes. DW and perfusion imaging offer simultaneous evaluation of multiple joints of

[a] Division of Musculoskeletal Imaging, Department of Radiology, UT Southwestern Medical Center, Dallas, TX, USA; [b] Iasis Diagnostic Centre, Kalamata, Greece; [c] Division of Rheumatic Disease, Department of Internal Medicine, UT Southwestern Medical Center, Dallas, TX, USA; [d] Department of Radiology, Max Multispeciality Centre, Panchsheel Park, New Delhi, India; [e] Department of Orthopedic Surgery, UT Southwestern Medical Center, UT Southwestern, 5323 Harry Hines Boulevard, Dallas, TX 75390-9178, USA; [f] Johns Hopkins University and Walton Centre for Neuroscience, UK

* Corresponding author. Department of Orthopedic Surgery, UT Southwestern Medical Center, UT Southwestern, 5323 Harry Hines Boulevard, Dallas, TX 75390-9178.
E-mail address: avneesh.chhabra@utsouthwestern.edu

Magn Reson Imaging Clin N Am 31 (2023) 239–253
https://doi.org/10.1016/j.mric.2023.02.001
1064-9689/23/© 2023 Elsevier Inc. All rights reserved.

the hand and wrist as well as the ability to perform both qualitative and quantitative assessments with objectively demonstrable maps of synovial blood flow reflecting the degree of active inflammation.[7] Disadvantages of the technique include high cost, longer scan time, and limited patient comfort. Contraindications to MR imaging are not infrequent.

The purpose of this article is to illustrate the role of Doppler US, DW MR imaging, and perfusion MR imaging in assessment of hand arthritis. After reviewing this work, the reader will be able to use these techniques and principles in their practices for improved diagnosis and multidisciplinary care of such patients.

CLINICAL PERSPECTIVE

Arthritis is a leading cause of morbidity in the United States,[8] with considerable financial and emotional burden on the patients, their families, and the health care system. It is estimated that 78.4 million adults will be affected by arthritis by 2040,[9] and the annual direct medical costs attributable to arthritis are approximately $81 billion in the United States.[10] The pain and discomfort from arthritis can result in physical inactivity, which in turn has a negative impact on the body with increased prevalence of other comorbidities, that is, prediabetes, diabetes mellitus, obesity, and heart disease. Limited function owing to arthritis can also lead to impaired daily activities, patient's inability to work, increased absence from work, and possible unemployment. Because of temporal heterogeneous dissemination of the symptoms and signs of different rheumatic disorders, the clinical diagnosis of the underlying disease is often challenging and takes longer to establish with several diagnostic and serologic tests required that increase the financial and emotional burden of the disease for the patients and their families. Therefore, it is imperative to use a prudent diagnostic modality that can help the clinician render timely diagnosis so that medical treatment can be initiated properly to prevent further damage and comorbidities. Conventional and advanced imaging plays a paramount role in this regard and can provide invaluable information in patients with atypical presentation. The common inflammatory conditions include erosive osteoarthrosis, rheumatoid arthritis (RA), gout, systemic lupus erythematosus (SLE), psoriasis, sarcoidosis, calcium pyrophosphate deposition disease (CPPD), calcium hydroxyapatite deposition, and reactive arthritis. Furthermore, the authors describe the role of different imaging modalities, including advanced imaging, in the assessment of wrist and hand arthritis.

IMAGING MODALITIES
Radiography

Among the several imaging modalities used in the evaluation of hand arthritis, conventional radiography remains the first choice for the initial imaging assessment and screening of inflammatory diseases of the hand owing to its low cost and wide availability.[4] Radiography provides adequate assessment of the distribution and extent of the disease but may be normal in the early stages of the inflammatory process, whereby osseous changes have not yet occurred. The findings of the various types of hand and wrist arthritis in conventional radiography are described in **Table 1** and shown in **Fig. 1**. Advanced imaging with US or MR imaging is helpful in early cases of inflammatory arthropathy, including RA (**Fig. 2**).

Ultrasound

Over the last couple of decades, US with Doppler assessment has established its role in musculoskeletal diseases by offering dynamic and real-time high-resolution imaging combined with low cost, wide availability, no radiation exposure, quick scan time, high patient acceptance, and ability to compare with the contralateral side.[6] In hand arthritis, US can easily detect joint effusion, synovial hypertrophy, juxta-articular soft tissue swelling and tenosynovitis chondrocalcinosis, bone erosions, and cartilage damage.[11] Doppler US depicts hyperemia and increased blood flow in synovium and soft tissues, which may be the only findings in early inflammatory arthritis (**Figs. 3 and 4**). In gout, the double cartilage sign may be evident owing to echogenic tophi layered over the cartilage surfaces (**Fig. 5**). US is however limited by its inherent operator dependency and requires experienced examiners. US has proven sensitive in detecting inflammation in the early stages of hand arthritis.[12–16] In some studies, the sensitivity of US in detecting synovitis was found equal or even greater than MR imaging.[17–19] However, in these studies, experienced investigators performed the US, and it is well known that results depend highly on the skill of the examiner.[20] US can also be used for image guidance for diagnostic and/or therapeutic joint and tendon aspirations, and synovial biopsies (**Fig. 6**). **Tables 2** present the US findings of the various types of hand and wrist arthritis.

MR Imaging

MR imaging is the reference standard in the imaging assessment of musculoskeletal diseases. It is a noninvasive imaging technique that can produce

Table 1
Radiographic findings of the various types of hand and wrist arthritis

Rheumatoid arthritis	• Periarticular (early stage) or diffuse osteoporosis (late stage)
	• Symmetrical soft tissue swelling in early stages and soft tissue atrophy in late stages
	• Uniform joint space narrowing in proximal interphalangeal joints (PIP), metacarpophalangeal joints (MCP), and wrist (radiocarpal and intercarpal) joints with decreased carpal height
	• Erosions of PIP, MCP, and wrist joints
	• Ulnar deviation of the 2nd to 5th MCP joints ("windswept hand")
	• Joint deformities
	  ○ Hyperextension of the PIP joint and flexion of the distal interphalangeal joints (DIP) joint ("swan neck" deformity)
	  ○ Flexion of the PIP joint and hyperextension of the DIP point (boutonnière deformity)
	• Fusion of carpal bones and other small joints (in advanced stages)

Systemic lupus erythematosus	• Periarticular osteopenia
	• Symmetrical soft tissue swelling
	• Joint deformities
	  ○ Most common at the PIP and MCP joints
	  ○ Hyperextension of the PIP joint and flexion of the DIP joint ("swan neck" deformity)
	  ○ Flexion of the PIP joint and hyperextension of the DIP point (boutonnière deformity)
	  ○ Hyperextension of the 1st interphalangeal joint, fixed flexion, and subluxation of the 1st MCP joint (hitchhiker's thumb)
	  ○ Ulnar deviation at MCP joints
	• Limited MCP joint extension

Psoriatic arthritis	• Most common as symmetric polyarthropathy at the PIP and DIP joints • Less common as asymmetric oligoarthropathy at the MCP and other large joints • Enthesitis and marginal bone erosions ("pencil-in-cup" deformity) • Irregular, "fuzzy" configuration of bones around the affected joints due to bone proliferation (rose thornlike perpendicular periostitis to the long axis of small bones of hand) • Periostitis appearing as irregular cortical thickening or a new periosteal bone layer • Diffuse soft tissue swelling due to dactylitis ("sausage digit") • Resorption of distal phalanges (acro-osteolysis) • Osteolysis and articular collapse resulting to "telescoping fingers" (arthritis mutilans) • Occasional joint subluxation or ankylosis
Gout	• Typical asymmetric uniarthropathy or polyarthropathy • Eccentric juxta-articular calcified soft tissue nodules (tophi, pathognomonic feature) • Well-defined marginal or juxta-articular "punched-out" erosions with sclerotic margins and overhanging edges • Joint space preserved until late stages • Absence of periarticular osteopenia
Erosive osteoarthritis	• Asymmetric or eccentric joint space narrowing in large joints and symmetric uniform narrowing and soft tissue swellings of PIP and DIP joints • Subchondral sclerosis • Subchondral erosions and cysts • Marginal osteophytes and bony lipping
CPPD arthropathy	• Chondrocalcinosis • MCP, radiocarpal, and intercarpal joint distribution is typical • Scattered subchondral cysts • Joint space is maintained till late

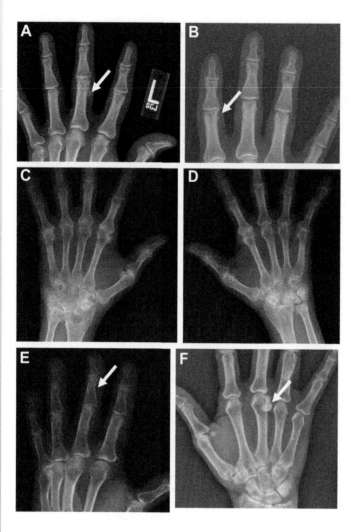

Fig. 1. Classic radiographic findings of hand and wrist arthritis. (*A*, *B*) Psoriatic arthritis with perpendicular enthesopathy and sausage-digit of left index finger (*arrows*). (*C*, *D*) Bilateral SLAC wrist of CPPD arthropathy. (*E*) Lacework pattern of sarcoidosis (*arrow*). (*F*) Calcium hydroxyapatite deposition in the long finger MCP joint (*arrow*).

cross-sectional images in any plane, without morphologic distortion or magnification. MR imaging noninvasively allows simultaneous examination of all components of the joints—soft tissues, synovium, tendons, articular cartilage, and bone, without ionizing radiation. MR imaging delivers all information obtained by US, more objectively and with higher contrast resolution (**Fig. 7**).[21] Advanced MR techniques include 3-dimensional (3D) isotropic precontrast imaging, DW imaging, and dynamic contrast-enhanced (DCE) imaging. The disadvantages of MR imaging are higher cost, reduced availability, and less accessibility than US and radiograph, and the occasional inability to perform owing to MR imaging because of unsafe body implants and devices.

Synovitis is a strong predictor of early RA and other active inflammatory arthropathy conditions and is best evaluated on fat-suppressed contrast-enhanced T1-weighted (T1W) images[22,23] (see **Fig. 7**). DCE imaging is also used

as a marker to assess synovitis and disease activity in such conditions. The early enhancement rate (EER) has been shown to correlate with other serologic disease activity markers, along with increased vascularity and perivascular edema, which can predict progression of osseous erosions over time.[24–30] EER has also been shown to be surrogate of response to treatment with steroids,[31] disease-modifying antirheumatic drugs,[24,25,31] and antitumor necrosis factor (anti-TNF) medications.[32,33] 3D maximum intensity projection (MIP) imaging has proven to be useful in detecting synovitis of the hands and wrists and can provide a whole overview of disease locations in a single image[34,35] (**Fig. 8**). In 1 study, the sensitivity, specificity, and accuracy of 3D MIP imaging in detecting synovitis was 91%, 98%, and 96%, respectively,[35] similar to what is recently shown in axial spondyloarthritis **Table 3**.[36]

Synovial volume can be measured directly by manually outlining the inflamed synovium, but it is

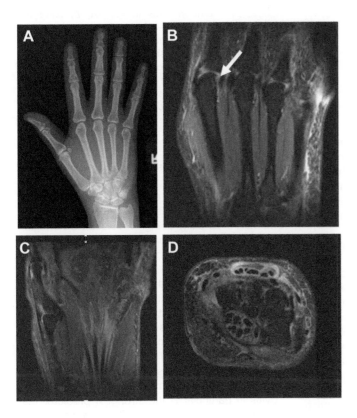

Fig. 2. A 44-year-old woman with known RA. (*A*) Hand radiograph did not reveal any significant findings. (*B*, *C*) Corresponding coronal MR imaging and axial MR imaging. (*D*) Fat-saturated T2W (fsT2W) images show erosions in the MCP joint (*arrow*), flexor and extensor tenosynovitis compatible with active RA.

time-consuming. Semiautomated techniques have been developed that allow such measurement in acceptable times, and this type of quantitation is purportedly more reproducible and sensitive than Outcome Measures in Rheumatology Clinical

Trials (OMERACT) scoring and correlates with histologic inflammation and response to treatment (**Fig. 9**).[37]

The semiquantitative RA MR imaging scoring system (RAMRIS) was developed by the OMERACT

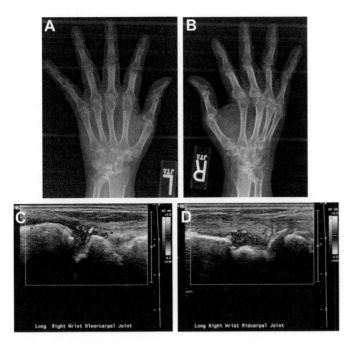

Fig. 3. A 45-year-old woman with RA. Radiographs and US done to evaluate activity. (*A*, *B*) Radiographs of both hands show long-term sequelae of RA with wrist erosions and finger deformities bilaterally. (*C*, *D*) US-color Doppler assessment shows synovial hypertrophy of the ulnocarpal and midcarpal joints with excessive hyperemia confirming activity of RA.

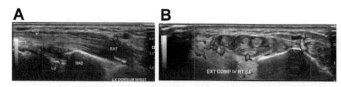

Fig. 4. Wrist synovitis and extensor tenosynovitis in RA. (*A*, *B*) Long-axis and short-axis power Doppler sonographic images of the dorsal recess of the wrist show mild isoechoic synovial proliferation (*arrows*) and tenosynovitis of the overlying extensor tendons. The increased power Doppler signal reflects inflammatory hyperemia. IV, intravenous; EXT, extensor tendon; RAD, radius; LU, Lunate.

to score synovitis, bone marrow edema, and bone erosions in clinical trials. This system has proven useful in detecting early synovitis in RA.[38] The RAM-RIS also has shown good interreader and intrareader reliability and has been suggested as a suitable system for monitoring joint inflammation and destruction in RA.[21,37]

Evaluation of synovitis in DCE imaging relies on the administration of contrast, which may be contraindicated in patients with renal failure or with a history of allergic reaction. Investigators have sought novel MR imaging techniques to diagnose synovitis without the need of intravenous contrast agent.[4] DW imaging focuses on intravoxel motion of water molecules and enables evaluation of microstructural changes in a tissue. It has been widely used to characterize the nature of osseous and soft tissue lesions, to monitor posttreatment response in oncology patients, and to differentiate residual active tumor from posttreatment changes that could be oftentimes challenging.[39,40] Some investigators have found promising evidence that DW imaging can reliably detect and characterize synovitis in the wrist and hand. ADC is mildly restricted in synovitis as compared with abscess of cellular tumor owing to free fluid motion in the joints; however, significant restriction can be seen with gouty tophi. Li and colleagues[4] evaluated MR imaging of 25 patients and found that DWI can detect synovitis with sensitivity, specificity, and accuracy of 76%, 89%, and 84%, respectively. Although the findings are optimistic and similar to what has been shown in axial spondyloarthritis,[41] further assessment with larger samples is required. The findings of the hand and wrist arthritis on advanced MR imaging are shown in **Table 2** and **Figs. 10–12**.

DISCUSSION

Early diagnosis of RA is essential to optimize treatment, decrease joint destruction, and improve function. Recognition of RA is challenging in patients who do not present with the classical hallmarks.[42] The utility of high-resolution US imaging and advanced MR imaging in early arthritis has been studied. Although there is evidence that power Doppler-positive findings in US correlate with radiograph-based prognosis, the data in using US to predict inflammatory arthritis remain sparse, and the current level of evidence is moderate.[43] Several studies on inflammatory markers depicted by MR imaging in undifferentiated arthritis have reported that bone marrow edema, synovitis, tenosynovitis, and erosions are associated with the development of RA. Flexor tenosynovitis in particular is the strongest predictor that independently associates with development of RA, whereas the lack of detected synovitis decreases probability of progression to RA.[42]

The synovial membrane is the principal site of inflammation in early RA, and symmetrical synovitis is the earliest abnormality to appear in the disease. Synovial proliferation exhibits low to medium signal in nonenhanced T1W images. In T2-weighted (T2W) images, pannus shows heterogeneous signal similar to the signal of joint fluid.

Synovial volumes measured using unenhanced images are larger than those measured from enhanced images owing to variable additional contributions from underlying connective tissue, poor vascularization, fibrous pannus, and joint fluid.[44] Gadolinium–diethylenetriamine pentaacetic acid is transported in the plasma as an unlinked molecule and diffuses freely to the expanded interstitial space or fibrosis. It allows differentiation of

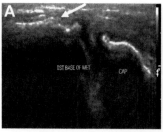
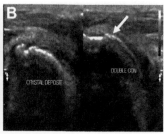

Fig. 5. US images (*A*, *B*) of a patient with gout demonstrate echogenic tophi (*arrows*) at the level of the first metatarsalphalangeal joint with double contour cartilage line sign, related to deposition of monosodium urate crystals on the surface of hyaline articular cartilage. CAP, capitate; DOUBLE CON, double contour.

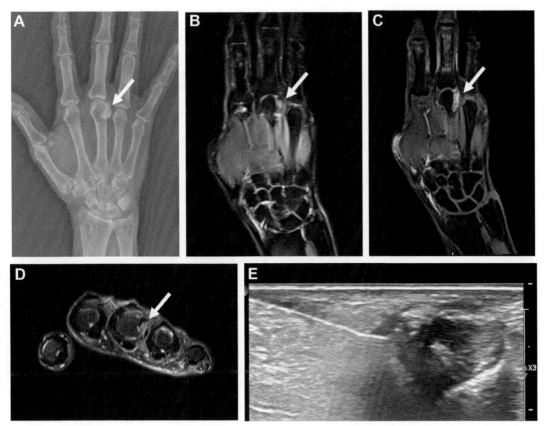

Fig. 6. (*A*) A 72-year-old woman with calcium hydroxyapatite deposition. Posteroanterior (PA) radiograph of hand and wrist. (*B*) Coronal fsT2W. (*C*) Coronal postcontrast fat-saturated T1W (fsT1W). (*D*) Axial fsT2W images show calcium hydroxyapatite deposition at the third MCP joint and associated enhancing inflammation (*arrows*). (*E*) US-guided attempted aspiration and needling of calcium hydroxyapatite deposits. Not much could be aspirated, and needle fenestration was performed.

the synovial membrane from the surrounding tissues through a marked increase of signal intensity on T1W images. Enhancing synovitis corresponds to active and inflamed tissue and is therefore expected to be a better marker of disease activity. Higher contrast doses improve synovial conspicuity and slightly increase the measured volume of enhancing tissue.[45] Strongly T1W sequences optimize contrast between the enhancing synovitis and the surrounding tissues. The delay between contrast administration and scanning is important, as the volume of enhancing synovitis increases initially before stabilizing after about 4 minutes. After 6 to 11 minutes of acquisition, contrast reaches the synovial fluid, obscuring the synovium/fluid interface. Therefore, imaging is best performed between these times. Isotropic 3D T1W gradient echo images are particularly useful for accurate identification of synovitis because of their speed of acquisition. In addition, subtraction images increase the conspicuity of enhancing synovitis, tenosynovitis, and bone erosions.[37]

In another study, synovitis of metacarpophalangeal joints measured by maximum level of synovial enhancement DCE MR imaging strongly correlated to local histologic inflammation. Besides conventional histologic criteria, the finding of CD68 staining is considered one of the best histologic markers for disease activity in RA.[46] Hodgson and colleagues[47] performed DCE MR imaging of the hand and wrist in patients with RA twice, before and once 2 weeks after treatment with anti-TNF therapy, and found a decrease of about 20% in volume transfer constant (K^{trans}) after treatment, proving the efficacy of the technique in evaluating the treatment response.

Registration of the time-dependent changes in signal intensity of the synovial membrane on contrast-enhanced images represents a marker of synovial inflammation and disease activity. It can be used to discriminate patients with active RA from those who are in remission or controls. Enhancement curves have also been associated not only with laboratory and clinical indicators of

Table 2
The ultrasound-Doppler findings of hand and wrist arthritis

Inflammatory arthropathies	• Synovitis 　○ Nondisplaceable and poorly compressible intra-articular tissue 　○ Usually hypoechoic and less commonly isoechoic or hypoechoic to subcutaneous fat 　○ May display increased Doppler flow signal in active state • Joint effusion 　○ Hypoechoic or anechoic intra-articular fluid 　○ Displaceable and compressible 　○ Lacks Doppler flow signal • Bone erosions 　○ Intra-articular discontinuities of the echogenic bone surface 　○ Visible in 2 orthogonal planes • Tendinopathy 　○ Tendon architectural distortion, altered signal, and/or intrasubstance tearing 　○ Less commonly shows increased Doppler flow signal • Tenosynovitis 　○ Tendon sheath distension, filled with anechoic or hypoechoic material 　○ Less common synovial hypertrophy and Doppler signal • Enthesitis 　○ Entheseal thickening and hypoechogenicity 　○ Usually shows increased Doppler flow signal
Gout	• Synovitis and tenosynovitis (nondisplaceable and poorly compressible intra-articular tissue, which is usually hypoechoic and less commonly isoechoic or hypoechoic to subcutaneous fat and may display increased Doppler flow signal) • Tophus 　○ Single or multiple intra-articular or extra-articular 　○ Hypoechoic peripheral rim/halo and hyperechoic/heterogeneous center 　○ Pathognomonic • Erosions 　○ Juxta-articular cortical irregularity and depression, usually with echogenic margins and overhanging edges 　○ Visible in 2 perpendicular planes 　○ Subjacent to the tophus • Cartilage involvement 　○ Deposits of monosodium urate crystals on articular cartilage surface 　○ See as anechoic curvilinear band paralleling the cortex ("double contour sign")

Table 3
Imaging findings of the various types of hand and wrist arthritis on dynamic contrast-enhanced perfusion and diffusion-weighted MR imaging

Inflammatory arthropathies and active gout	• Synovitis 　○ Rapid and increased contrast enhancement of thickened synovium reflects active synovitis. Typically, the enhancement progressively increases and persists in delayed scans 　○ The maximum level of synovial enhancement corresponds to the degree of synovial inflammation 　○ Delayed contrast enhancement of thickened synovium indicates synovial fibrosis 　○ Synovial areas of restricted diffusion correspond to synovitis

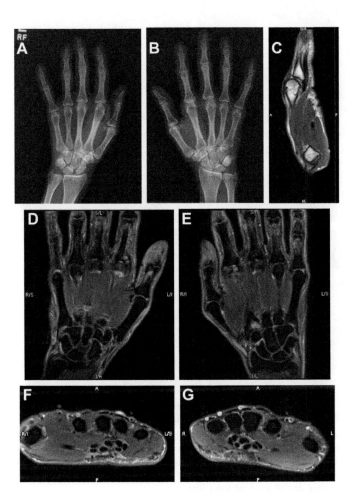

Fig. 7. A 55-year-old woman with SLE. (*A–C*) Hand and wrist radiographs bilaterally and sagittal T1W MR imaging show mild finger deformities and volar subluxation at the MCP joint without bone erosions. (*D–G*) Coronal and axial fsT2W MR images show multifocal joint synovitis and flexor tenosynovitis bilaterally consistent with active SLE arthropathy.

inflammation but also with the Health Assessment Questionnaire, a functional index that is one of the best predictors of outcome in RA.[28]

On contrast-enhanced T1W images, synovial proliferation exhibits significant signal increase and discloses variable morphologic patterns, which vary from homogeneous layers along the joint cavities to irregular nodularity of the wall with homogeneous and solid areas.[48] Contrast-enhanced MIP images provide clear visualization of synovitis and enable differentiation of articular synovitis and tenosynovitis anatomically. A single MIP image of the hands allows observation of the whole of both hands, like plain radiographs.[34]

The best quantitative method to assess the inflammatory activity and the volume of inflamed synovium is DCE MR imaging using 3D sequences with high spatial resolution.[35] Because the quantitative technique for measuring synovitis (particularly synovial volume measurement) usually involves a skilled operator outlining the synovial tissue on each slice of an MR data set, which is very time consuming, 3D MIP can be used to visualize high-intensity structures within volumetric data.[49] At each pixel, the highest data value encountered along a corresponding viewing ray is depicted in 3D, thus allowing clear visualization and easy diagnosis with 1 image.[35]

In addition to synovitis, bone marrow edema has also been reported as an imaging finding that predicts joint destruction. It has been shown that the progress of joint destruction is significantly greater in bone marrow edema–positive joints than in bone marrow edema–negative joints.[34]

DW imaging presents a noninvasive approach to contrast-free imaging of synovitis in the hands of RA. Although synovial proliferation is often less bright on DWI as well as on short tau inversion recovery (STIR) images compared with joint effusion, these cannot be easily differentiated. Because DW imaging is based on a T2W sequence, the signal intensity in b-value images depends not only on the diffusivity of water molecules but also on the T2 relaxation properties of the tissue leading to T2 shine-through effect. Although high b-value images can decrease the influence of the T2 shine-through, they may cause image distortion and

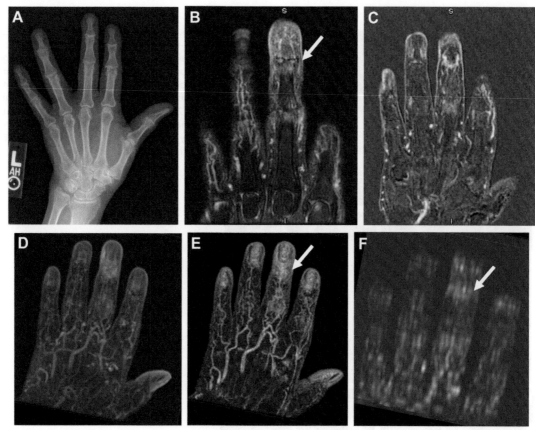

Fig. 8. A 62-year-old woman with erosive osteoarthritis (OA). (*A*) Hand and wrist radiograph shows typical findings of erosive OA of PIP and DIP joints. MR imaging was ordered to assess activity. (*B, C*) Coronal fsT2W and post-contrast fsT1W images show synovitis of small joints of fingers, most pronounced at DIP joint of the long finger (*arrows*). Coronal MIP reconstructions from fsT1W image (*D*), heat MIP map (*E*), and DWI MIP map (*F*) show the full extent of multifocal joint synovitis, most active at DIP joint of long finger.

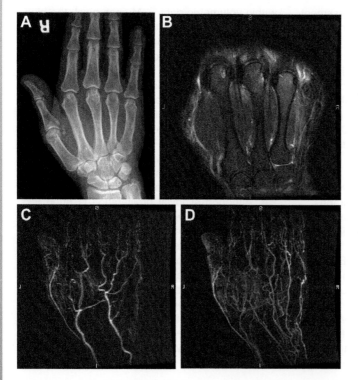

Fig. 9. A 57-year-old man with known RA on treatment. (*A, B*) Coronal hand and wrist radiograph and fsT2W MR imaging show chronic erosions and cysts of MCP joints. (*C, D*) DCE images show no significant uptake at MCP joints consistent with good response to treatment and absent active synovitis.

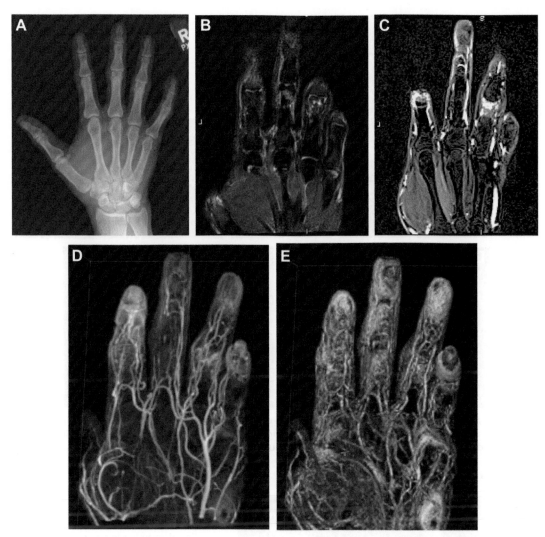

Fig. 10. A 36 year-old man with gout. (*A–C*) PA hand and wrist radiograph, coronal fsT2W and fsT1W postcontrast images show finger deformities and periarticular erosions–cystic changes of the PIP joints. (*D*) MIP image from DCE and (*E*) corresponding heat map show the full extent of the lesions at PIP and DIP joints with lumpy-bumpy appearance of classic gouty arthropathy and tophi.

weaken the signal-to-noise ratio because the phase shift by the stronger diffusion gradient results in greater dephasing. In addition, the longer time to echo for higher b-value DW imaging decreases the MR signals.[50]

In the study by Li and colleagues,[4] DW imaging proved reliable in detecting and characterizing synovitis of wrist and hand. Inflamed lesions appeared hyperintense relative to the surrounding presumably normal tissues on DW images owing to the infiltration of the inflammatory cells, which could demonstrate impeded molecular water mobility. In addition, DW images were more sensitive in detecting positive lesions compared with T2W images with STIR technique. The major

disadvantage of DW images for imaging both wrists and hands at the same time was the image artifacts produced by substantial magnetic susceptibility variations, which occurred mainly around both adjacent thumbs and had bad influence on observing the first carpometacarpal and metacarpophalangeal joints.

In another study, Tanaka and colleagues[50] used a computed technique to differentiate synovial proliferation from joint effusion. In this mathematical method, DW images at higher b values were mathematically derived from directly measured lower b-value DW imaging using the apparent diffusion coefficient (ADC) without direct image acquisition. The data can be obtained without

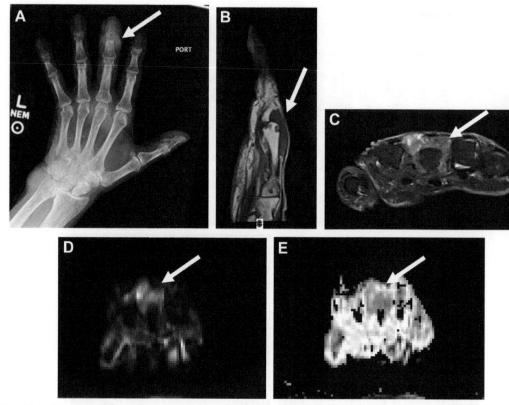

Fig. 11. A 69-year-old man with gout. (*A–C*) PA hand and wrist radiograph, sagittal T1W, and fsT2W images show finger deformities and periarticular erosions–cystic changes with tophi (*arrows*) apparent on MR imaging. (*D*) Axial DWI and (*E*) corresponding ADC map show the gouty tophus with ADC of 0.96×10^{-3} mm^2/s.

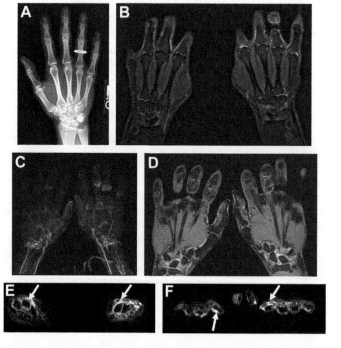

Fig. 12. (*A*) Radiograph of a young woman who presented with pain in the wrists and metacarpophalangeal joints. Clinical examination raised suspicion of erosive osteoarthritis. Her antinuclear antibody test was positive, and radiograph was negative for any significant findings. (*B–D*) Coronal fsT2W, DCE, and postcontrast delayed fsT1W images show multifocal synovitis, especially of the wrists, also apparent on corresponding DWI images (*arrows* in *E*, *F*).

additional scanning and the distortion of the images in higher b-value DW images, and it has the potential to improve the lesion-to-background contrast ratio compared with directly acquired lower b-value DW images. The investigators showed that DW imaging with optimal b value based on optimal combination of b values detects the difference of synovial proliferation and joint effusion, which cannot be differentiated by measured DWI and ADC values. They found that DW imaging with b value of 2000 s/mm^2 based on b values of 400 and 1000 s/mm^2 had the potential of an alternative method of contrast-enhanced MR imaging for differentiating synovial proliferation from joint effusion.

To conclude, radiograph represents the initial screening method for hand and wrist arthritis. Doppler US and MR imaging with diffusion and perfusion imaging aid in problem solving cases for the initial diagnosis, for timely assessment of activity, and for follow-up on medical management for the assessment of treatment response.

CLINICS CARE POINTS

- Radiograph remains the initial screening method for hand and wrist arthritis. In problem solving cases, Doppler ultrasound and MR imaging with diffusion and perfusion are recommended for the initial diagnosis, assessment of activity, and monitoring of treatment response.

- In Doppler US and MR imaging, synovitis, tenosynovitis, and bone marrow edema are indicative of active inflammation. Bone and cartilage erosions indicate long-standing disease.

DISCLOSURES

A. Chhabra: Consultant: ICON Medical and TREACE Medical Concepts Inc; Book Royalties: Jaypee, Wolters; Speaker: Siemens; Medical advisor, and research grant: Image biopsy Inc. Others: None.

CONFLICTS OF INTEREST

None.

REFERENCES

1. Hsu ES, Argoff C, Galluzzi E, et al. Hand and wrist arthritis. In: Problem-based pain management. Cambridge: Cambridge University Press; 2013. p. 97–101.
2. Botha-Scheepers S, et al. Progression of hand osteoarthritis over 2 years: a clinical and radiological follow-up study. Ann Rheum Dis 2009;68(8): 1260–4.
3. Andersen M, et al. Ultrasound colour Doppler is associated with synovial pathology in biopsies from hand joints in rheumatoid arthritis patients: a cross-sectional study. Ann Rheum Dis 2014;73(4): 678–83.
4. Li X, et al. Diffusion-weighted MR imaging for assessing synovitis of wrist and hand in patients with rheumatoid arthritis: a feasibility study. Magn Reson Imaging 2014;32(4):350–3.
5. Sewerin P, et al. Assessing associations of synovial perfusion, cartilage quality, and outcome in rheumatoid arthritis using dynamic contrast-enhanced magnetic resonance imaging. J Rheumatol 2020;47(1): 15–9.
6. Lin J, et al. An illustrated tutorial of musculoskeletal sonography: part I, introduction and general principles. AJR Am J Roentgenol 2000;175(3):637–45.
7. Sudol-Szopinska I. L. Jans, and J. Teh, Rheumatoid arthritis: what do MRI and ultrasound show. J Ultrason 2017;17(68):5–16.
8. Centers for Disease C. and Prevention, Prevalence of doctor-diagnosed arthritis and arthritis-attributable activity limitation–United States, 2010-2012. MMWR Morb Mortal Wkly Rep 2013;62(44): 869–73.
9. Hootman JM, et al. Updated projected prevalence of self-reported doctor-diagnosed arthritis and arthritis-attributable activity limitation among US Adults, 2015-2040. Arthritis Rheumatol 2016;68(7): 1582–7.
10. Yelin E, et al. Medical care expenditures and earnings losses among persons with arthritis and other rheumatic conditions in 2003, and comparisons with 1997. Arthritis Rheum 2007;56(5):1397–407.
11. Filippucci E, et al. Ultrasound imaging in rheumatoid arthritis. Radiol Med 2019;124(11):1087–100.
12. Szkudlarek M, et al. Ultrasonography of the metacarpophalangeal and proximal interphalangeal joints in rheumatoid arthritis: a comparison with magnetic resonance imaging, conventional radiography and clinical examination. Arthritis Res Ther 2006;8(2): R52.
13. Szkudlarek M, et al. Ultrasonography of the metatarsophalangeal joints in rheumatoid arthritis: comparison with magnetic resonance imaging, conventional radiography, and clinical examination. Arthritis Rheum 2004;50(7):2103–12.
14. Hmamouchi I, et al. A comparison of ultrasound and clinical examination in the detection of flexor tenosynovitis in early arthritis. BMC Muscoskel Disord 2011;12:91.

15. Backhaus M, et al. Prospective two year follow up study comparing novel and conventional imaging procedures in patients with arthritic finger joints. Ann Rheum Dis 2002;61(10):895–904.

16. Milosavljevic J, Lindqvist U, Elvin A. Ultrasound and power Doppler evaluation of the hand and wrist in patients with psoriatic arthritis. Acta Radiol 2005; 46(4):374–85.

17. Backhaus M, et al. Arthritis of the finger joints: a comprehensive approach comparing conventional radiography, scintigraphy, ultrasound, and contrast-enhanced magnetic resonance imaging. Arthritis Rheum 1999;42(6):1232–45.

18. Weidekamm C, et al. Diagnostic value of high-resolution B-mode and doppler sonography for imaging of hand and finger joints in rheumatoid arthritis. Arthritis Rheum 2003;48(2):325–33.

19. Terslev L, et al. Doppler ultrasound and magnetic resonance imaging of synovial inflammation of the hand in rheumatoid arthritis: a comparative study. Arthritis Rheum 2003;48(9):2434–41.

20. Zikou AK, et al. Magnetic resonance imaging quantification of hand synovitis in patients with rheumatoid arthritis treated with adalimumab. J Rheumatol 2006;33(2):219–23.

21. Haavardsholm EA, et al. Reliability and sensitivity to change of the OMERACT rheumatoid arthritis magnetic resonance imaging score in a multireader, longitudinal setting. Arthritis Rheum 2005;52(12): 3860–7.

22. Narvaez JA, et al. MR imaging of early rheumatoid arthritis. Radiographics 2010;30(1):143–63 [discussion: 163-5].

23. Boutry N, et al. Early rheumatoid arthritis: a review of MRI and sonographic findings. AJR Am J Roentgenol 2007;189(6):1502–9.

24. Lee J, et al. Magnetic resonance imaging of the wrist in defining remission of rheumatoid arthritis. J Rheumatol 1997;24(7):1303–8.

25. Huang J, et al. A 1-year follow-up study of dynamic magnetic resonance imaging in early rheumatoid arthritis reveals synovitis to be increased in shared epitope-positive patients and predictive of erosions at 1 year. Rheumatology 2000;39(4):407–16.

26. Ostergaard M, et al. Quantitative assessment of the synovial membrane in the rheumatoid wrist: an easily obtained MRI score reflects the synovial volume. Br J Rheumatol 1996;35(10):965–71.

27. Konig H, Sieper J, Wolf KJ. Rheumatoid arthritis: evaluation of hypervascular and fibrous pannus with dynamic MR imaging enhanced with Gd-DTPA. Radiology 1990;176(2):473–7.

28. Cimmino MA, et al. Dynamic gadolinium-enhanced magnetic resonance imaging of the wrist in patients with rheumatoid arthritis can discriminate active from inactive disease. Arthritis Rheum 2003;48(5): 1207–13.

29. Gaffney K, et al. Quantitative assessment of the rheumatoid synovial microvascular bed by gadolinium-DTPA enhanced magnetic resonance imaging. Ann Rheum Dis 1998;57(3):152–7.

30. Palosaari K, et al. Contrast-enhanced dynamic and static MRI correlates with quantitative 99Tcm-labelled nanocolloid scintigraphy. Study of early rheumatoid arthritis patients. Rheumatology 2004;43(11): 1364–73.

31. Reece RJ, et al. Comparative assessment of leflunomide and methotrexate for the treatment of rheumatoid arthritis, by dynamic enhanced magnetic resonance imaging. Arthritis Rheum 2002;46(2): 366–72.

32. Kalden-Nemeth D, et al. NMR monitoring of rheumatoid arthritis patients receiving anti-TNF-alpha monoclonal antibody therapy. Rheumatol Int 1997;16(6): 249–55.

33. Tam LS, et al. Rapid improvement in rheumatoid arthritis patients on combination of methotrexate and infliximab: clinical and magnetic resonance imaging evaluation. Clin Rheumatol 2007;26(6):941–6.

34. Akai T, et al. Prediction of radiographic progression in synovitis-positive joints on maximum intensity projection of magnetic resonance imaging in rheumatoid arthritis. Clin Rheumatol 2016;35(4):873–8.

35. Li X, et al. Diagnostic performance of three-dimensional MR maximum intensity projection for the assessment of synovitis of the hand and wrist in rheumatoid arthritis: a pilot study. Eur J Radiol 2014;83(5):797–800.

36. Gupta A, Ratakonda R, Boraiah G, Xi Y, Chhabra A. Three-Dimensional Isotropic Versus Conventional Multisequence 2-Dimensional Magnetic Resonance Imaging of Sacroiliac Joints in Suspected Axial Spondyloarthritis. J Comput Assist Tomogr 2022 Sep-Oct 01;46(5):755–61. https://doi.org/10.1097/RCT.0000000000001328. Epub 2022 Apr 27. PMID: 35483114.

37. Hodgson RJ, O'Connor P, Moots R. MRI of rheumatoid arthritis image quantitation for the assessment of disease activity, progression and response to therapy. Rheumatology 2008;47(1):13–21.

38. Axelsen MB, et al. Differentiation between early rheumatoid arthritis patients and healthy persons by conventional and dynamic contrast-enhanced magnetic resonance imaging. Scand J Rheumatol 2014;43(2):109–18.

39. Malayeri AA, et al. Principles and applications of diffusion-weighted imaging in cancer detection, staging, and treatment follow-up. Radiographics 2011;31(6):1773–91.

40. Bonekamp S, Corona-Villalobos CP, Kamel IR. Oncologic applications of diffusion-weighted MRI in the body. J Magn Reson Imaging 2012;35(2): 257–79.

41. Chhabra A, et al. Three tesla and 3D multiparametric combined imaging evaluation of axial spondyloarthritis and pelvic enthesopathy. Eur J Radiol 2020; 126:108916.

42. Sidhu N, et al. MRI-detected synovitis of the small joints predicts rheumatoid arthritis development in large joint undifferentiated inflammatory arthritis. Rheumatology 2022;61(SI):SI23–9.

43. van den Berg R, et al. What is the value of musculoskeletal ultrasound in patients presenting with arthralgia to predict inflammatory arthritis development? A systematic literature review. Arthritis Res Ther 2018;20(1):228.

44. Savnik A, et al. MRI of the arthritic small joints: comparison of extremity MRI (0.2 T) vs high-field MRI (1.5 T). Eur Radiol 2001;11(6):1030–8.

45. Oliver C, et al. Advantages of an increased dose of MRI contrast agent for enhancing inflammatory synovium. Clin Radiol 1996;51(7):487–93.

46. Vordenbaumen S, et al. Dynamic contrast-enhanced magnetic resonance imaging of metacarpophalangeal joints reflects histological signs of synovitis in rheumatoid arthritis. Arthritis Res Ther 2014;16(5):452.

47. Hodgson RJ, et al. Pharmacokinetic modeling of dynamic contrast-enhanced MRI of the hand and wrist in rheumatoid arthritis and the response to anti-tumor necrosis factor-alpha therapy. Magn Reson Med 2007;58(3):482–9.

48. Reiser MF, et al. Gadolinium-DTPA in rheumatoid arthritis and related diseases: first results with dynamic magnetic resonance imaging. Skeletal Radiol 1989;18(8):591–7.

49. Choo HJ, et al. Ankle MRI for anterolateral soft tissue impingement: increased accuracy with the use of contrast-enhanced fat-suppressed 3D-FSPGR MRI. Korean J Radiol 2008;9(5):409–15.

50. Tanaka Y, et al. Computed diffusion-weighted imaging for differentiating synovial proliferation from joint effusion in hand arthritis. Rheumatol Int 2019;39(12):2111–8.

Brachial Plexus Nerve Injuries and Disorders
MR Imaging—Ultrasound Correlation

Sirisha Koneru, MBBS, DO[a], Vinh T. Nguyen, MD[b],
Jacques H. Hacquebord, MD[c], Ronald S. Adler, MD, PhD[a],*

KEYWORDS

• Brachial plexus • Magnetic resonance neurography • Ultrasound • Neurolymphomatosis
• Neurogenic thoracic outlet syndrome

KEY POINTS

• Ultrasound and MR imaging are complementary imaging modalities for evaluating the brachial plexus pathology.
• Ultrasound is superior in delineating internal architecture of the nerves, traumatic neuromas, and dynamic evaluation in thoracic outlet syndrome and useful in patients with contraindications for MR imaging.
• MR imaging is superior in areas not amenable for ultrasound such as preganglionic injuries, evaluating global picture, and denervation edema.

 Video content accompanies this article at http://www.mri.theclinics.com.

INTRODUCTION

Brachial plexus imaging is challenging due to complex anatomy. Multimodality imaging can be beneficial to accurately localize and characterize the pathology or site of injury. Although there are no standard imaging guidelines, a combination of computed tomography (CT), ultrasound (US), and MR imaging in conjunction with history, physical examination, nerve conduction studies, and electromyography (EMG) findings are helpful to obtain an accurate diagnosis.[1,2] US and magnetic resonance neurography (MRN) are often complementary and in combination are effective in diagnosing various causes such as entrapment, injury, focal or diffuse neuritis/neuropathy, and tumor infiltration/entrapment. The purpose of this review is to compare and correlate high-resolution ultrasonography and MRN imaging for detection of brachial plexus pathology, correlating with clinical findings and surgical pathology.

NORMAL ANATOMY AND IMAGING TECHNIQUE

A complete understanding of normal anatomical relationships of the brachial plexus is essential for identification and interpretation of the pathology. Although considerable morphological and anatomical variations have been described, the brachial plexus is commonly formed from the anterior rami of C5 to T1 nerve roots (**Fig. 1**). The plexus is further categorized into 4 major components as it passes through the upper extremity bounded by distinct anatomical structures. The anterior rami of the roots coalesce into 3 major trunks as they pass between the anterior and middle scalene muscles: C5 and C6 forming the upper

a NYU Grossman School of Medicine, New York, NY 10016, USA; b Department of Radiology, NYU Grossman School of Medicine, New York, NY 10016, USA; c Department of Orthopedic Surgery, NYU Grossman School of Medicine, New York, NY 10016, USA
* Corresponding author. Langone Orthopedic Center, 333 East 38th Street, Room 6-209, New York, NY 10016.
E-mail address: Ronald.Adler@nyulangone.org

Magn Reson Imaging Clin N Am 31 (2023) 255–267
https://doi.org/10.1016/j.mric.2023.01.006
1064-9689/23/© 2023 Elsevier Inc. All rights reserved.

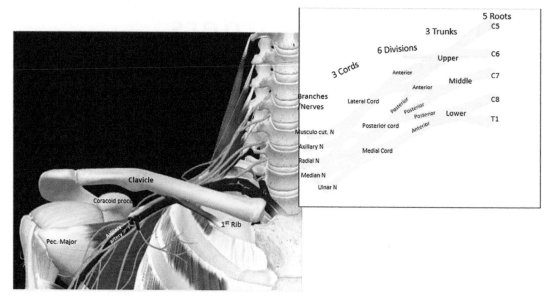

Fig. 1. Image courtesy–Complete anatomy. Images provided courtesy of Thanks@3D Formatica. Anatomy of the Brachial plexus with individual components labeled. Formed by ventral rami of C5 to T1 and forms 4 components, 3 trunks, 6 divisions, 3 cords, and terminal branches. C5 and C6 forming the upper trunk, C7 the middle trunk, C8 and T1 forming the inferior trunk (also called the lower trunk). Each trunk divides into anterior and posterior divisions at the level of first rib for a total of 6 divisions. These 6 divisions pass posterior to the middle one-third of the clavicle through the cervicoaxillary canal and coalesce once again to form 3 cords—medial, posterior, and lateral cords, which contribute to the 5 terminal branches (musculocutaneous, axillary, radial, median, and ulnar nerves) that provide motor and sensory innervation to the upper extremity.

trunk, C7 the middle trunk, and C8 and T1 forming the inferior trunk. Each trunk divides into anterior and posterior divisions at the level of first rib for a total of 6 divisions. These 6 divisions pass posterior to the middle one-third of the clavicle through the cervicoaxillary canal and coalesce once again to form 3 cords. Cords are visualized in the infraclavicular cervicoaxillary canal and are named based on their position relative to the axillary artery. The lateral cord (lateral to the axillary artery) consists of anterior divisions of upper and middle trunk; medial cord (medial to the axillary artery) as continuation of anterior division of inferior trunk; and posterior cord (posterior to the axillary artery) formed from the posterior divisions of all 3 trunks. These 3 cords contribute to the 5 terminal branches providing sensory and motor innervation to the upper extremity. The *musculocutaneous nerve* (C5, C6, C7) arises from the lateral cord supplying the coracobrachialis, biceps brachii, and brachialis musculature and to the skin of the lateral forearm. The lateral cord (C5–C7) and medial cord (C8–T1) both contribute to the formation of the *median nerve*, which innervates anterior forearm muscles and thenar half of the skin and muscles of the palm. The *ulnar nerve* is a branch of the medial cord (C7–T1) and supplies the forearm and hand medial half of the ring finger. The shoulder joint

and lateral skin, over the deltoid muscle, are innervated by the *axillary nerve* that originates from the posterior cord. Finally, the largest branch of the posterior cord gives rise to the *radial nerve* (C5–T1), which supplies all the posterior compartment muscles and most of the posterior skin of the arm.

ULTRASOUND TECHNIQUE

High-resolution ultrasonography using the current generation of linear high-frequency phased array transducers and scanners can visualize much of the brachial plexus and the peripheral nerves. The examination should be performed with patient in supine position, arm by the side, with neck resting on a flat pillow slightly rotated to the opposite side using a linear transducer of at least 10 MHz varying with patient's body habitus, imaging depth, and accessibility. Normal nerves in short axis are round or oval shaped, uniform contour with characteristic uniform honeycomb appearance reflecting intact fascicular architecture.[3] Normal nerve fascicles are hypoechoic surrounded by hyperechoic internal epineurium. Both short and long axis imaging of the nerve are performed to demonstrate nerve continuity, course, and pathology. Continuous scanning in short axis (acquiring a cine loop) can be helpful in tracing nerve continuity, particularly when the nerve follows a complex course. Primary findings of nerve injury are visualized as focal or diffuse nerve enlargement and hypoechogenicity with loss of normal fascicular architecture. Nerve discontinuity, mass effect, scarring, and neuroma formation are also readily identified on US. Secondary signs of nerve injury such as muscle denervation and fatty atrophy with increased echogenicity and reduced muscle bulk are also characterized on US as soon as 2 weeks after nerve injury.[4,5]

Interscalene triangle is the easiest part of the brachial plexus to visualize with US, and the examination of the brachial plexus can begin at this location. The anterior and middle scalene muscles can be identified in a transverse plane in relation to the thyroid. At the entry into the interscalene triangle, roots C5, C6, and C7 are seen stacked one on the other, with the C8 and T1 roots lying deeper in the triangle (**Fig. 2**A). The 3 trunks are also visualized in the interscalene triangle (**Fig. 2**B). The costoclavicular space is usually inaccessible with US, and evaluation is limited in this area. The infraclavicular portion of the cords along-side the axillary artery are imaged by placing the transducer medial to the coracoid process. When so aligned, it looks like a 3-point star with the artery in the middle (**Fig. 3**). The 5 terminal branches are visualized in the axillary region with axillary approach with abduction of the shoulder and placement of the transducer in transverse plane across the axillary artery. Dynamic imaging and comparison to the contralateral side may be helpful.

MAGNETIC RESONANCE NEUROGRAPHY

Direct multiplanar imaging capabilities and superior soft tissue contrast have established MR imaging of the nerves as a primary imaging tool. Advanced magnetic resonance scanner, pulse sequences, and 3-dimensional acquisitions have enabled the performance of high-quality imaging of brachial plexus with neurography of the peripheral nerves. Imaging is typically performed using 3T scanners for higher signal-to-noise ratio and better spatial resolution with selection of appropriate imaging coils. Classic neurography technique relies predominantly on T2-weighted fat-suppressed sequences and T1-weighted spin echo type sequences along with selective maximum intensity projections of multiple successive sections along the course of the nerves. Gadolinium contrast agents are used for neoplastic, inflammatory, infectious, postradiation, and postoperative cases. Normal anatomy of brachial plexus roots and trunks on coronal images are depicted in **Fig. 4**. Brachial plexus cords in the infraclavicular portion in relationship to the axillary vessels on axial images are depicted in **Fig. 5**.

CLINICAL APPLICATIONS

Brachial plexopathies are divided broadly into traumatic and nontraumatic causes, and timely diagnosis with accurate history is essential. Nontraumatic plexopathy is a broad category including congenital, inflammatory, infectious, postradiation, compression/entrapment, and benign and malignant neoplasms. Patterns of nerve injury are classified as neuropraxia, axonotmesis, and neurotmesis depending on the disruption of the nerve layers, which correspond to the likelihood of functional recovery. Most severe injury is neurotmesis with nerve transection or neuroma in continuity, requiring surgical intervention. Acute neurogenic muscle denervation edema can be difficult to evaluate on US. There is subtle increased echogenicity with normal or slightly increased muscle bulk with maintained muscle morphology. Chronic denervation atrophy is seen as diminished volume, loss of normal fascicular morphology, and increased echogenicity. Atrophy on MR imaging is visualized in 1 or 2 groups of muscles with resolution of changes after symptom improvement and is less conspicuous on US.

Traumatic Pseudomeningocele

Traumatic plexus injuries can result in severe functional and mechanical disability as well as chronic pain. Traumatic traction of the brachial plexus can be partial or complete, leading to proximal/preganglionic nerve root avulsion or stretching as well as distal rupture. MR imaging is advantageous over US in identifying the preganglionic injuries. The authors present a case of an 18-year-old's status after all-terrain-vehicle accident with multiple fractures, splenic laceration, pneumothorax, and brachial plexus injury. MR imaging showed pan-plexus injury with preganglionic nerve root avulsions of the left C7, C8, and T1 nerve roots as well as avulsion of the C6 dorsal rootlets with pseudomeningocele formation (**Fig. 6**A, B). Postganglionic injury near the expected location of the formation of the upper trunk with upper trunk transection and scar tissue about the displaced first rib fracture is shown on sagittal (**Fig. 6**C) and coronal images with associated denervation edema and fatty infiltration of the rotator cuff musculature (**Fig. 6**D). Additional atrophy of the teres major, serratus anterior, pectoralis as well as the paraspinal muscles at the level of the nerve root avulsions was also seen. On US, there is diffuse thickening of the brachial plexus roots,

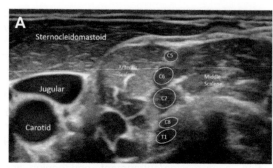
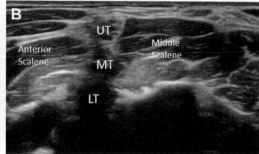

Fig. 2. (*A*) C5-T1 roots of the brachial plexus in the interscalene triangle. T1 root may not be readily visualized. (*B*) Upper, middle, and lower trunks in the interscalene triangle between anterior and middle scalene as labeled. LT, lower trunk; MT, middle trunk; UT, upper trunk.

trunks up to the supraclavicular region appearing as thickened and heterogeneous with loss of normal fascicular architecture and appearing as conglomerate masses due to retraction (**Fig. 6E, F**). Intraoperatively, postganglionic injury involving the upper and middle trunks predominantly with preservation of dorsal scapular nerve and some preservation of lower trunk was found.

Avulsion/Stretch Injury

Traumatic traction can result in avulsion or stretch injury of the brachial plexus. Incidental findings such as hematomas at the site of avulsion, denervation injuries with fatty infiltration, atrophy on US, edema, and enhancement on MR imaging involving the shoulder girdle musculature can occur. Visualized nerves may again seem thickened and heterogeneous or hypoechoic with loss of fascicular architecture. Perineural scarring or neuroma formation appears as hypoechoic infiltration of the perineural fat or discrete hypoechoic nodules in continuity with the nerve. The authors

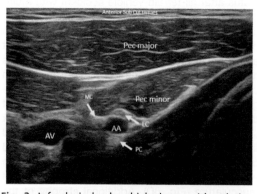

Fig. 3. Infraclavicular brachial plexus with relationship of the cords to the axillary artery with normal fascicular architecture and honeycomb appearance. AA, axillary artery; AV, axillary vein; LC, lateral cord; MC, medial cord; PC, posterior cord.

present a case of a 28-year-old with history of motor vehicle accident and stretch injury of the brachial plexus with nonfunctioning right arm and inability to move shoulder, elbow, and fingers. US of the brachial plexus demonstrated profound thickened enlarged nerve roots, trunks, divisions, and cords as well as enlargement of the median, radial nerve and its branches, and ulnar nerves (**Fig. 7A**) with loss of fascicular architecture. MR imaging demonstrated extensive edema/hematoma within the fat planes of the right supraclavicular/neck planes compressing the brachial plexus (**Fig. 7B**). Associated atrophy of the rotator cuff musculature comparing MR imaging from March 2019 and January 2020 (**Fig. 7C, D**) along with denervation edema of the triceps and flexor compartment forearm musculature (not included in the pictures).

Penetrating Trauma

Motor vehicle accidents, penetrating trauma, and gunshot wounds are other causes of traumatic cause, owing to combination of high kinetic energy with either direct penetrating injury or secondary blast injury from the ensuing shock wave. Posttraumatic neuromas are seen as focal hypoechoic and nodular thickening on US and that enhance on MR following contrast administration. Following is the case of a 22-year-old man with laceration injury in the axilla injuring the brachial artery status post repair with continued numbness and tingling in the arm. US showed diffuse median nerve neuritis with localized 1.3 × 0.7 cm neuroma involving the proximal median nerve (**Fig. 8A**) with a discrete intrasubstance longitudinal fissure in the nerve at the site of laceration injury (**Fig. 8B**). Incidental note was made of atrophy of pronator quadratus, suggesting neuritis involving the anterior interosseous nerve (not shown). MR shows focal change in caliber of the median nerve just below the axilla with perineural scarring along

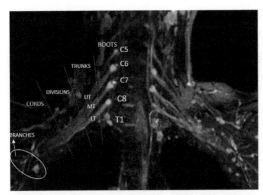

Fig. 4. Coronal T2 fat-saturated images demonstrate C5-T1 roots forming upper, middle, and lower trunks. Labeled image shows roots, trunks, cords, and divisions of the brachial plexus.

with denervation changes in the flexor forearm musculature (**Fig. 8**C). Infraclavicular brachial plexus exploration was performed demonstrating extensive scar tissue forming a neuroma around the median nerve with partial laceration of the nerve (**Fig. 8**D).

Ballistic Injury

Gunshot wounds are other causes of traumatic cause, owing to combination of high kinetic energy or secondary blast injury from the ensuing shock wave. A 34-year-old man with multiple gunshot wounds to both upper extremities presented with numbness, tingling, and hypersensitivity in bilateral upper extremities. US of the median nerves at the level of axilla demonstrated an approximately 3 cm neuroma at the axilla on the left with diffuse median nerve neuritis and loss of normal

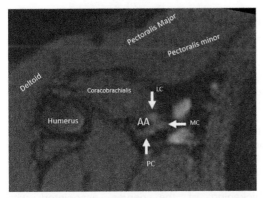

Fig. 5. MR axial fat-saturated images in the infraclavicular portion demonstrate relationship of the brachial plexus cords and divisions to the axillary vessels. AA, axillary artery; LC, lateral cord; MC, medial cord; PC, posterior cord.

fascicular architecture (**Fig. 9**A–C). MR of the brachial plexus did not demonstrate the neuroma due to the limited field of view. Additional gunshot wound tract at the volar forearm extending from the median nerve to the skin surface with T2 hyperintense signal and irregularity of the superficial fascicles and associated soft tissue edema were present (not included). Intraoperative exploration and neurolysis of left infraclavicular brachial plexus with neurolysis of the musculocutaneous nerve and the median nerve was performed. Interfascicular dissection and excision of the neuroma was performed creating a 4 cm gap (**Fig. 9**D), subsequently reconstructed with sural nerve autograft.

Erb's Palsy

Neonatal brachial plexus palsy occurs in approximately 0.2% of live births. Erb-Duchenne palsy, traction of the superior plexus (C5-C7), is more common than Klumpke palsy involving the inferior C8 and T1 plexus.[6,7] These injuries are usually managed conservatively with surgery reserved for those with poor functional recovery and suspected preganglionic injury on imaging.[8] **Fig. 10**A shows imaging from a 54-year-old woman with Erb's palsy at birth with persistent and worsening pain radiating down the left arm with weakness and loss of grip. US was performed demonstrating prominent soft tissue in the supraclavicular region of the brachial plexus involving the C5 and C6 nerve roots/upper trunk, sequela of combination of old avulsion injury and secondary posttraumatic neuroma formation (see **Fig. 10**A). MR imaging shows marked enlargement of the upper trunk of the brachial plexus along the inferolateral margin of the scalene triangle with sparing of the middle and inferior trunks (**Fig. 10**B). Moderate diffuse fatty atrophy of the deltoid, particularly the middle head, was seen in **Fig. 10**B. Patient underwent brachial plexus neurolysis with partial release of the anterior and middle scalene musculature with intraoperative visualization of a 4 cm neuroma of the upper trunk just distal to the C5 nerve root with scarring and encasement.

Radiation

Postradiation brachial plexopathy in patients with breast cancer, apical lung cancer, or cervical head and neck cancer receiving high radiation doses was first reported in 1966.[9,10] Most common metastatic lesions causing brachial plexopathy occur with breast, lung, head and neck cancers either due to direct tumor infiltration or due to mass effect.[11] Most common site for breast or lung cancer is the medial cord with

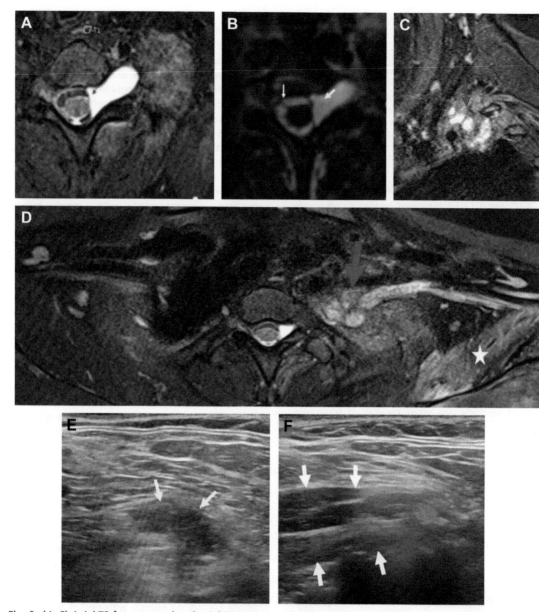

Fig. 6. (*A*, *B*) Axial T2 fat-saturated and axial T1 images with preganglionic left C8 avulsion injury and formation of traumatic pseudomeningocele (*yellow arrow*). Normal C8 nerve roots on the right in (*B*) (*white arrow*). (*C*) Sagittal T2 fat-saturated images demonstrate transected and retracted nerve roots and trunks (*red arrow*) forming a conglomerate in the scalene triangle. (*D*) Coronal T2 fat-saturated images showing clumped and retracted roots and trunks forming conglomerate on the left (*red arrow*). Edema in the rotator cuff musculature (*star*). (*E*) Short axis view demonstrates loss of normal fascicular architecture and echogenicity with conglomerate appearance of the retracted roots and trunks with scarring (*yellow arrows*) in the interscalene triangle. (*F*) Long axis imaging in the supraclavicular region shows diffuse thickening and increased echogenicity of the upper trunk (*white arrows*) and middle trunk (*yellow arrows*) in the scalene triangle with loss of normal fascicular architecture.

symptoms of ulnar neuropathy. Radiation-induced brachial plexopathy on US is seen as hyperechoic thickening of the nerves with adjacent soft tissue changes. On MR, radiation changes mostly involve smooth longitudinal thickening of the nerves associated with increased T2 signal intensity and uniform contrast enhancement with associated perineural fibrosis. A 31-year-old woman with breast cancer status post mastectomy and radiation therapy was

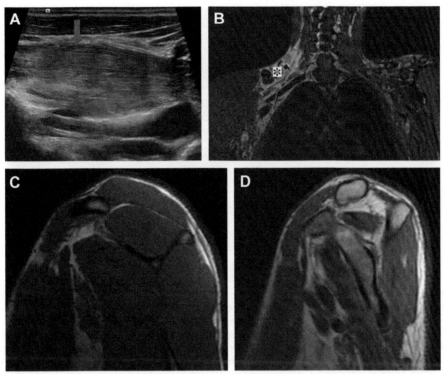

Fig. 7. (*A*) Long axis ultrasound showing markedly enlarged and thickened plexus with loss of identification of individual trunks. (*B*) Coronal T2 fat-saturated MR images with extensive edema and hematoma in the right neck soft tissues (*asterisk*) with mass effect on the plexus (*red arrow*). (*C* and *D*) Denervation atrophy of the rotator cuff musculature in January 2020 (*right*) compared with March 2019 (*left*).

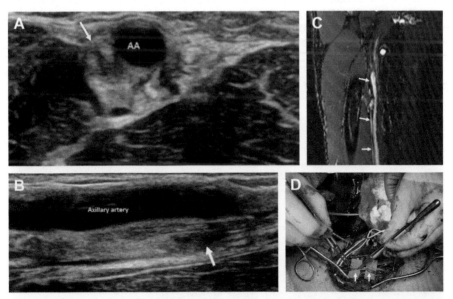

Fig. 8. (*A*) Short axis ultrasound showing diffuse medial nerve neuritis with thickened and enlarged nerve with a localized intrasubstance fissure (*yellow arrow*). AA, axillary artery. (*B*) Long axis ultrasound showing diffuse thickened scar encased median nerve with loss of normal architecture and intrasubstance longitudinal fissure in the nerve at the site of laceration injury (*yellow arrow*). (*C*) Coronal MR shows thickened and hyperintense median nerve in the axilla and proximal arm (*yellow arrows*). (*D*) Intraoperative images demonstrate change in caliber of the median nerve in the axilla and proximal arm (*white arrows*) with a longitudinal split tear.

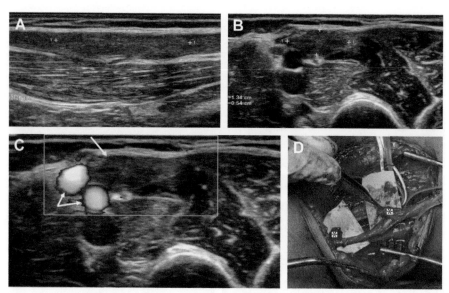

Fig. 9. (A) Long axis view of median nerve at the level of axilla demonstrates diffuse thickening of nerve with loss of normal fascicular architecture with formation of a 3 cm localized neuroma (+marks). (B) Short axis view of median nerve at the level of axilla demonstrates diffuse thickening of nerve (+marks) with loss of normal fascicular architecture with formation of a 3 cm localized neuroma. (C) Power Doppler ultrasound of the median nerve at the level of axilla demonstrates neuroma formation (yellow arrow) with adjacent axillary vessels (white arrows). (D) Intraoperative picture demonstrates 4 cm gap in the nerve after neuroma resection between the distal and proximal resected margins (between 2 asterisks), which was reconstructed with sural nerve auto graft.

unable to use right hand with complaints of pain and swelling. US showed C7 and C8 nerve root thickening with diffuse hypoechogenicity and thickening of the infraclavicular portion of the brachial plexus (Fig. 11A–C). MR imaging showed thickening and T2 hyperintensity of the right brachial plexus throughout its course with extension into the median, ulnar, and radial nerves to the level of the elbow (Fig. 11D). Associated mild atrophy and fatty infiltration of the deltoid and to a lesser degree triceps muscles was present. Patient had right infraclavicular and supraclavicular brachial plexus exploration and neurolysis, right coracoid, clavicular osteotomies, and right pectoralis major superior third tendon release. Intraoperative preneurolysis images demonstrate extensive scarring in the soft tissues tethering the brachial plexus, with postneurolysis pictures demonstrating resection of the scar tissue and visualization of the plexus (Fig. 11E, F).

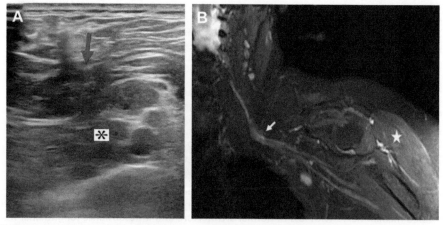

Fig. 10. (A) Short axis ultrasound shows thickened upper trunk (asterisk) with loss of fascicular morphology and neuroma formation (red arrow). (B) Coronal T2 fat-saturated images show thickened and enlarged upper trunk (yellow arrow) with associated atrophy of the deltoid (star).

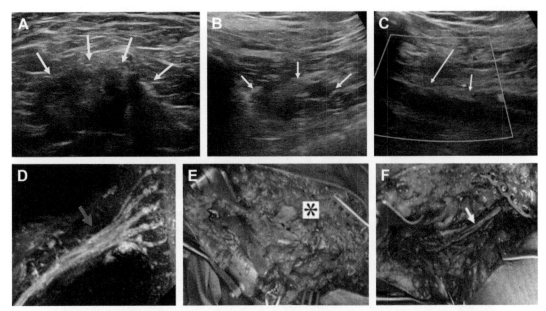

Fig. 11. (*A*) Short axis ultrasound images demonstrate diffuse thickening with indistinctness and loss of normal architecture of the infraclavicular brachial plexus (*arrows*). Dense posterior acoustic shadowing due to scar formation obscures the axillary artery. (*B*) Short axis ultrasound images demonstrate diffuse thickening with indistinctness and loss of normal architecture of the supraclavicular plexus (*arrows*). (*C*) Power Doppler ultrasound long axis view shows thickened and enlarged trunks, divisions and cords (*yellow arrows*) with indistinctness and loss of normal fascicular architecture. A small segment of the axillary artery in this image (*orange*). (*D*) Coronal MIP MR showing diffuse thickened and hyperintense plexus involving roots, trunks, and cords extending into the branches in the axilla (*red arrow*). (*E* and *F*) Intraoperative preneurolysis (*E*) shows extensive scar tissue (*asterisk*) encasing the brachial plexus. Postneurolysis (*F*) status after resection of scar tissue with visualization of plexus (*white arrow*).

Neurolymphomatosis

In contrast to radiation, tumor or metastases are more likely to appear as nodular thickening with enhancement. Leukemic involvement of the peripheral nerves also can occur but is rare. Imaging is particularly important for assessing the extent of disease because lymphoma of the central nervous system may require intrathecal chemotherapy and potentially radiation therapy.[12–14] The authors present the case of a 61-year-old woman with history of relapsing acute myeloid leukemia with leukemic infiltration of the right brachial plexus. US of the brachial plexus shows enlarged hypoechoic ill-defined soft tissue inseparable from the right supra- and infraclavicular brachial plexus interposed between multiple vascular structures as well as multiple unaffected nerve branches (**Fig. 12A**). MR imaging of the brachial plexus showed diffuse masslike enlargement and enhancement of the right brachial plexus (**Fig. 12B**) with increased fluorodeoxyglucose uptake on PET/CT on the right compared with the left (**Fig. 12C**). Percutaneous biopsy was requested, which was deferred secondary to the complex anatomic relationship between these structures and adjacent vessels.

Three months after allogenic bone marrow transplant/chemotherapy, there is decreased masslike enhancement with improved visualization of the perineural fat planes of the brachial plexus.

Neoplasms

The brachial plexus may be affected by primary or secondary neoplasms. Primary tumors of the plexus are rare. Peripheral nerve sheath tumors including schwannomas and neurofibromas are the most common benign primary tumors. They can occur sporadically or as part of neurofibromatosis type 1 and type 2. A neurofibroma has a classic target sign of central T2 hypointensity and peripheral T2 hyperintensity, with reversal of the target sign following contrast administration.[15] Plexiform neurofibromas are mostly congenital in cause manifesting as tortuous and multinodular expansion of the nerve. On US, nerve sheath tumors appear as oval hypoechoic masses involving the fascicles with limited flow on color or power Doppler.[3] On MR imaging, they appear as T2 hyperintense homogenously enhancing oval lesions with circumscribed margins along the longitudinal axis of the nerve. Primary neural tumors are

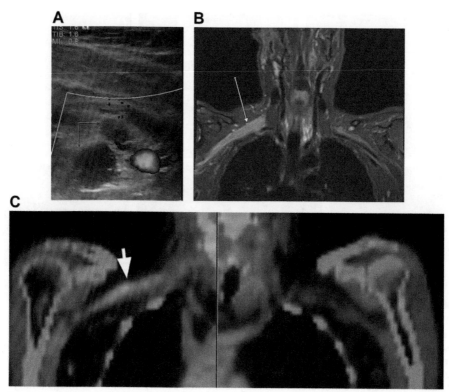

Fig. 12. (*A* [*left*], [*right*]) Power Doppler ultrasound (*left*) and gray scale images (*right*) show enlarged hypoechoic ill-defined soft tissue inseparable from the right brachial plexus interposed between medial and posterior cords (*red arrows*). (*B*) Coronal T2 fat-saturated image showing diffuse masslike enlargement and hyperenhancement of the right brachial plexus (*yellow arrow*). (*C*) PET/CT with increased fluorodeoxyglucose uptake on the right (*white arrow*) compared with the left. AA, axillary artery.

rare with a spectrum ranging from neurofibromas to malignant peripheral nerve sheath tumor (MPNST). Approximately 50% of the nerve sheath tumors are associated with neurofibromatosis type 1 and the remainder occur sporadically. Imaging is useful for identifying suspicious features that may help direct biopsy or resection; however, benign versus MPNST cannot be reliably differentiated with imaging alone.[15] The authors present a 38-year-old man with a palpable left neck mass with a hypoechoic solid mass with internal vascularity on US (**Fig. 13A**). MR imaging demonstrates a heterogeneously enhancing tumor originating in contiguity with left brachial plexus trunks (**Fig. 13B**). Intraoperative images show the mass in the left brachial plexus arising from left upper trunk and anterior division; neurolysis was performed with excision of the peripheral nerve sheath tumor (**Fig. 13C**) with pathological diagnosis of benign schwannoma. The patient also had multiple nerve sheath tumors both in forearms and hands, and a genetic workup for schwannomatosis was performed showing alterations in the INI-1/SMARCB1 pathway with partial loss of INI-1 expression. No atypia was identified.

Neurogenic Thoracic Outlet Syndrome

Thoracic outlet syndrome (TOS) is secondary to chronic mechanical injury of the neurovascular structures mainly at 3 sites—interscalene triangle, costoclavicular space, and retropectoral space with various structural abnormalities such as variant rib anatomy and scarring/atrophic muscles.[16] Neurogenic TOS is the most common type with pain or paresthesia of the upper extremity exacerbated by provocative shoulder movements such as abduction and external rotation. Dynamic high-frequency US can be used to assess for brachial plexus compression, with the patient performing dynamic maneuvers (eg, neck rotation, tilting, arm abducted and externally rotated) to reproduce symptoms.[17] US yields important information as variant anatomy is common, particularly at the level of the interscalene triangle.[18] The real-time nature of US makes it particularly useful in assessing dynamic compression. MR is used for evaluating soft-tissue structures that may contribute to compression, such as fibrous bands, abnormal scalene muscular attachments, and supernumerary muscles (eg, scalene minimus). MR imaging with

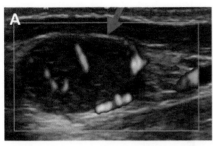
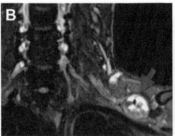
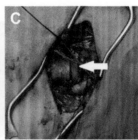

Fig. 13. (A) Ultrasound demonstrating hypoechoic solid vascular mass on power Doppler in contiguity with the superior trunk of the brachial plexus. (B) Coronal T2 fat-saturated post contrast MR imaging showing an oval heterogeneously enhancing mass in contiguity with upper trunk (*red arrow*). (C) Intraoperative picture showing oval mass corresponding to the ultrasound and MR imaging findings (*white arrow*).

the arm imaged in a neutral position and in overhead positions may depict brachial plexus impingement manifesting as loss of the normal perineural fat planes and T2 signal changes of the nerves.[19] The authors present a 25-year-old woman with bilateral upper extremity pain and neuropathy with painful shockwave signals down the arms during exercise in **Fig. 14**A, B. Dynamic MR imaging was performed without compression of bilateral subclavian vessels on abduction. An incidental note of asymmetrically prominent right C6-7 and C7-T1 transforaminal veins without significant compression of the exiting right C7 or C8 nerve roots was made (**Fig. 14**C). US of brachial plexus showed no morphological abnormality. Dynamic maneuvering demonstrated mild compression of the inferior brachial plexus cords at coracoid process at the insertion of pectoralis minor on abduction of the arm, bilaterally, left greater than right (Video 1). Patient was referred for physiotherapy.

Parsonage-Turner Syndrome

US findings of Parsonage-Turner syndrome includes segmental nerve enlargement or focal nerve constriction, with the suprascapular nerve most commonly affected.[17] The suprascapular nerve can be visualized anteriorly or posteriorly. The anterior approach identifies the nerve lateral

to the supraclavicular brachial plexus as a branch of the upper trunk. Assessment of spinoglenoid notch should be included in the US protocol as a common location for nerve compression.[11] The suprascapular nerve is formed by the upper trunk of the brachial plexus (**Fig. 15**), enters the suprascapular notch, running through the suprascapular canal, and exits via the spinoglenoid notch into the infraspinatus fossa. The nerve provides motor innervation to the supraspinatus before entering the suprascapular canal and to infraspinatus after emerging from the spinoglenoid notch. The authors present a 22-year-old demonstrating sudden onset of pain and weakness in the distribution of the radial nerve. US demonstrated focal strictures within the nerve fascicles, described as segmental constrictions in Parsonage Turner syndrome (see **Fig. 15**A). Intraoperative preneurolysis images also demonstrate focal circumferential constriction along the course of the nerve (see **Fig. 15**B). Patient had marked clinical improvement after neurolysis release of the constrictions (see **Fig. 15**C). The authors present a different patient, a 22-year-old with sudden onset of left shoulder weakness and pain with MR findings of diffuse thickening and hyperintense signal of all the cords and trunks (see **Fig. 15**D) with denervation-related muscle edema and atrophy (see **Fig. 15**E).

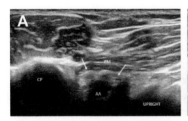
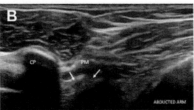
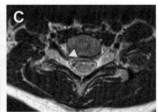

Fig. 14. (A [*left*], B [*right*]) Dynamic ultrasound demonstrating mass effect with flattening of the brachial plexus (*white arrows*) against coracoid process (CP) on abduction of arm (*right*) when compared with upright image (*left*). (C) Axial MR showing thickened nerve root with increased hyper intense signal on the right (*yellow arrow*) when compared with the left. AA, axillary artery; CP, coracoid process; PM, pectoralis minor.

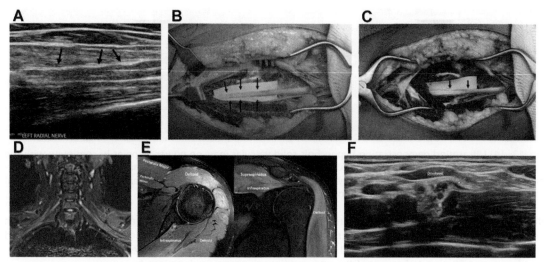

Fig. 15. (*A*) Long axis sonographic view of the left radial nerve demonstrates focal narrowing with formation of strictures (*arrows*) within the nerve fascicles. (*B*) Preneurolysis intraoperative image demonstrating 3 focal circumferential constrictions in the radial nerve (*black arrows*). (*C*) Postneurolysis intraoperative image after release of the constrictions with normal appearance of the nerve (*black arrows*). Patient had full recovery clinically after neurolysis. (*D*) Coronal T2 fat-saturated images show diffuse thickening and hyperintensity of the trunks and cords on the left (*white arrows*) with clinical symptoms of Parsonage-Turner syndrome. (*E*) Axial T2 (*left*) and coronal T2 (*right*) fat-saturated images of the left shoulder with diffuse edema in deltoid, supraspinatus, infraspinatus, and pectoralis musculature. (*F*) Normal origin of suprascapular nerve from the upper trunk of brachial plexus (*white arrow*), at the level of omohyoid.

Other causes that affect multiple peripheral nerves systemically with symmetric or asymmetric distribution including hereditary or acquired mechanisms, include diabetic peripheral neuropathy, alcohol-related neuropathy, chronic inflammatory demyelinating polyneuropathy, and Guillain-Barre syndrome with acute inflammatory demyelinating polyneuropathy. However, compared with acquired polyneuropathies, hereditary conditions such as demyelinating-type Charcot-Marie-Tooth disease are more likely to manifest with symmetric nerve changes.[15] Acute inflammatory or infectious brachial plexopathy is mostly dependent on the clinical factors with good history, physical examination, and EMG findings.

SUMMARY

Multimodality imaging of brachial plexus with a combination of MR imaging and US is essential for identifying the normal anatomy and associated pathology. A multitude of lesions may occur involving the brachial plexus including trauma, neoplasms, and inflammatory lesions. US has advantage in identifying the nerve architecture with partial or intrasubstance tears, identification of neuromas as well as for dynamic imaging. MR is advantageous over US in identifying the preganglionic injuries and associated muscle changes.

Accurate reporting of the pathology with dedicated MR imaging protocols in conjunction with Doppler US and dynamic imaging is paramount to provide practical and useful information to help the referring physicians and surgeons to optimize medical or surgical exploration.

DISCLOSURES

Dr J.H. Hacquebord has financial disclosures with Consulting Synthes, Tissium, and Checkpoint. No financial conflicts of interest or commercial disclosures or funding sources for other authors.

SUPPLEMENTARY DATA

Supplementary data related to this article can be found online at https://doi.org/10.1016/j.mric. 2023.01.006.

REFERENCES

1. Amrami KK, Port JD. Imaging the brachial plexus. Hand Clin 2005;21(1):25–37.
2. Caporrino FA, Moreira L, Moraes VY, et al. Brachial plexus injuries: diagnosis performance and reliability of everyday tools. Hand Surg 2014;19(1): 7–11.
3. Griffith JF. Ultrasound of the Brachial Plexus. Semin Muscoskel Radiol 2018;22(3):323–33.

4. Brown JM, Yablon CM, Morag Y, et al. US of the peripheral nerves of the upper extremity: a landmark approach. Radiographics 2016;36(2):452–63.

5. Yablon CM, Hammer MR, Morag Y, et al. US of the peripheral nerves of the lower extremity: a landmark approach. Radiographics 2016;36(2):464–78.

6. Chauhan SP, Blackwell SB, Ananth CV. Neonatal brachial plexus palsy: incidence, prevalence, and temporal trends. Semin Perinatol 2014;38(4):210–8.

7. Mollberg M, Hagberg H, Bager B, et al. High birth-weight and shoulder dystocia: the strongest risk factors for obstetrical brachial plexus palsy in a Swedish population-based study. Acta Obstet Gynecol Scand 2005;84(7):654–9.

8. Mikityansky I, Zager EL, Yousem DM, et al. MR Imaging of the brachial plexus. Magn Reson Imaging Clin N Am 2012;20(4):791–826.

9. Chen AM, Hall WH, Li J, et al. Brachial plexus-associated neuropathy after high-dose radiation therapy for head-and-neck cancer. Int J Radiat Oncol Biol Phys 2012;84(1):165–9.

10. Bruzzi JF, Komaki R, Walsh GL, et al. Imaging of non-small cell lung cancer of the superior sulcus: part 2: initial staging and assessment of resectability and therapeutic response. Radiographics 2008; 28(2):561–72.

11. Lapegue F, Faruch-Bilfeld M, Demondion X, et al. Ultrasonography of the brachial plexus, normal appearance and practical applications. Diagn Interv Imaging 2014;95(3):259–75.

12. Grisariu S, Avni B, Batchelor TT, et al. Neurolymphomatosis: an International Primary CNS Lymphoma Collaborative Group report. Blood 2010;115(24): 5005–11.

13. Bowen BC, Pattany PM, Saraf-Lavi E, et al. The brachial plexus: normal anatomy, pathology, and MR imaging. Neuroimaging Clin N Am 2004;14(1): 59–viii.

14. Chhabra A. MR neurography. Neuroimaging Clin N Am 2014;24(1):xvii.

15. Martín Noguerol T, Barousse R, Gómez Cabrera M, et al. Functional MR neurography in evaluation of peripheral nerve trauma and postsurgical assessment. Radiographics 2019;39(2):427–46.

16. Sanders RJ. Anatomy of the Thoracic Outlet and Related Structures. Thoracic Outlet Syndrome 2021;17:24.

17. Nwawka OK. Ultrasound imaging of the brachial plexus and nerves about the neck. Ultrasound Q 2019;35(2):110–9.

18. Leonhard V, Smith R, Caldwell G, et al. Anatomical variations in the brachial plexus roots: implications for diagnosis of neurogenic thoracic outlet syndrome. Ann Anat 2016;206:21–6.

19. Raptis CA, Sridhar S, Thompson RW, et al. Imaging of the patient with thoracic outlet syndrome. Radiographics 2016;36(4):984–1000.

Acute and Chronic Elbow Disorders
MR Imaging–Ultrasonography Correlation

Steven P. Daniels, MD[a], Jan Fritz, MD, PD, RMSK[b],*

KEYWORDS

• Elbow • MR imaging • Ultrasonography

KEY POINTS

- Both MR imaging and ultrasonography can be used to evaluate the many important soft-tissue structures about the elbow.
- MR imaging and ultrasonography findings often correlate though each modality has advantages and disadvantages depending on the clinical indication.
- MR imaging is valuable in cases of complex injury where multiple structures are likely involved and often provides a more accurate evaluation of difficult-to-evaluate structures such as the distal biceps tendon.
- Ultrasonography is excellent for the targeted evaluation of small structures due to its superior spatial resolution and in cases where dynamic evaluation is essential, such as evaluation of the ulnar nerve in the cubital tunnel.

INTRODUCTION

The elbow is a complex joint encompassing three articulations and containing numerous important surrounding ligaments and tendons. The elbow articulations include the ulnotrochlear joint functioning as a hinge joint, the proximal radioulnar joint allowing for rotation, and the radiocapitellar joint allowing for both hinge and rotational motions. The complex anatomy of the elbow joint and the surrounding ligaments allow for elbow flexion, elbow extension, forearm protonation, and forearm supination. In addition, the distal humerus serves as the attachment site for multiple muscle-tendon units, allowing for wrist and finger flexion and extension. The radial, median, and ulnar nerves all travel within the soft tissues of the elbow and can be involved in many pathologic conditions.

Elbow pain is common, and patients with pain present in a variety of clinical settings.[1,2] In most clinical scenarios, radiographs will be the initial imaging study obtained. If further imaging is necessary, ultrasonography (US) and/or MR imaging can be performed, with each modality having advantages and disadvantages depending on the suspected pathologic condition. This article will review the use of both MR imaging and US in evaluating the elbow joint and its surrounding structures. We review techniques for performing MR imaging and US of the elbow, highlight the advantages and disadvantages of each modality, and illustrate important structures and common pathologic conditions of the elbow.

MR IMAGING TECHNIQUE

Protocols for MR imaging of the elbow vary depending on the institution though they generally include imaging in all three planes using a combination of T1-weighted, proton-density- and intermediate-weighted, and T2-weighted sequences with and

a Department of Radiology, New York University Grossman School of Medicine, 660 1st Avenue, 3rd Floor, New York, NY 10016, USA; b Department of Radiology, Musculoskeletal Radiology, New York University Grossman School of Medicine, 660 1st Avenue, 3rd Floor, Room #313, New York, NY 10016, USA
* Corresponding author.
E-mail address: Jan.Fritz@nyulangone.org

Magn Reson Imaging Clin N Am 31 (2023) 269–284
https://doi.org/10.1016/j.mric.2023.01.007
1064-9689/23/© 2023 Elsevier Inc. All rights reserved.

without fat suppression using a field of view of 12 to 15 cm. The standard MR imaging protocol at our institution is included in **Table 1**. Distally, the anatomic coverage should extend beyond the biceps tendon insertion to include the radial tuberosity. Proximally, the triceps muscle-tendon junction should be included. In cases with suspected retracted biceps tendon rupture, an extended field-of-view sagittal pulse sequence should include the retracted tendon end to aid surgical planning.

The epicondylar line, which connects the medial and lateral epicondyles and is often rotated about 5° from the flexion axis in the axial plane, should be used as the coronal plane prescription allowing for optimal evaluation of the flexor-pronator and extensor tendons. The sagittal plane should be prescribed perpendicular to the epicondylar line.

MR imaging can either be performed with the patient prone (superman position) or supine (reverse superman position) and the arm positioned overhead, or with the patient supine and the arm adducted and extended at the patient's side. Imaging the patient in the superman position is advantageous as it places the region of interest at the magnet isocenter and requires less phase oversampling due to eliminating anatomic structure next to the field of view. In addition, knee coils can be used. However, superman positions can be difficult for patients to tolerate and ultimately lead to motion artifacts and degraded images. MR imaging in a supine position with the arm adducted and extended at the patient's side places the region of interest away from the isocenter of the magnet, which reduces signal and increases noise. In addition, substantial phase-oversampling is needed for coronal and often sagittal image planes, depending on the elbow rotation, which adds acquisition time and image artifacts. However, this position is easiest to tolerate and produces the least motion artifacts.

Our preference is to perform MR imaging of the elbow at 3.0 T with 15- and 18-channel knee coils or multichannel blanket coils to maximize signal-to-noise ratios while taking advantage of simultaneous multislice and parallel imaging techniques to decrease examination time.[3–6] MR arthrography of the elbow is rarely performed at our institution though it can provide a more accurate assessment of the collateral ligaments and can be used when conventional MR imaging findings are discordant with the physical examination.[7] Some institutions have performed MR arthrography with axial traction in the hopes of better evaluating the articular cartilage though this is not performed at our institution.[8,9]

ULTRASONOGRAPHY TECHNIQUE

US of the elbow is best performed with a high-frequency linear transducer, ideally of 10 to 18 MHz, for high spatial resolution evaluation of the soft-tissue structures about the elbow. The examination can be performed with the patient in the sitting, supine, prone, or decubitus positions with the arm at the patient's side or overhead. The arm can be extended or flexed to highlight specific structures. A major advantage of US is the ability to interact with the patient in real-time and correlate the imaging findings with the area of pain. Dynamic images and/or images of the contralateral elbow can also highlight certain pathology and draw attention to what would otherwise be a subtle abnormality.[10]

Table 1
Elbow MR imaging protocol

Sequence Parameters	Axial PD	Axial PDFS	Coronal PD	Coronal PDFS	Sagittal PDFS
Pulse sequence type	TSE	TSE	TSE	TSE	TSE
Repetition time (ms)	4300	3800	4000	3800	5000
Echo time (ms)	30	38	30	38	46
Receiver bandwidth (Hz/pixel)	350	300	350	300	300
Acceleration factor	2	2	2	2	2
Turbo factor	11	11	11	11	11
Field of view (mm)	120 × 120	120 × 120	120 × 120	120 × 120	120 × 120
Matrix (pixel)	336 × 252	288 × 216	336 × 248	288 × 216	288 × 216
Slice thickness (mm)	3	3	2.8	2.8	3
Interslice distance factor (%)	10	10	10	10	10
Imaging time (min:ss)	1:04	1:57	1:24	2:32	1:30

Abbreviations: FS, spectral fat suppression; PD, proton-density weighting; TSE, turbo spin echo.

US of the elbow requires practice and expertise in scanning techniques to evaluate the small but important anatomic structures accurately. To avoid anisotropy, which can cause normal ligaments and tendons to appear hypoechoic and spuriously abnormal, one must be careful to direct the ultrasound beam perpendicular to the insonated structure. Subtle adjustment of the probe can help differentiate this artifact from true tendon abnormalities but requires a thorough understanding of the often curvilinear ligament and tendon anatomy of the elbow.

We prefer to perform an ultrasound of the elbow as a targeted examination focused on the anterior, medial, posterior, or lateral elbow and/or individual nerves in cases with a specific clinical concern. Less commonly, we perform a complete evaluation of all elbow structures in patients with generalized pain who cannot undergo MR imaging. Unlike with MR imaging, there are no contraindications to undergoing US. The examinations are well tolerated, and many patients prefer musculoskeletal US to MR imaging.[11]

COMPARING ULTRASONOGRAPHY AND MR IMAGING FINDINGS

MR imaging and US are exquisitely accurate in evaluating the integrity of tendons. Normal and abnormal tendons have overlapping and differentiating imaging and signal characteristics (**Table 2**).

On MR imaging, normal tendons, and ligaments show a smooth contour and homogenous low signal on all pulse sequences without evidence of fiber discontinuity. In US, normal tendons and ligaments show a smooth hyperechoic fibrillar pattern.[12] On MR imaging, abnormal tendons can appear thickened and signal hyperintense in degenerative tendinosis and show fiber discontinuity and fluid signal with tendon tearing. Corresponding findings in US include a thickened and hypoechoic appearance in tendinosis and fiber discontinuity and an anechoic fluid gap in tendon tearing. Scar-remodeled ligaments due to degeneration and prior partial tearing often appear with irregular surfaces and heterogenous internal substance signals. On MR imaging, T2 signal hyperintense joint fluid can be difficult to differentiate from a thickened synovium in the setting of synovitis. In US, joint fluid often appears anechoic and compressible, allowing for differentiation from hyperechoic synovium.

Nerves are highly ordered structures made up of fascicles, connective tissue, and surrounding fat. On MR imaging, normal nerves show intermediate T1 and T2 signal with smooth contour and travel in expected anatomic locations. In US, normal nerves show round internal hypoechoic fascicle-like structures and bundles, which are separated by hyperechoic septae. Nerve abnormalities on MR imaging are represented by T2 signal hyperintensity, nerve and internal fascicular enlargement, loss of the normal internal fascicular-type architecture, perineural scarring, and blurring of the perifascicular fat. Corresponding findings in US include a hypoechoic nerve appearance, loss of the normal fascicular-type architecture, intraneural hypervascularity, and nerve enlargement.

ANTERIOR ELBOW

The structures of interest when evaluating patients with anterior elbow pain include the distal biceps tendon, the bicipitoradial bursa, the anterior elbow joint, the brachialis muscle and tendon, and the median nerve (**Table 3**).

Normal anatomy

The distal biceps tendon forms approximately 7 cm proximal to the elbow joint as a continuation

---

Table 2
Tendon appearances on MR imaging and ultrasonography

Characteristic	MR imaging	US
Normal tendon surface	Smooth, uniform, and continuous	
Normal tendon substance	Dark and uniform on all pulse sequences	Hyperechoic fibrillar pattern
Degenerative tendinosis	Tendon thickening. Hyperintense internal signal.	Tendon thickening. Hypoechoic appearance
Tendon tearing	Tendon attenuation. Internal T2 hyperintense fluid signal.	Tendon attenuation. Internal anechoic fluid gap.
Healed and scar-remodeled tendons	Smooth or irregular surface, irregular caliber changes, and heterogeneous internal signal	

Table 3
Quadrant checklist

Anterior Quadrant	Medial Quadrant	Lateral Quadrant	Posterior Quadrant
Distal biceps tendon	Common flexor tendon	Common extensor tendon	Triceps insertion
Bicipitoradial bursa	Ulnar collateral ligament	Lateral collateral ligament complex	Olecranon bursa.
Brachialis muscle and tendon	Ulnar nerve	Radiocapitellar articulation	Posterior joint capsule and recess
Median nerve	Ulnotrochlear articulation	Radial nerve	Ulanr nerve

of the long and short muscle heads. The tendon often appears as two distinct parts, a short head contribution, and a long head contribution, and averages approximately 9 cm in length.[13] As the tendon forms, the long head contribution is located laterally, whereas the short head contribution is located medially. As the tendon courses distally, it rotates 90°, so the lateral head contribution is posterior, and the short head contribution is anterior. The tendon courses obliquely to insert at the radial tuberosity over a distance of approximately 2.5 cm, with the long head contribution inserting proximal to the short head contribution.[14] The biceps aponeurosis, also known as the "lacertus fibrosus," is important in stabilizing the distal biceps tendon (**Fig. 1**). The lacertus fibrosus extends from the fascia of the medial flexor/pronator muscles superficial to the brachial artery and medial nerve and attaches to the distal biceps tendon proximal to its insertion. The lacertus

fibrosus may be considered the fibrous head of the distal biceps tendon. In distal biceps tendon injuries, a preserved lacertus fibrosus prevents a torn distal biceps tendon from retracting proximally to the elbow joint line. The biciptoradial bursa is a bursal space between the distal biceps tendon and the radial tuberosity that often wraps around the distal biceps tendon.

The brachialis muscle originates at the anterior distal humerus and courses deep and lateral to the biceps muscle and tendon. The muscle crosses just anterior to the ulnohumeral joint before forming a short distal tendon that inserts over a distance of 2 to 4 cm at the ulnar tuberosity.[15] Although it was previously thought that the deep muscle fibers of the brachialis muscle attached directly to the anterior elbow joint capsule, histologic evaluation has shown a thin layer of loose connective tissue separating these structures (**Fig. 2**).[16]

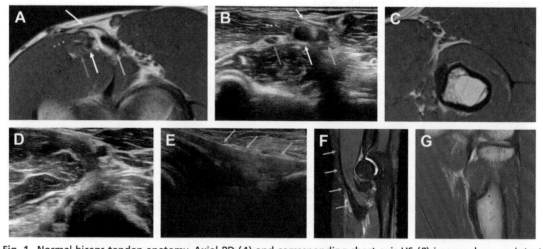

Fig. 1. Normal biceps tendon anatomy. Axial PD (*A*) and corresponding short-axis US (*B*) images show an intact lacertus fibrosus (*yellow arrows*) extending from the medial flexor/pronator muscles (*white asterisks*) to the intact distal biceps tendon (*blue arrow*). At this level, the brachial artery (*white arrow*) and median nerve (*gray arrow*) are medial to the distal biceps tendon. More distal axial PD (*C*) and corresponding short-axis US (*D*) images show an intact distal biceps tendon at the radial tuberosity (*blue arrow*). Long-axis US (*E*) and corresponding sagittal T2 fat-suppressed (*F*) images show an intact distal biceps tendon (*blue arrows*) which is also well seen on a coronal PD image (*blue arrow*, G).

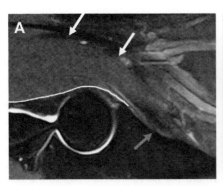 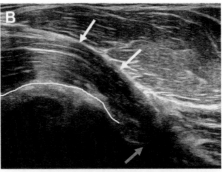

Fig. 2. Normal brachialis muscle and tendon. Sagittal T2 fat-suppressed (*A*) and corresponding long-axis US (*B*) images show an intact brachialis muscle (*white arrows*) and tendon (*gray arrow*). The brachialis muscle closely approximates the anterior elbow joint capsule (*curved white lines*).

The median nerve is a terminal branch nerve of the brachial plexus formed from the medial and lateral cords. The nerve travels through the medial aspect of the upper arm along with the brachial artery. Just proximal to the elbow joint, the median nerve courses deep to the lacertus fibrosis and between the humeral head of the pronator teres (superficial) and the brachialis muscle and ulnar head of the pronator teres (deep) to enter the forearm (**Fig. 3**). In the proximal forearm, the nerve courses deep to the fibrous arch formed by the two heads of the flexor digitorum superficialis muscle, a potential site of nerve compression.

Pathologic conditions

The most common indication for anterior elbow imaging is concern for a distal biceps tendon injury.[17] Distal biceps tendon tears account for about 10% of biceps tendon injuries and often occur in the dominant arm of middle-aged men. They often occur during an eccentric contraction, such as in lifting a heavy object, and in middle-aged and older patients are often preceded by degenerative tendinosis.[18] In the clinical evaluation of distal biceps tendon injury, it is sometimes difficult to differentiate between partial and complete tears, especially when an intact lacertus fibrosus prevents significant tendon retraction. Also, in the setting of complete, retracted tears, it can sometimes be difficult to predict the degree of tendon retraction accurately with clinical tests. Therefore, the purpose of imaging in distal biceps tendon injury is to verify the injury site, differentiate partial from complete tendon tears, and quantify the degree of tendon retraction.

We perform MR imaging of the distal biceps tendon using our standard MR imaging protocol (see **Table 1**). Some institutions add MR images in flexed abducted supinated (FABS) position, described in 2004, to visualize the distal biceps tendon in profile (**Fig. 4**).[19] However, published data on the clinical utility of the FABS view is mixed. A 2021 study showed that additional FABS position MR images did not change the radiologist's impression in most cases and did not change diagnostic accuracy when using a surgical reference standard.[20] A 2020 study showed that

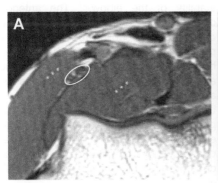 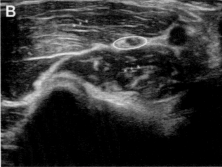

Fig. 3. Normal median nerve anatomy. Axial PD (*A*) and corresponding short-axis US (*B*) images just proximal to the ulnotrochlear articulation show the median nerve (*white oval*) coursing between the humeral head of the pronator teres (*white asterisks*) and brachialis (*yellow asterisks*) muscles.

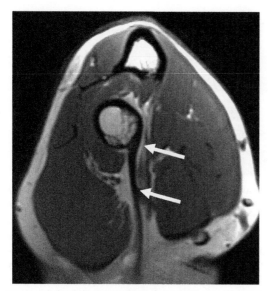

Fig. 4. FABS view. PD image using FABS view in a 36-year-old with anterior elbow pain shows an intact biceps tendon (*white arrows*) inserting at the radial tuberosity.

adding FABS MR images did not change sensitivity or specificity in identifying distal biceps tendon tears, though it did improve inter-rater reliability and accuracy in describing the extent of partial tearing compared with surgical findings.[21] In our experience, adding FABS MR images provides little additional information in most cases. The FABS requirements for patient repositioning, coil change, and acquisition of new scout images prolong MR imaging exam times substantially. We rarely add FABS position MR images, predominantly in challenging cases or if specifically requested by the ordering surgeon.

US evaluation of the distal biceps tendon can involve anterior, medial, lateral, and posterior approaches.[22,23] The distal biceps tendon can be difficult to evaluate due to the oblique tendon course, which predisposes it to anisotropy. We commonly perform US in the short-axis anterior and long-axis anteromedial planes to evaluate tendon continuity and the degree of tendon injury. MR imaging and US accurately identify complete tears, especially when the tendons are retracted proximally from the radial tuberosity.[24–26] Both imaging examinations are less accurate in identifying partial tears and describing the cross-sectional extent of tendon tearing, though MR imaging appears to be the more accurate examination in many settings.[25,26] With both MR imaging and ultrasound, it can be difficult to differentiate tendinosis from tendon tearing (Fig. 5).

Brachialis muscle and tendon injuries are rare and can mimic biceps injuries. Owing to the proximity of the brachialis muscle to the anterior joint capsule, it is at risk for injury during elbow hyperextension and elbow dislocation.[27,28] Median nerve entrapment at the elbow can mimic compression at the wrist and contribute to a confusing clinical presentation.[29] Potential sites of median nerve compression about the elbow include at the distal humerus by a ligament of Struthers, at the elbow by a thickened lacertus fibrosis, between the superficial and deep heads of the pronator teres, and in the proximal forearm where the nerve travels deep to the flexor digitorum superficialis arch.[30]

MEDIAL ELBOW

The structures of interest when evaluating the medial elbow are the common flexor tendon, ulnar collateral ligament, ulnar nerve, and ulnotrochlear articulation (see **Table 3**).

Normal anatomy

The common flexor tendon origin comprises the flexor digitorum superficialis, flexor carpi radialis, palmaris longus, and flexor carpi ulnaris tendons and originates at the medial epicondyle (**Fig. 6**). The pronator teres also originate at the medial humerus with its origin at the medial supracondylar ridge, just proximal to the medial epicondyle, and at the proximal portion of the medial epicondyle.

The ulnar collateral ligament is just deep to the flexor-pronator muscle group and has its humeral attachment just anteroinferior to the common flexor tendon on the anterior inferior undersurface of the medial epicondyle. The ulnar collateral ligament is just superficial to and contiguous with the medial elbow joint capsule.[31] The ligament is composed of anterior, posterior, and transverse bundles, with the anterior bundle being the most important component contributing to the valgus stability of the elbow.[32] The anterior bundle courses from the undersurface of the medial epicondyle to the subline tubercle of the coronoid process of the ulna (**Fig. 7**). The posterior bundle has its humeral attachment just posterior to the anterior bundle and broadly attaches to the ulna at the semilunar notch. Importantly, the posterior bundle forms the floor of the cubital tunnel and provides secondary valgus stability when the elbow is in flexion.[33] The transverse bundle does not cross the ulnotrochlear articulation and does not contribute to the valgus stability of the elbow.

The ulnar nerve is the terminal branch of the medial cord of the brachial plexus, receiving contributions from the C8 and T1 nerve roots. The

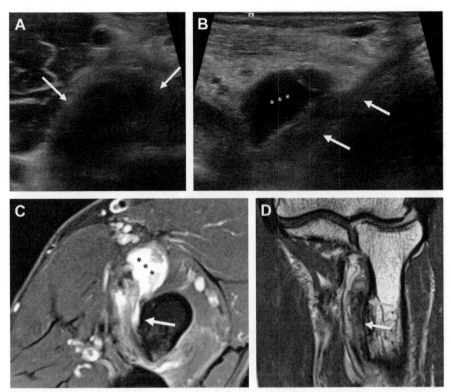

Fig. 5. Partial distal biceps tendon tear. An 81-year-old man with anterior left elbow pain after lifting a heavy object. On the initial short-axis US image (*A*), it is difficult to differentiate tendinosis, tendon tearing, and probable bicipitoradial bursitis adjacent to the radial tuberosity (*white arrows*). Long-axis US image (*B*) shows some intact biceps tendon fibers (*white arrows*) and bicipitoradial bursitis (*white asterisks*). MR imaging was performed 6 weeks later. Axial PD image (*C*) shows partial tearing at the radial tuberosity (*white arrow*) and bicipitoradial bursitis (*black asterisks*). Coronal PD image (*D*) shows tearing to predominantly involve the short head fibers (*yellow arrow*) with some intact long head fibers (*blue arrow*).

nerve travels in the posterior portion of the anterior compartment of the upper arm, posteromedial to the brachial vessels, before piercing the intermuscular septum and entering the posterior compartment, where the nerve travels adjacent to the medial head of the triceps muscle. Just proximal to the elbow joint, the nerve travels posterior to the medial epicondyle within the cubital tunnel. The roof of the cubital tunnel is Osborne's ligament, and the floor is formed by the posterior bundle of the UCL (**Fig. 8**). After exiting the cubital tunnel, the ulnar nerve travels between the humeral and ulnar heads of the flexor carpi ulnaris muscle to enter the forearm.

The ulnotrochlear articulation forms the medial aspect of the elbow joint and acts as a hinge joint. The joint can become degenerated in all portions, but special attention should be paid to the posterior portion of the joint where the posterior trochlea articulates with the olecranon, as this area can become degenerated early in overhead throwers in the setting of valgus extension overload.[34,35]

Pathologic conditions

Abnormalities of the medial elbow soft-tissue structures can occur in a variety of clinical settings, including acute trauma such as in elbow dislocations and chronic conditions such as valgus extension overload syndrome in overhead throwers, chronic flexor tendinosis, and cubital tunnel syndrome. In the setting of elbow dislocation and subluxation, injury can occur to many of the surrounding soft-tissue structures with or without fractures. Surgeons at our institution commonly order computed tomography (CT) of the elbow after radiographs in such cases to better document the extent, comminution, and displacement of fractures. They then sometimes order MR imaging to delineate better the extent of soft-tissue injury (**Fig. 9**). Owing to the variety of structures that can be injured in this setting, MR imaging is favored over US to identify all components of these often complex injuries more effectively.[36,37]

The high valgus load of the late cocking and acceleration phases of overhead throwing place

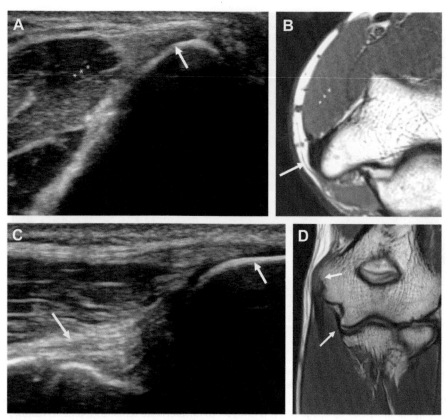

Fig. 6. Normal common flexor tendon anatomy. Short-axis US (*A*) and corresponding axial PD (*B*) images show an intact common flexor tendon (*white arrow*) posterior to the humeral head of the pronator teres muscle (*white asterisks*). Long-axis US (*C*) and corresponding coronal PD (*D*) images show an intact common flexor tendon (*white arrow*) and a partially imaged, intact distal portion of the ulnar collateral ligament (*yellow arrow*).

tremendous strain on the medial soft-tissue structures of the elbow.[38] The ulnar collateral ligament, common flexor tendon, and flexor-pronator muscles are at risk for acute injury and can weaken over time.[39] Weakening of the medial soft-tissue structures can lead to the abutment of the medial olecranon with the olecranon fossa and ultimately cartilage loss, osteophyte formation, synovitis,

and olecranon stress injury.[34,35] In addition, weakened medial soft-tissue structures and abnormal contact at the posterior ulnotrochlear articulation can lead to ulnar nerve symptoms.[40] MR imaging and US can be used to evaluate overhead throwers with medial elbow pain as both modalities can show injuries to the common flexor tendon and ulnar collateral ligament. MR imaging

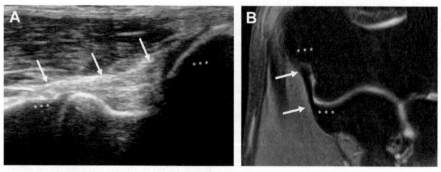

Fig. 7. Normal ulnar collateral ligament. Long-axis US (*A*) and corresponding coronal PD fat-suppressed (*B*) images show an intact ulnar collateral ligament (*white arrows*) attaching proximally at the medial epicondyle (*yellow asterisks*) and distally at the subline tubercule (*white asterisks*).

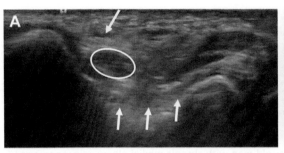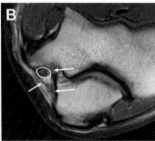

Fig. 8. Normal ulnar nerve. Short-axis US (*A*) and corresponding axial PD (*B*) images show an intact ulnar nerve (*white oval*) deep to the ligament of Osborne (*yellow arrow*) and superficial to the posterior bundle of the ulnar collateral ligament (*white arrows*), which forms the floor of the cubital tunnel.

and MR arthrography have the advantage of being able also to evaluate the elbow joint cartilage and identify patterns of bone marrow edema that suggest valgus instability, whereas ultrasound allows for dynamic assessment for the ulnotrochlear articulation, which widens with valgus stress in the setting of ulnar collateral ligament injury.[7,41,42] In a 2016 paper evaluating both MR arthrography and US in 144 baseball players, MR arthrography showed a sensitivity, specificity, and accuracy of 81%, 91%, and 88% in identifying ulnar collateral ligament tears versus 96%, 81%, and 87% for dynamic US. Importantly, a combined approach

using both modalities showed a sensitivity, specificity, and accuracy of 96%, 99%, and 98% suggesting both modalities provide important, complementary information.[42] Recently, MR imaging using the flexed elbow valgus external rotation (FEVER) position was piloted in Major League Baseball pitchers, showing promise in identifying more ulnar collateral ligament injuries than traditional MR imaging.[43]

Chronic flexor tendinosis (medial epicondylitis) is a degenerative condition that occurs more frequently in golfers and can be diagnosed clinically when patients exhibit pain over the medial

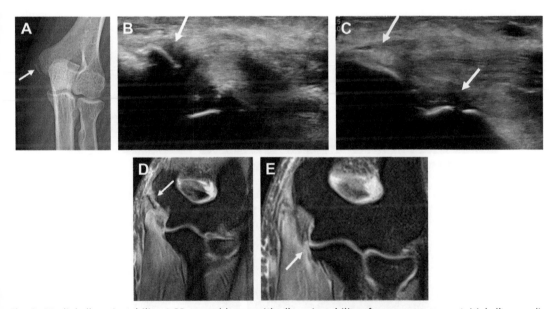

Fig. 9. Medial elbow instability. A 33-year-old man with elbow instability after recent trauma. Initial elbow radiograph (*A*) shows a mildly displaced avulsion fracture adjacent to the medial epicondyle (*white arrow*). Long-axis US images from 1 week later show the avulsion fracture involving the posterior portion of the common flexor tendon origin (*white arrow, B*) with the anterior portion of the common flexor tendon intact (*yellow arrow, C*). The ulnar collateral ligament is ill-defined and possibly injured distally (*white arrow, C*). Coronal PD fat-suppressed image (*D*) from MR imaging performed 1 week later shows the avulsion fracture involving the posterior common flexor tendon (*white arrow*). A more anterior coronal PD fat-suppressed image (*E*) shows a complete tear of the distal ulnar collateral ligament from the sublime tubercle (*white arrow*).

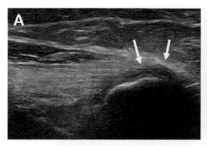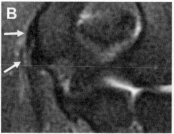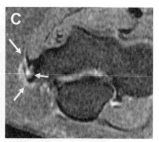

Fig. 10. Common flexor tendinosis. A 52-year-old man with chronic medial elbow pain. Long-axis US image (*A*) shows hypoechoic tissue at the common flexor tendon origin consistent with tendinosis. Coronal (*B*) and axial (*C*) PD fat-suppressed images from MR imaging performed 6 weeks later show thickened, hyperintense common flexor tendon (*white arrows*) with areas of interstitial tearing (*yellow arrow, C*).

epicondyle and pain with resisted forearm pronation and wrist flexion.[44,45] If advanced imaging is necessary to verify the suspected clinical diagnosis, MR imaging and US can accurately delineate the extent of tendinosis and tendon tearing (**Fig. 10**).

Ulnar neuropathy at the elbow, or cubital tunnel syndrome, is the second most common upper extremity peripheral neuropathy and can occur as an isolated entity or secondary to elbow instability, as previously described. MR imaging and US can accurately assess the ulnar nerve to evaluate for masses along the nerve course, including accessory muscles, nerve enlargement, and loss of the fascicular architecture (**Fig. 11**).[46] Referring physicians at our institution prefer US as this allows for dynamic evaluation to diagnose anterior subluxation/dislocation and a snapping medial head of the triceps muscle.[47]

LATERAL ELBOW

The structures of interest when evaluating the lateral elbow include the common extensor tendon, lateral collateral ligament complex, radiocapitellar articulation, and the radial nerve and its branches (see **Table 3**).

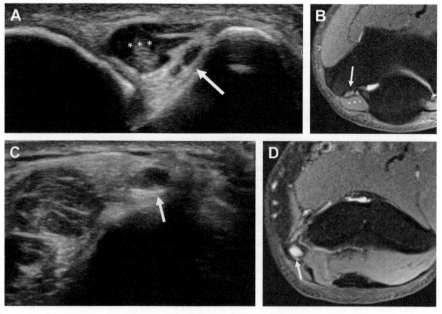

Fig. 11. Ulnar nerve compression. A 35-year-old woman with intermittent hand numbness. Short-axis US (*A*) and corresponding axial PD fat-suppressed (*B*) images at the level of the cubital tunnel show compression of the ulnar nerve (*white arrow*) by an anconeus epitrochlearis accessory muscle (*white asterisks*). Slightly more proximal short-axis US image (*C*) shows a hypoechoic, enlarged ulnar nerve (*yellow arrow*). Corresponding axial PD fat-suppressed image (*D*) shows an enlarged, hyperintense ulnar nerve (*yellow arrow*) consistent with the ultrasound findings.

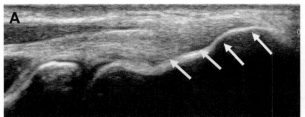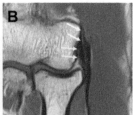

Fig. 12. Normal common extensor tendon and lateral collateral ligament complex. Long-axis US (*A*) and corresponding coronal PD (*B*) images show an intact common extensor tendon (*white arrow*) and lateral collateral ligament complex (*yellow arrow*) at the lateral epicondyle.

Normal anatomy

The common extensor tendon comprises the extensor carpi radialis brevis, extensor digitorum communis, extensor digiti minimi, and the extensor carpi ulnaris tendons and originates at the lateral epicondyle. The extensor carpi radialis brevis tendon is just deep to the extensor carpi radialis longus muscle belly and is the most prominent extensor tendon originating at the lateral epicondyle.

The humeral attachment of the lateral collateral ligament complex is just distal to the common extensor tendon and intimately associated with the tendon undersurface (**Fig. 12**). The humeral attachment is composed anteriorly of the radial collateral ligament and posteriorly of the lateral ulnar collateral ligament. The annular ligament is the third component of the lateral collateral ligament complex. The annular ligament wraps around and stabilizes the radial head at the proximal radioulnar joint with attachments at the anterior and posterior margins of the radial notch of the ulna. The radial collateral ligament attaches distally onto the annular ligament, whereas the lateral ulnar collateral ligament wraps around the humeral head posteriorly to attach at the supinator crest of the ulna.

The radial nerve is the terminal branch of the posterior cord of the brachial plexus. After traveling through the upper arm, the nerve courses

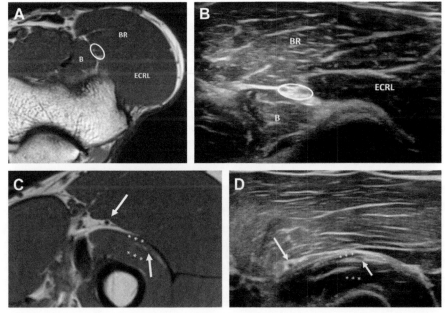

Fig. 13. Normal radial nerve. Axial PD (*A*) and corresponding short-axis US (*B*) images show a normal radial nerve (*white oval*) at the level of the radiocapitellar articulation traveling deep to the brachioradialis (BR) and extensor carpi radialis longus (ECRL) muscles and superficial to the brachialis (*B*) muscle. More distal axial PD (*C*) and corresponding short-axis US (*D*) images show the superficial branch of the radial nerve (*white arrow*) and the deep branch of the radial nerve/posterior interosseous nerve (*yellow arrow*), which travels between the superficial (*yellow asterisks*) and deep (*white asterisks*) heads of the supinator muscle.

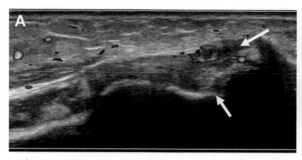
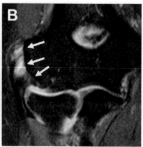

Fig. 14. Lateral epicondylitis. A 72-year-old man with chronic lateral elbow pain. Long-axis power Doppler US image (*A*) shows a hypoechoic common extensor tendon with areas of interstitial tearing (*white arrow*) and surrounding hyperemia as well as an intact humeral attachment of the lateral ulnar collateral ligament (*yellow arrow*). Coronal T2 fat-suppressed image (*B*) shows a thickened, hyperintense signal common extensor tendon with areas of interstitial tearing (*white arrows*) and an intact humeral attachment of the lateral ulnar collateral ligament (*yellow arrow*).

anterior to the lateral epicondyle and passes through the radial tunnel. At the level of the radiocapitelar joint, the nerve divides into a superficial sensory branch and a deep motor branch (**Fig. 13**). The deep motor branch travels under the arcade of Frohse and between the superficial and deep heads of the supinator, where it becomes the posterior interosseous nerve. The posterior interosseous nerve then exits the supinator and innervates the posterior compartment muscles in the forearm.

Pathologic conditions

As with the medial-sided soft-tissue structures, injury to the lateral-sided soft-tissue structures can occur acutely, often in the elbow dislocation/subluxation setting, or may be the result of chronic degeneration such as in lateral epicondylitis (common extensor tendinosis). In the setting of acute injury to the lateral-sided soft-tissue structures, MR imaging is commonly performed at our institution to assess the status of the common extensor tendon, lateral collateral ligament complex, and

articular cartilage. In the acute setting as well as in the setting of recurrent instability, the status of the lateral ulnar collateral ligament is a key factor in guiding surgical management.[48]

Degenerative common extensor tendinosis, or lateral epicondylitis, is very common, affecting about 1% to 2% of the population.[44] Patients commonly present with tenderness anterior and distal to the lateral epicondyle and pain with wrist and finger extension.[49] The diagnosis is usually made clinically, and initial treatment is initiated. In cases where the diagnosis is in question or initial treatment is unsuccessful, either MR imaging or US can be performed with both modalities capable of demonstrating the extent of disease and evidence of alternative diagnoses (**Fig. 14**). Involvement of the humeral attachment of the lateral collateral ligament complex has been shown to correlate with worse pain as well as a poor response to non-surgical management.[50,51]

In patients with chronic lateral-sided elbow pain, abnormality of the radial or posterior interosseous nerves is an important differential diagnostic consideration. We commonly perform US to

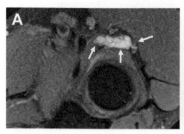
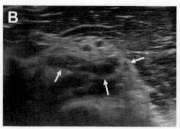
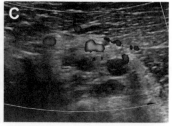

Fig. 15. Radial tunnel syndrome. A 52-year-old woman with 2 months of left elbow pain. Axial PD fat-suppressed image (*A*) shows a hyperintense mass (*yellow arrows*) adjacent to the deep branch of the radial nerve (*white arrow*) within the radial tunnel. Short-axis image (*B*) from US performed 3 weeks later shows a predominantly hypoechoic mass (*yellow arrows*) adjacent to the deep branch of the radial nerve (*white arrow*). The mass did not show flow on power Doppler imaging (*C*). Imaging findings were suspicious for a slow-flow vascular malformation.

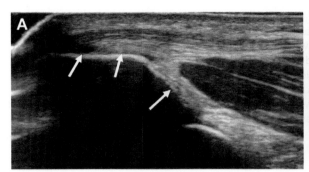
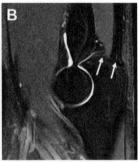

Fig. 16. Normal triceps tendon anatomy. Long-axis US (*A*) and sagittal T2 fat-suppressed (*B*) images show an intact superficial tendinous portion of the triceps attachment (*white arrow*) as well as an intact deep muscular portion (*yellow arrow*). The superficial tendinous portion consists mainly of contributions from the lateral and long heads of the triceps muscle, whereas the deep muscular portion consists of the medial head fibers.

evaluate the radial nerve and its branches to take advantage of the excellent spatial resolution. We rely on short-axis images in such cases and often see a focal enlargement of the deep branch of the radial nerve at the arcade of Frohse.[52] Mass lesions in the radial tunnel are a less common cause of symptoms and can be well evaluated with both US or MR imaging (**Fig. 15**).

POSTERIOR ELBOW

Structures of interest when evaluating the posterior elbow include the triceps insertion onto the olecranon and the olecranon bursa (see **Table 3**).

Normal anatomy

The triceps muscle has a complex attachment to the olecranon. The superficial tendinous portion of the triceps attachment is formed predominantly by the lateral and long heads of the triceps muscle and has a length of approximately 15 cm. The deeper muscular portion of the attachment is formed by the medial head muscle and is closely approximated to the posterior elbow joint capsule (**Fig. 16**).[53] The olecranon bursa is a bursal space within the subcutaneous tissues directly overlying

the proximal ulna. In normal patients, it is not perceptible on imaging.

Pathologic conditions

Injuries to the distal triceps tendon are uncommon. The most commonly reported mechanism is a fall on the hand with the elbow in extension though injuries have also been reported in weightlifters (possibly due to the potential use of anabolic steroids) and soccer players.[54] In such injuries, MR imaging or ultrasound can be used to show the degree of tendon tearing and tendon retraction, as well as other associated injuries about the elbow.[55,56] Complete triceps tendon injuries require surgical repair, whereas the most effective treatment of partial injuries is more controversial.[54] Although some surgeons advocate for nonoperative management of partial tears, others advocate for early surgical management of high-grade injuries using a threshold of 50% to 75% of the tendon thickness.[57,58]

Olecranon bursitis can occur due to various causes, including mechanical irritation, inflammation, gout, rheumatoid arthritis, or infection.[59] Although the diagnosis is often made clinically, MR imaging and US can help identify the extent

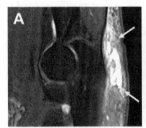
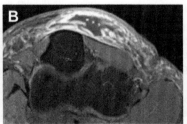
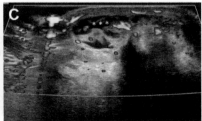

Fig. 17. Olecranon bursitis. A 60-year-old man with elbow pain, redness, and swelling. Sagittal T2 fat-suppressed image (*A*) shows edema and probable fluid posterior to the olecranon in the olecranon bursa (*yellow arrows*). Axial post-contrast T1 fat-suppressed image (*B*) better defines the rim-enhancing fluid in the olecranon bursa (*white asterisks*). Short-axis power Doppler US image (*C*) performed 1 day later shows hypoechoic fluid in the olecranon bursa (*white asterisks*) with surrounding hyperemia.

of surrounding soft-tissue abnormality, size of the fluid component, and potential alternative diagnoses **(Fig. 17)**.[60,61] At our institution, we prefer to use US to better differentiate the fluid component from the thickened bursal lining, which often requires contrast with MR imaging, and for guiding potential aspiration. When scanning with US, it is important to minimize transducer pressure which can collapse the fluid component.

SUMMARY

Elbow pain is common and can be due to pathologic conditions of the elbow joint and the many surrounding soft-tissue structures. MR imaging and US allow for excellent characterization of the injured structures of the elbow. It is important for musculoskeletal radiologists to be comfortable with both modalities in evaluating elbow pain as each has advantages and disadvantages in certain clinical scenarios. Understanding these advantages and disadvantages and how imaging findings correlate between modalities allows radiologists to provide accurate diagnoses and help best guide patient management.

CLINICS CARE POINTS

- When evaluating the distal biceps tendon, we prefer MR imaging over ultrasonography (US) in cases where there is a suspected partial tendon tear. We do not routinely perform imaging in the flexed abducted supinated position.

- In patients who present after elbow subluxation/dislocation, we prefer MR imaging over US to evaluate the multiple components of these complex injuries.

- When evaluating the ulnar nerve at the elbow, we prefer US over MR imaging as US allows for dynamic evaluation to diagnose anterior subluxation/dislocation and a snapping medial head of the triceps muscle.

- In patients with lateral epicondylitis, the status of the lateral collateral ligament complex is an important factor in predicting response to non-surgical management and in guiding potential surgery.

- Abnormality of the radial or posterior interosseous nerve is an important differential diagnostic consideration in patients with chronic lateral elbow pain. We rely on short-axis US images and commonly see focal enlargement of the deep branch of the radial nerve at the arcade of Frohse.

DISCLOSURES

Dr Daniels has no disclosures.

REFERENCES

1. Villarin LA, Belk KE, Freid R. Emercency department evaluation and treatment of elbow and forearm injuries. Emerg Med Clin 1999;17(4):843–58.
2. Javed M, Mustafa S, Boyle S, et al. Elbow pain: a guide to assessment and management in primary care. Br J Gen Pract 2015;65(640):610–2.
3. Fritz J, Guggenberger R, Del Grande F. Rapid Musculoskeletal MRI in 2021: Clinical Application of Advanced Accelerated Techniques. Am J Roentgenol 2021;216(3):718–33.
4. Fritz J, Fritz B, Zhang J, et al. Simultaneous Multislice Accelerated Turbo Spin Echo Magnetic Resonance Imaging: Comparison and Combination With In-Plane Parallel Imaging Acceleration for High-Resolution Magnetic Resonance Imaging of the Knee. Invest Radiol 2017;52(9):529–37.
5. Del Grande F, Rashidi A, Luna R, et al. Five-Minute Five-Sequence Knee MRI Using Combined Simultaneous Multislice and Parallel Imaging Acceleration: Comparison with 10-Minute Parallel Imaging Knee MRI. Radiology 2021;299(3):635–46.
6. Khodarahmi I, Fritz J. The Value of 3 Tesla Field Strength for Musculoskeletal Magnetic Resonance Imaging. Invest Radiol 2021;56(11):749–56.
7. Magee T. Accuracy of 3-T MR Arthrography Versus Conventional 3-T MRI of Elbow Tendons and Ligaments Compared With Surgery. Am J Roentgenol 2014;204(1):W70–5.
8. Lee RKL, Griffith JF, Yuen BTY, et al. Elbow MR arthrography with traction. Br J Radiol 2016;89(1064):20160378.
9. Kohyama S, Tanaka T, Shimasaki K, et al. Effect of elbow MRI with axial traction on articular cartilage visibility—a feasibility study. Skeletal Radiol 2020;49(10):1555–66.
10. Nazarian LN. The top 10 reasons musculoskeletal sonography is an important complementary or alternative technique to MRI. Am J Roentgenol 2008;190(6):1621–6.
11. Middleton WD, Payne WT, Teefey SA, et al. Sonography and MRI of the Shoulder: Comparison of Patient Satisfaction. Am J Roentgenol 2004;183(5):1449–52.
12. Daniels SP, de Tolla JE, Azad A, et al. Imaging Evaluation of Medial and Lateral Elbow Pain: Acute and Chronic Tendon Injuries of the Humeral Epicondyles. Semin Muscoskel Radiol 2021;25(4):589–99.
13. Eames MHA, Bain GI, Fogg QA, et al. Distal Biceps Tendon Anatomy: A Cadaveric Study. JBJS 2007;89(5):1044–9.
14. Bhatia DN, Kandhari V, DasGupta B. Cadaveric Study of Insertional Anatomy of Distal Biceps

Tendon and its Relationship to the Dynamic Proximal Radioulnar Space. J Hand Surg 2017;42(1):e15–23.

15. Kamineni S, Bachoura A, Behrens W, et al. In: Sarikcioglu L, editor. Distal insertional Footprint of the brachialis muscle: 3D Morphometric study. Anatomy Research International, 2015. 2015. p. 786508.

16. Sanal HT, Chen L, Negrao P, et al. Distal Attachment of the Brachialis Muscle: Anatomic and MRI Study in Cadavers. Am J Roentgenol 2009;192(2):468–72.

17. Fritz B, Parkar AP, Cerezal L, et al. Sports Imaging of Team Handball Injuries. Semin Muscoskel Radiol 2020;24(03):227–45.

18. Sutton KM, Dodds SD, Ahmad CS, et al. Surgical Treatment of Distal Biceps Rupture. JAAOS - Journal of the American Academy of Orthopaedic Surgeons 2010;18(3):139–48.

19. Giuffrè BM, Moss MJ. Optimal Positioning for MRI of the Distal Biceps Brachii Tendon: Flexed Abducted Supinated View. Am J Roentgenol 2004;182(4):944–6.

20. Tiegs-Heiden CA, Frick MA, Johnson MP, et al. Utility of the FABS MRI sequence in the evaluation of distal biceps pathology. Skeletal Radiol 2021;50(5):895–902.

21. Schenkels E, Caekebeke P, Swinnen L, et al. Is the flexion-abduction-supination magnetic resonance imaging view more accurate than standard magnetic resonance imaging in detecting distal biceps pathology? J Shoulder Elbow Surg 2020;29(12):2654–60.

22. Al-Ani Z, Lauder J. Ultrasound assessment in distal biceps tendon injuries: Techniques, pearls and pitfalls. Clin Imag 2021;75(July 2021):46–54.

23. de la Fuente J, Blasi M, Martínez S, et al. Ultrasound classification of traumatic distal biceps brachii tendon injuries. Skeletal Radiol 2018;47(4):519–32.

24. Lobo LDG, Fessell DP, Miller BS, et al. The Role of Sonography in Differentiating Full Versus Partial Distal Biceps Tendon Tears: Correlation With Surgical Findings. Am J Roentgenol 2013;200(1):158–62.

25. Lynch J, Yu CC, Chen C, et al. Magnetic resonance imaging versus ultrasound in diagnosis of distal biceps tendon avulsion. J Orthop Traumatol: Surgery & Research 2019;105(5):861–6.

26. Festa A, Mulieri PJ, Newman JS, et al. Effectiveness of Magnetic Resonance Imaging in Detecting Partial and Complete Distal Biceps Tendon Rupture. J Hand Surg 2010;35(1):77–83.

27. Krych AJ, Kohen RB, Rodeo SA, et al. Acute brachialis muscle rupture caused by closed elbow dislocation in a professional American football player. J Shoulder Elbow Surg 2012;21(7):e1–5.

28. Wasserstein D, White L, Theodoropoulos J. Traumatic Brachialis Muscle Injury by Elbow Hyperextension in a Professional Hockey Player. Clin J Sport Med 2010;20(3):211–2.

29. Lee MJ, LaStayo PC. Pronator Syndrome and Other Nerve Compressions That Mimic Carpal Tunnel Syndrome. J Orthop Sports Phys Ther 2004;34(10):601–9.

30. Bilecenoglu B, Uz A, Karalezli N. Possible anatomic structures causing entrapment neuropathies of the median nerve: an anatomic study. Acta Orthop Belg 2005;71(2):169–76.

31. O'Driscoll SW, Jaloszynski R, Morrey BF, et al. Origin of the medial ulnar collateral ligament. J Hand Surg 1992;17(1):164–8.

32. Morrey BF, An KN. Articular and ligamentous contributions to the stability of the elbow joint. Am J Sports Med 1983;11(5):315–9.

33. Regan WD, Korinek SL, Morrey BF, et al. Biomechanical study of ligaments around the elbow joint. Clin Orthop Relat Res 1991;(271):170–9.

34. Dugas JR. Valgus extension overload: diagnosis and treatment. Clin Sports Med 2010;29(4):645–54.

35. Ahmad CS, Park MC, ElAttrache NS. Elbow Medial Ulnar Collateral Ligament Insufficiency Alters Posteromedial Olecranon Contact. Am J Sports Med 2004;32(7):1607–12.

36. Schnetzke M, Ellwein A, Maier D, et al. Injury patterns following simple elbow dislocation: radiological analysis implies existence of a pure valgus dislocation mechanism. Arch Orthop Trauma Surg 2021;141(10):1649–57.

37. Lenich A, Pfeifer C, Proier P, et al. Reattachment of the flexor and extensor tendons at the epicondyle in elbow instability: a biomechanical comparison of techniques. BMC Muscoskel Disord 2018;19(1):432.

38. Werner SL, Fleisig GS, Dillman CJ, et al. Biomechanics of the Elbow During Baseball Pitching. J Orthop Sports Phys Ther 1993;17(6):274–8.

39. Kancherla VK, Caggiano NM, Matullo KS. Elbow Injuries in the Throwing Athlete. Orthop Clin N Am 2014;45(4):571–85.

40. Chen FS, Rokito AS, Jobe FW. Medial elbow problems in the overhead-throwing athlete. J Am Acad Orthop Surg 2001;9(2):99–113.

41. Lurie B, Fritz J, Potter HG. MR Imaging in Patients with Ulnar Collateral Ligament Injury. In: Dines JS, Altchek DW, editors. Elbow ulnar collateral ligament injury: a guide to diagnosis and treatment. Springer US; 2015. p. 67–77.

42. Roedl JB, Gonzalez FM, Zoga AC, et al. Potential Utility of a Combined Approach with US and MR Arthrography to Image Medial Elbow Pain in Baseball Players. Radiology 2016;279(3):827–37.

43. Lund P, Waslewski GL, Crenshaw K, et al. FEVER: The Flexed Elbow Valgus External Rotation View for MRI Evaluation of the Ulnar Collateral Ligament in Throwing Athletes—A Pilot Study in Major League Baseball Pitchers. Am J Roentgenol 2021;217(5):1176–83.

44. Shiri R, Viikari-Juntura E, Varonen H, et al. Prevalence and Determinants of Lateral and Medial

Epicondylitis: A Population Study. Am J Epidemiol 2006;164(11):1065–74.

45. Taylor SA, Hannafin JA. Evaluation and management of elbow tendinopathy. Sports Health 2012;4(5):384–93.

46. Miller TT, Reinus WR. Nerve Entrapment Syndromes of the Elbow, Forearm, and Wrist. Am J Roentgenol 2010;195(3):585–94.

47. Jacobson JA, Jebson PJL, Jeffers AW, et al. Ulnar Nerve Dislocation and Snapping Triceps Syndrome: Diagnosis with Dynamic Sonography—Report of Three Cases. Radiology 2001;220(3):601–5.

48. Camp CL, Sanchez-Sotelo J, Shields MN, et al. Lateral Ulnar Collateral Ligament Reconstruction for Posterolateral Rotatory Instability of the Elbow. Arthroscopy Techniques 2017;6(4):e1101–5.

49. Calfee RP, Patel A, DaSilva MF, et al. Management of Lateral Epicondylitis: Current Concepts. JAAOS - Journal of the American Academy of Orthopaedic Surgeons 2008;16(1):19–29.

50. Bredella MA, Tirman PF, Fritz RC, et al. MR imaging findings of lateral ulnar collateral ligament abnormalities in patients with lateral epicondylitis. Am J Roentgenol 1999;173(5):1379–82.

51. Dones VC, Grimmer K, Thoirs K, et al. The diagnostic validity of musculoskeletal ultrasound in lateral epicondylalgia: a systematic review. BMC Med Imag 2014;14(1):10.

52. Kim Y, Ha DH, Lee SM. Ultrasonographic findings of posterior interosseous nerve syndrome. Ultrasonography 2017;36(4):363–9.

53. Barco R, Sánchez P, Morrey ME, et al. The distal triceps tendon insertional anatomy-implications for surgery. JSES Open Access 2017;1(2):98–103.

54. Tom JA, Kumar NS, Cerynik DL, et al. Diagnosis and Treatment of Triceps Tendon Injuries: A Review of the Literature. Clin J Sport Med 2014;24(3):197–204.

55. Tagliafico A, Gandolfo N, Michaud J, et al. Ultrasound demonstration of distal triceps tendon tears. Eur J Radiol 2012;81(6):1207–10.

56. Koplas MC, Schneider E, Sundaram M. Prevalence of triceps tendon tears on MRI of the elbow and clinical correlation. Skeletal Radiol 2011;40(5):587–94.

57. Strauch RJ. Biceps and triceps injuries of the elbow. Orthop Clin N Am 1999;30(1):95–107.

58. Mair SD, Isbell WM, Gill TJ, et al. Triceps Tendon Ruptures in Professional Football Players. Am J Sports Med 2004;32(2):431–4.

59. Blackwell JR, Hay BA, Bolt AM, et al. Olecranon bursitis: a systematic overview. Shoulder Elbow 2014;6(3):182–90.

60. Blankstein A, Ganel A, Givon U, et al. Ultrasonographic Findings in Patients with Olecranon Bursitis. Ultraschall der Med 2007;27(6):568–71.

61. Floemer F, Morrison WB, Bongartz G, et al. MRI Characteristics of Olecranon Bursitis. Am J Roentgenol 2004;183(1):29–34.

Musculoskeletal Soft-tissue Masses

MR imaging–Ultrasonography Correlation, with an Emphasis on the 2020 World Health Organization Classification

Christopher J. Burke, MBChB*, Jan Fritz, MD, Mohammad Samim, MD

KEYWORDS

• Ultrasound • MRI • Soft-tissue masses • Tumor • Classification

KEY POINTS

- Musculoskeletal soft-tissue masses reflect a heterogeneous group of benign, intermediate, and malignant entities predominantly arising from mesenchymal non-epithelial extraskeletal tissues.
- Evaluation of soft-tissue masses is a common clinical practice indication for imaging with both ultrasound and MR imaging.
- UltrasonographyUS) and MR imaging can have complementary roles in tumor characterization, staging, planning percutaneous biopsy and surgical excision, and surveillance.
- US is excellent for the characterization of superficial masses due to its high axial and spatial resolution, allowing evaluation of tissue architecture, layers, and vascularity.
- MR imaging allows improved characterization of anatomic detail with respect to the compartmental location, soft-tissue contrast, and resolution of deep structures.
- Focused ultrasound can be used as an adjunct to non-contrast MR imaging to evaluate masses for the presence of internal vascularity, avoiding the need for intravenous contrast agents. Targeted ultrasound can confirm the cystic nature of T2 signal hyperintense lesions on MR imaging.
- Advances in molecular genetics and their surrogate immunohistochemical markers have created a paradigm shift in the diagnosis and management of soft-tissue masses, leading to reclassification and prognostication of existing tumor entities in the 2020 World Health Organization (WHO) update.
- As radiologists play an increasingly important role in diagnosing, treating, and following soft-tissue masses, they should integrate updates and WHO reclassifications into their US and MR imaging practice.

INTRODUCTION

Soft-tissue masses (STMs) within the musculoskeletal system reflect a pathologically diverse group of lesions presenting at all ages, predominantly arising from mesenchymal non-epithelial extraskeletal tissues.[1,2] These can occur within the extremities and trunk, head, and neck, involving adipose, muscle, tendons and fibrous tissues, peripheral nerves, and blood vessels. Benign masses far outnumber malignant entities, with soft-tissue sarcomas comprising only approximately 1%.[3]

Evaluation of such masses has become a common indication for imaging with ultrasonography (US) and MR imaging in everyday clinical practice, with both modalities offering various strengths. It may be possible to narrow the differential

NYU Langone Orthopedic Hospital, 301 East 17th Street, New York, NY 10003, USA
* Corresponding author.
E-mail address: Christopher.Burke@nyulangone.org

Magn Reson Imaging Clin N Am 31 (2023) 285–308
https://doi.org/10.1016/j.mric.2022.10.001
1064-9689/23/© 2022 Elsevier Inc. All rights reserved.

diagnosis substantially based on age, location, and radiological characteristics. However, overlapping imaging features are common and may prevent a specific diagnosis. Such lesions often undergo biopsy for histopathological examination, increasingly supplemented with immuno-histochemistry.

The fifth edition of the World Health Organization (WHO) classification of soft-tissue tumors published in 2020 represents an updated consensus for evaluation.[4] This categorizes lesions based on histologic differentiation with newly introduced entities, incorporating biological behavior, genetics and morphology.[5]

This review illustrates US and MR imaging correlations of common STMs based on histopathological subtype classification. We discuss various categories of benign and malignant masses, including adipocytic tumors, fibroblastic, fibrohistiocytic, vascular lesions such as hemangiomas, pericytic and perivascular tumors, peripheral nerve sheath tumors, smooth muscle, and skeletal muscle masses. Cases and discussions highlight pertinent sonographic and MR imaging features and relevant aspects of the updated WHO classification. Finally, we present a combined US-MR imaging flowchart approach for evaluating STMs.

ULTRASOUND AND MR IMAGING IN THE EVALUATION OF MUSCULOSKELETAL SOFT-TISSUE MASSES

The role of the US as the primary screening tool in evaluating STMs within the musculoskeletal system is now well established.[6,7] US is excellent for the characterization of superficial STMs due to its high axial resolution, allowing evaluation of tissue architecture, offering excellent spatial resolution. It is cost-effective, widely accessible, and allows for the characterization of internal cystic or vascularized contents without requiring intravenous contrast administration. In this regard, focused US can be performed as an adjunct for additional characterization of lesions that are indeterminate or incompletely characterized on MR imaging.[5]

MR imaging affords its own set of unique benefits, including precise characterization of anatomic detail with respect to the lesion location, soft-tissue contrast, and resolution of deep structures. It can enable characterization depending on the signal characteristics and accurately show the lesion margins, extent, and involvement with the surrounding structures. This allows for accurate tumor staging and preoperative planning.

Ultrasound Technique

Ultrasound assessment is generally performed using a high-frequency probe, usually a linear 9 to 18 MHz transducer, depending on the depth of the STM. Small foot-plate "hockey stick" transducers can be used to image small STMs. Both gray-scale and Doppler imaging is performed with attention to internal echogenicity and vascularity, respectively. Power Doppler is particularly useful in musculoskeletal imaging as it is more sensitive in detecting low levels of internal vascularity at the expense of directional information.[8] Spectral Doppler can further evaluate any internal vascularity by looking for arterial or venous waveforms. Although mostly a research tool, contrast resolution can also be improved through compression-based or shear wave elastography.[9,10] Extended field-of-view imaging can scan a larger field incorporating it into a single "panoramic" sonographic image. Parameters must be properly optimized, including gain, time gain compensation, depth and number of focal zones, frequency, gray scales, and dynamic range.[11] For superficial STMs, it is important not to distort the lesion by applying sufficient amounts of gel as a "stand off" and avoiding excessive pressure. Dynamic sonography can assess fixation to mobile structures such as tendons using active or passive maneuvers. US may be useful where MR imaging cannot be obtained due to certain implants or issues related to patient tolerance, such as claustrophobia. US can also be used to guide real-time percutaneous biopsy adjacent to critical structures and target regions within a mass to avoid necrotic or highly vascularized areas.

MR Imaging Technique

Markers placed on the overlying skin can delineate and bracket the symptomatic region of concern without distorting the more superficial mass. Images can be performed at 1.5 or 3 T field strength.[12] Most protocols include T1-weighted, fluid-sensitive sequences such as T2-weighted or short tau inversion recovery (STIR) and fat-suppressed T1-weighted sequences with and without contrast.[13] Multiple acceleration techniques are available for rapid tumor MR imaging protocols.[14–20] Two-dimensional or three-dimensional turbo spin-echo and gradient echo pulse sequences may be used for STM characterizations.[17,21–26] In the presence of metallic orthopedic implants, dedicated metal artifact reduction techniques may be incorporated into tumor MR imaging protocols.[27–35] Synthetic contrast techniques may aid in T1 and T2 quantification and improve fat suppression.[36–39]

Intravenous contrast is used to distinguish non-enhancing cystic or necrotic components from enhancing solid tissue, to show internal vascularity, and evaluate tissue planes for the extent of invasion into neurovascular and other structures. Contrast can also aid in helping to identify tumor nodules in cystic, lipomatous, or hemorrhagic masses.

Sequences obtained pre and post-contrast administration should ideally be obtained with identical imaging parameters to allow adequate assessment of enhancement and enable obtaining subtraction images. A pitfall is that some masses may appear T1 hyperintense simply because fat suppression has been applied, which may be erroneously interpreted as gadolinium enhancement.

Restricted diffusion on diffusion-weighted imaging (DWI) can play a role in evaluating masses and response to therapy.[13,40,41] Longitudinal tumor dimension, central enhancement, and ADC values may indicate histology grades in musculoskeletal soft-tissue malignancies.[42] Adding physiologic sequences to the conventional protocols can increase the sensitivity for determining treatment response in soft-tissue sarcomas.[43] Chemical shift MR imaging can be performed to detect microscopic fat. MR spectroscopy has also been used to characterize STMs, although it remains an investigational tool.[44]

THE WORLD HEALTH ORGANIZATION 2020 CLASSIFICATION

The hallmark of the new WHO classification of soft-tissue tumors is the inclusion of multiple novel genetic alterations and their surrogate immunohistochemical markers to provide reliable diagnostic and prognostic markers.[45] A full discussion is beyond the scope of this article; however, the updated classification describes soft-tissue tumors under eleven categories which are subcategorized based on the biological behavior into benign (those that do not recur after resection), intermediate/locally aggressive (locally infiltrative with a high rate of recurrence but do not metastasize), intermediate/rarely metastasizing (in <2% cases) and malignant (those with a high risk of metastasis) (**Table 1**).[4] Undifferentiated small round cell sarcomas are now described in a new separate category.

SUBTYPES OF SOFT-TISSUE MASSES

The most common benign STMs are adipocytic neoplasms, specifically lipoma, followed by fibroblastic and fibrohistiocytic tumors. Liposarcoma, leiomyosarcoma, and undifferentiated pleomorphic sarcomas are the most common sarcomas in adults, whereas rhabdomyosarcoma, Ewing sarcoma, and synovial sarcoma are common in children. Extremities are the most common site of soft-tissue sarcomas (75%), followed by the retroperitoneum and the trunk wall.

ADIPOCYTIC TUMORS

The spectrum of adipocytic tumors ranges from benign lipomas, lipoblastoma, and lipomatosis to intermediate atypical lipomatous tumors with liposarcomas at the malignant end.[46,47]

Lipomas

Lipomas are the most common benign fat-containing mass with a reported incidence of up to 2.1%. They are made up of tissue histologically identical to adipose fat and show a characteristic appearance on US and MR imaging, typically resembling subcutaneous fat, often with a few thin septa and a capsule.[48,49] Lipomas are usually well-vascularized tumors, though plump adipocytes often compress the tenuous vessels.[50,51]

Lipomas are isointense relative to subcutaneous adipose tissue on MR imaging obtained on all pulse sequences, without areas of nodularity or thickened septations. Typical sonographic appearances of a simple lipoma are of a mass within the subcutaneous adipose tissue, lower in echogenicity than muscle but more reflective than adjacent subcutaneous fat, without posterior acoustic enhancement. Although most are hyperechoic, a significant proportion can also be hypoechoic or isoechoic.[52] Intramuscular lipomas may show well-defined or infiltrative margins and internal septae due to interspersed muscle fibers. These fibers should be isointense to normal muscle on both T1-and T2-weighted pulse sequences and maintain their native architecture without nodularity or irregular thickening. The subcutaneous versus intramuscular location of the lipoma is relevant for surgical planning. A significant number of benign lipomas show nonadipose features, with 31% demonstrating nonfatty content, which may be attributed to fat necrosis and associated calcification, fibrosis, inflammation, and myxoid changes.[49]

Other Benign Fat-Containing Masses

Less common benign fat-containing STMs include lipoblastoma, angiolipoma, spindle cell lipoma/pleomorphic lipoma, myolipoma, chondroid lipoma, lipomatosis of nerve, lipomatosis, hibernoma, and fat necrosis. Most of these variants

Table 1
2020 World Health Organization classification of soft-tissue tumors, including the main tumors under each category. New entities and changes are highlighted in italics and bold fonts

Category	Benign	Locally Aggressive	Rarely Metastasising	Malignant
Adipocytic	Lipoma Lipomatosis lipoblastoma Angiolipoma Myolipoma Chondroid lipoma, spindle cell lipoma *Atypical spindle Cell/pleomorphic Lipomatous tumor* Hibernoma	Atypical lipomatous tumor		Liposarcoma (well-differentiated, dedifferentiated, and myxoid pleomorphic *Myxoid pleomorphic*)
Fibroblastic and myofibroblastic	Nodular fasciitis Proliferative fasciitis Proliferative myositis Elastofibroma fibroma Hamartoma of infancy Fibroma of tendon sheath Desmoplastic fibroblastoma Myofibroblastoma Calcifying aponeurotic fibroma *Ewsr1-Smad3 positive fibroblastic tumor* Angiomyofibroblastoma Cellular angiofibroma *Angiofibroma of soft tissue* Nuchal fibroma Acral fibromyxoma gardner fibroma	Solitary fibrous tumor fibromatosis (palmar, plantar, and desmoid type) lipofibromatosis Giant cell fibroblastoma	Dermatofibrosarcoma protuberans Solitary fibrous tumor inflammatory myofibroblastic tumor Myofibroblastic sarcoma *Superficial Cd34-positive fibroblastic tumor* Myxoinflammatory fibroblastic sarcoma Infantile fibrosarcoma	Solitary fibrous tumor Fibrosarcoma Myxofibrosarcoma Low-grade fibromyxoid sarcoma sclerosing epitheloid fibrosarcoma
So-called fibrohistiocytic tumors	Tenosynovial giant cell tumor Deep benign fibrous histiocytoma	Plexiform fibrohistiocytic tumor giant cell tumor of soft parts		Malignant tenosynovial giant cell tumor

Vascular tumors	Hemangioma Epithelioid hemangioma Acquired tufted hemangioma	Kaposiform hemangioendothelioma	Retiform Hemangioendothelioma Papillary intralymphatic Angioendothelioma composite Hemangioendothelioma Kaposi sarcoma Pseudomyxogenic Hemangioendothelioma	Epithelioid Hemangioendothelioma ***Epithelioid Hemangioendothelioma with Yap1- Tfe3 fusion*** Angiosarcoma
Pericytic tumors	Glomus tumor Myopericytoma Angioleiomyoma			Malignant glomus tumor
SMOOTH MUSCLE TUMORS	Leiomyoma	Smooth muscle tumor of uncertain malignant potential		Leiomyosarcoma ***Inflammatory leiomyosarcoma***
Skeletal muscle tumors	Rhabdomyoma			Rhabdomyosarcoma (embryonal, alveolar, pleomorphic, and spindle cell) ***Ectomesenchymoma***
Gastrointestinal stromal tumor				
Chondro-osseous tumors	Chondroma			Extraskeletal osteosarcoma
Peripheral nerve sheath tumors	Schwannoma neurofibroma Plexiform neurofibroma Perineurioma Granular cell tumor nerve Sheath myxoma solitary Circumscribed neuroma Meningioma Hybrid nerve sheath tumor			Malignant peripheral sheath tumor ***melanotic malignant Nerve sheath tumor*** Malignant granular cell tumor ***Malignant perineurioma***

(continued on next page)

Table 1
(continued)

Category	Benign	Locally Aggressive	Rarely Metastasising	Malignant
Tumors of uncertain differentiation	Myxoma Aggressive angiomyxoma Pleomorphic hyalinizing Angiectatic tumor Phosphaturic mesenchymal tumor perivascular epitheloid tumor ***Angiomyolipoma***	***Epithelioid angiomyolipoma*** Hemosiderotic fibrolipomatous tumor	Atypical fibroxanthoma Angiomatoid fibrous Histiocytoma Ossifying fibromyxoid Tumor Myoepithelioma	***NTRK rearranged spindle cell neoplasm*** Synovial sarcoma Epithelioid sarcoma Alveolar soft part sarcoma Clear cell sarcoma Extraskeletal myxoid chondrosarcoma desmoplastic small round cell tumor Rhabdoid tumor Malignant perivascular Epithelioid tumor Intimal sarcoma Malignant ossifying fibromyxoid tumor ***Undifferentiated sarcoma*** ***Undifferentiated spindle cell sarcoma*** ***Undifferentiated pleomorphic sarcoma***
Undifferentiated small cell sarcoma of bone and soft-tissues				***Ewing's sarcoma*** ***Round cell sarcoma with EWSR1-non ETS fusion*** ***CIC rearranged sarcomas*** ***Sarcoma with BCOR genetic alterations***

The 2020 WHO classification of soft-tissue tumors with a list of main tumors under each category. New changes and entities are highlighted in italics and bold.

show macroscopic fat; however, few entities like chondrolipoma and spindle cell lipoma (**Fig. 1**) may not show evidence of macroscopic or microscopic fat on MR imaging when the predominant portion of the mass is from chondroid or spindle cell component, respectively.[48,53]

Lipoma variants, such as angiolipoma and myolipoma, are another group of tumors that are predominantly fat-containing thin-walled blood vessels and varying amounts of smooth muscle, respectively. Benign lipomatous tumors typically should not have thick, irregular, enhancing septa and nonfatty components. However, benign lipomatous lesions and well-differentiated liposarcomas/atypical lipomatous tumors may exhibit overlapping imaging findings.

Liposarcoma

Liposarcoma is the second most common soft-tissue sarcoma accounting for approximately 16% to 18% of all soft-tissue tumors.[54] Liposarcoma has a wide spectrum of imaging appearances reflecting the diverse and heterogenous histologic subtypes, though certain imaging generalizations can be made for its varying subtypes. Liposarcoma subtypes include well-differentiated, dedifferentiated, myxoid, pleomorphic, and the newly added myxoid pleomorphic subtype.[4]

The more differentiated the tumor, the more tissue with adipose imaging features is visible. Features favoring malignant liposarcoma include lesion size greater than 10 cm, presence of thick (>2 mm) septae (either diffuse or focal), presence of globular and nodular nonadipose tissue, and lesion composition of less than 75% fat. Although more well-differentiated liposarcomas show a predominant fat component, more aggressive liposarcoma subtypes (dedifferentiated, myxoid, and pleomorphic) may contain minimal or no visible fat.

Atypical Lipomatous Tumors and Well-Differentiated Liposarcomas

Originally designated as well-differentiated liposarcoma (WDL), atypical lipomatous tumors (ALT) was introduced to describe a subtype of lipomatous tumor which can be locally aggressive with no propensity to metastasize. In the past, a distinction was made between atypical lipomatous tumors and well-differentiated liposarcomas. Although histopathologically identical, they were described as ALT in the extremities and well-differentiated liposarcomas in the retroperitoneum and mediastinum. This distinction was made to reflect the low morbidity and low incidence of recurrence in the extremities, where wide excision is usually achievable as opposed to that of retroperitoneal and mediastinal tumors, where complete excision is more often technically difficult.

This distinction has been removed so both entities are now considered to be the same. Imaging features in favor of ALT/WDL are predominant fatty components of a mass (75% adipose tissue) with thin septa that are uniform in thickness and less than 2 mm thick. Although ALT/WDL and lipomas have overlapping MR imaging features, patient age over 60 years, maximum lesion dimension >10 cm, location in the lower limb, and presence of nonfatty (solid or amorphous) components are more suggestive of ALT/WDL. Ultimately, discrimination of lipoma and ALT/WDL should be based on tissue sampling and histologic examination with MDM2 amplification status.[55] Most qualitative MR imaging features can help distinguish ALT from

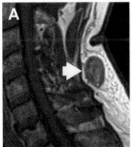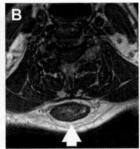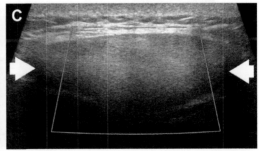

Fig. 1. Atypical spindle cell lipomatous tumor in a 68-year-old man presenting with a posterior neck mass. (*A*) Sagittal and axial (*B*) T1-weighted MR images show an encapsulated, mildly heterogeneous, subcutaneous mass in the subcutaneous soft-tissues of the posterior neck (*white arrows*) containing internal foci of fat. (*C*) Transverse ultrasound image with power Doppler before biopsy demonstrating an encapsulated lobular soft-tissue mass, mildly hyperechoic to the surrounding adipose tissue and without substantial internal vascularity on power Doppler imaging. Biopsy showed a mixture of prominent spindle cells with ropey collagen and adipocyte vacuoles with some variation in size; however, the tissue was negative for high-grade features.

lipomas; however, the additional value of contrast enhancement may be more limited than previously assumed.[47]

FIBROBLASTIC AND MYOFIBROBLASTIC TUMORS

Fibroblastic and myofibroblastic soft-tissue tumors encompass a broad spectrum of lesions. Tumors in this category include benign entities like nodular fasciitis, proliferative myositis, elastofibroma and malignant lesions such as fibrosarcoma and myxofibrosarcoma. Desmoid tumors (**Fig. 2**) and dermatofibrosarcoma protuberans (**Fig. 3**) are included in the intermediate group. Hemangiopericytoma was previously removed as a separate entity and is now rather recognized as a histologic pattern of staghorn-shaped branching blood vessels which can be seen in many tumors like solitary fibrous tumor (**Fig. 4**), synovial sarcoma, and malignant peripheral nerve sheath tumors.

The tumors in this category are usually homogeneous, demonstrating low T2 signal due to their fibrous content, and delayed contrast enhancement. Fibromatosis is an aggressive lesion that can occur in superficial or deep locations. They are usually T2 hypointense due to mature collagen, whereas the more cellular tumors can be T2 hyperintense.

Desmoid-Type Fibromatosis

Desmoid-type fibromatoses, also known as desmoid tumors, are a biologically heterogeneous group of locally aggressive fibroblastic neoplasm.[56] These tumors typically affect the fascia, septa, and aponeuroses between muscles, although they can infiltrate the subcutaneous tissues. The estimated incidence of these lesions is approximately 2 to 4 per million in the United States.[57] They are more common in women (3:1 ratio).[51] Deep fibromatoses can occur anywhere, though 70% of cases occur in the extremities.[51] The biological behavior ranges from indolent to aggressive, with deep fibromatosis having no potential to metastasize but frequently recurring locally.[58] Histologically, they are poorly circumscribed and infiltrative, composed of dense collagenous stroma and long fascicles of band, uniform fibroblasts with low cellularity.

Sonographically, desmoid tumors are visualized as an oval, solid STM with smooth or poor margins and variable echogenicity depending on tumor composition. The collagenous and fibrotic mass is typically hypoechoic, whereas tumors with cellular components are usually hyperechoic. Doppler US can show variable degrees of internal vascularity (see **Fig. 2**).

MR imaging usually shows a heterogeneous appearance with variable T2 signal and isointense signal on T1-weighted images. The variability in signal intensity has been attributed to three stages of histologic evolution.[59–61] The first stage includes more cellularity with large extracellular spaces, therefore showing an increased T2 signal. During the second and third stages, collagenation progresses and becomes more diffuse, resulting in decreased cellularity, extracellular space volume, water content, and overall decreased T2 signal intensity. Contrast enhancement is variable, with up to 90% of lesions demonstrating moderate-to-

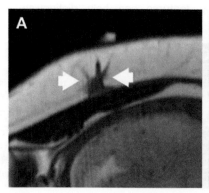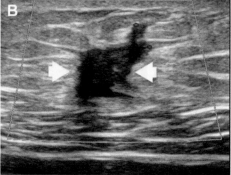

Fig. 2. Desmoid tumor in a 35-year-old woman within the right lower abdominal wall. (*A*) Axial HASTE image shows a spiculated low signal lesion within the subcutaneous fat (*white arrows*), which broadly abuts but does not extend into the underlying rectus abdominis musculature. Corresponding transverse ultrasound image (*B*) with power Doppler showing a hypoechoic, minimally vascularized soft-tissue mass with irregular posterior shadowing and spiculated borders extending through the subcutaneous adipose tissue (*white arrows*). Subsequent biopsy showed a low-grade low-moderate cellularity spindle cell tumor with prominent fibrotic changes. Morphology and immunohistochemistry staining was compatible with a Desmoid tumor/fibromatosis.

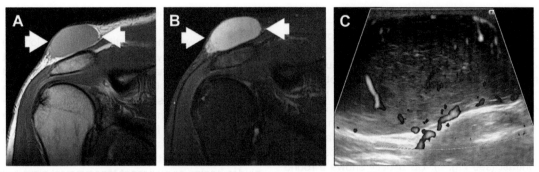

Fig. 3. Dermatofibrosarcoma Protuberans in a 53-year-old man presenting with a shoulder mass. Coronal (A) proton density and (B) STIR images show a well-circumscribed subcutaneous ovoid lesion initially interpreted as a fluid collection superior to the acromioclavicular joint (*white arrows*). Corresponding ultrasound image with power Doppler (C) shows a vascularized soft-tissue mass. Histologic evaluation showed characteristic sheets of tumor cell proliferation in storiform, cartwheel, and focally herringbone patterns with increased cellularity, atypia, increased mitotic activity, and decreased staining for CD34.

marked enhancement, corresponding to the cellular portions of the lesion.[62,63]

The "Staghorn sign" represents intramuscular finger-like extensions representing local invasion from the deeper tumor along fibrous septa into the subcutaneous fat. The "fascial tail sign" corresponds to linear extension along fascial planes, as a thin beak or linear extension along the orientation of the involved muscle fibers or aponeurosis. However, this sign is useful, though not pathognomonic, as it also occurs in sarcomas that may arise in the fascia, especially myxofibrosarcoma and malignant fibrous histiocytoma.[64]

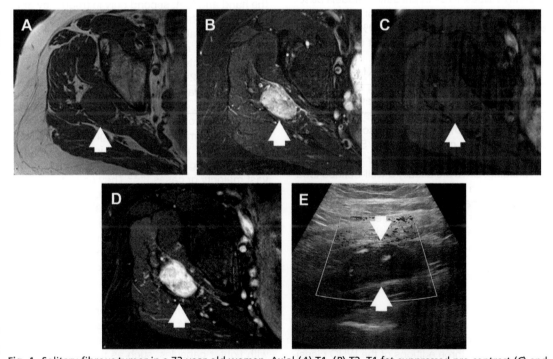

Fig. 4. Solitary fibrous tumor in a 73-year-old woman. Axial (A) T1, (B) T2, T1 fat-suppressed pre-contrast (C) and post-contrast (D) MR images show a T2 hyperintense, T1 isointense diffusely enhancing ovoid intramuscular mass interposed between the right gluteus medius and minimus muscles (*white arrows*). Sagittal ultrasound image (E) with power Doppler shows internal vascularity (*white arrows*). Histopathology showed characteristic appearances of a solitary fibrous tumor with well-demarcated hypercellular nodules, tumor cells showing overlapping and prominent cytologic atypia, and brisk mitotic activity.

Dermatofibrosarcoma Protuberans

Dermatofibrosarcoma protuberans is a low-grade malignant tumor arising from dermal and subcutaneous tissues. It is the most common cutaneous sarcoma. Dermatofibrosarcoma protuberans occur most commonly in the trunk and proximal extremities.[65] MR imaging usually shows T1 hypointense signal and T2 hyperintense signal, often higher than the adjacent subcutaneous fat, which can be misdiagnosed as a cyst in the absence of contrast (see **Fig. 3**). US usually shows a round or ovoid vascularized mass in the subcutaneous region, with well-defined margins, mildly lobulated border, and heterogeneously hypoechoic matrix.

Solitary Fibrous Tumor

Solitary fibrous tumor (SFT) is a fibroblastic tumor characterized by NAB2-STAT6 gene rearrangement. It can occur in any anatomic location, including extremities and deep soft-tissues. Unlike other soft-tissue tumors, it is difficult to predict the biologic behavior of SFT only based on the conventional grading and cancer staging systems.[66] The 2020 WHO classification introduced locally aggressive and malignant varieties of SFT. Recently validated risk stratification models based on age, tumor size in increments of 5 cm, mitotic activity score, and necrosis >10% have been included to help delineate those at higher risk for aggressive behavior.[67]

With variable and nonspecific US features, SFTs may be predominantly hypoechoic, although both benign and malignant lesions can also be heterogeneous owing to intralesional cystic or myxoid degeneration.[68] Owing to low vascular flow, the staghorn vessels characteristic of SFTs may not be that apparent on color Doppler images.[69] On MR imaging, SFTs are usually a well-defined lobulated mass with heterogeneous contrast enhancement and variable T2 signal corresponding to fibrous, cellular, and myxoid areas (see **Fig. 4**). There may be feeding vessels and foci of calcification. Diffuse nuclear expression of STAT6 and diffuse CD34 expression are diagnostic on immunohistochemistry.

FIBROHISTIOCYTIC TUMORS

The fibrohistiocytic group lost several entities through the last three editions of the WHO classification. The "fibrohistiocytic" designation does not necessarily denote lineage differentiation, as in most cases, the histiocytic component is actually non-neoplastic. However, the histiocytic component contributes substantially to the development of the lesion, as in the giant cell tumor.[70]

The most well-known entity formerly belonging to this subcategory was the family of malignant fibrous histiocytoma (MFH), which was removed in 2013. This accounted for approximately 50% of sarcoma diagnoses until early 2000.[71] Undifferentiated pleomorphic sarcoma (UPS) is now the terminology used for the prototypical storiform and pleomorphic variant of MFH.[70]

This fibrohistiocytic tumor category now also includes benign or malignant tenosynovial giant cell tumor (TSGCT), deep benign fibrous histiocytoma, plexiform fibrohistiocytic tumor, and giant cell tumor of soft-tissue. TSGCT is a benign tumor in this group that can occur in either a localized or diffuse form. The localized form typically presents as a well-defined encapsulated nodular or polypoid mass around the tendons, most commonly in the wrist and hand (**Fig. 5**). The diffuse form of TSGCT is rare and usually occurs adjacent to large weight-bearing joints.[72] The intraarticular tumor counterpart of the TSGCT is pigmented villonodular synovitis (PVNS), with an identical histologic appearance to its extraarticular counterpart.

TSGCT is one of the most common STMs of the hand and feet, second only in frequency after ganglion.[73] They are typically adjacent to an interphalangeal joint, manifesting as a small, slow-growing mass. On MR imaging, they are typically isointense or hypointense to muscle on T1-and T2-weighted MR images owing to abundant collagen and hemosiderin, often with enhancement. Some may not contain enough hemosiderin to be T1 and T2 hypointense or to cause a blooming artifact on gradient-echo images. TSGCT typically shows intense enhancement following gadolinium administration in the vast majority of cases.[74,75] They can cause pressure erosions of the adjacent bone in approximately 15% of cases.[76] TSGCT has a variable appearance on US and has been described as homogenously or heterogeneously hypoechoic to hyperechoic.[77] On Doppler, these tumors typically show hypervascularity. Posterior acoustic enhancement is present in about 33% of cases.[78]

PVNS most commonly involves the large joints, with almost 75% to 80% of cases involving the knee. Bone erosions are more common in joints with tighter capsules, such as the hip and shoulder.[79] The joint space is usually preserved, as is bone mineralization.[79] It usually presents as a heterogeneous synovial-based mass that may extend along the synovial surface. On T1 and T2-weighted MR images, the overall signal intensity of the mass

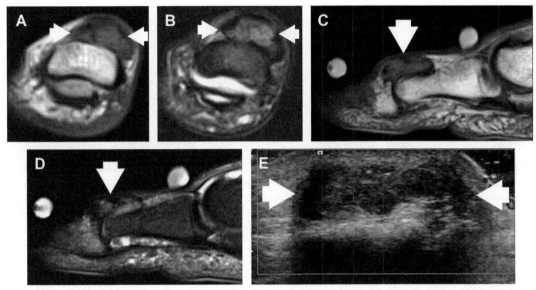

Fig. 5. Tenosynovial giant cell tumor in a 42-year-old woman. Axial (*A*) T1 and (*B*) fat-suppressed T2, sagittal (*C*) T1, and (*D*) fat-suppressed T2 MR images show a circumscribed mass (*white arrows*) at the dorsal medial aspect of the first interphalangeal joint, which shows intermediate-to-low T1 signal and intermediate to high T2 signal with a hypointense rim. The mass contacts the medial aspect of the extensor hallucis longus. (*E*) Transverse US image with power Doppler demonstrating heterogeneously hypoechoic mass (*white arrows*) with minimal vascularity over the dorsal aspect of the first interphalangeal joint. The mass was excised. Histopathology confirmed a tenosynovial giant cell tumor.

is similar to or less than skeletal muscle, although scattered areas of high T2 signal may be present. Decreased T2 signal intensity suggests hemosiderin contents.[80,81]

VASCULAR TUMORS

Vascular tumors arise from the proliferation of endothelial cells, with lesions exhibiting a spectrum of clinical behavior. The spectrum includes benign lesions such as hemangiomas (**Fig. 6**); kaposiform (**Fig. 7**) and other hemangioendotheliomas, and Kaposi sarcoma in the intermediate category; and angiosarcoma and epithelioid hemangioendothelioma in the malignant group.

Hemangiomas

Hemangiomas comprise 7% of all benign tumors and are the most common tumor in infancy and childhood.[82] In addition to vessels, hemangiomas can contain fat, smooth muscle, hemosiderin, and phleboliths. Congenital hemangiomas are present at birth and are classified based on their behaviors as rapidly involuting, non-involuting, or partially involuting.

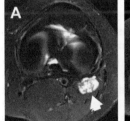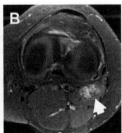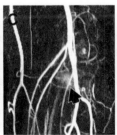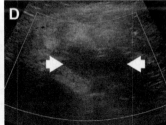

Fig. 6. Intramuscular hemangioma in a 33-year-old woman. Axial (*A*) fat-suppressed T2 and (*B*) fat-suppressed T1 post-contrast MR images show a T2 hyperintense heterogeneously enhancing mass (*white arrows*) along the posterolateral knee joint capsule. Coronal (*C*) MR angiogram performed concurrently shows a slow flow vascular malformation with minimal internal vascularity (*white arrow*), which was not clearly apparent on Doppler ultrasound (*white arrows* in D). The mass was excised. Histopathology confirmed an intramuscular hemangioma with metaplasia at the tissue edges.

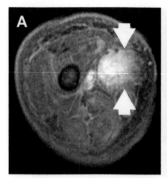 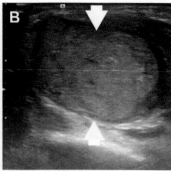 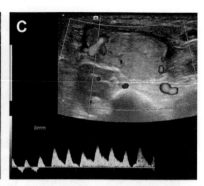

Fig. 7. Kaposiform hemangioendothelioma in a 16-month-old girl. (*A*) Axial fat-suppressed T1 post-contrast MR image demonstrating a homogeneously enhancing mass (*white arrows*) within the medial soft-tissues of the right thigh. Corresponding transverse gray-scale ultrasound image (*B*) demonstrating a mass centered in the deep distal thigh (*white arrows*). Spectral Doppler waveform analysis (*C*) reveals a low-resistance arterial waveform pattern within the lesion. Surgical excision showed a kaposiform hemangioendothelioma.

Imaging is generally indicated for large or deep-seated masses. These appear as solid lobulated lesions with intense vascularity. The presence of phleboliths, which are focal dystrophic mineralization in a thrombus, can aid characterization. Periosteal reaction, cortical and medullary remodeling, and overgrowth can occur reactively.

US typically reveals a complex heterogenous mass, and acoustic shadowing may be seen in the presence of phleboliths.[83] Doppler may show no abnormality, although low resistance arterial pattern with forward flow during both systole and diastole indicative of abnormal low vascular resistance can be present.[84,85] Compared with the infantile variant, congenital hemangiomas more often show inhomogeneous echogenicity with relatively large intralesional vessels, visible on gray-scale sonographic imaging. During the proliferative phase, infantile hemangiomas usually appear as a well-defined mass in the subcutaneous tissue, showing variable echogenicity and increased Doppler signal indicating internal vascularity.

Hemangiomas may be well-circumscribed or have poorly defined margins, with varying amounts of hyperintense T1 signal owing to either reactive fat overgrowth or hemorrhage. Areas of slow flow typically have high T2 signal, whereas rapid flow can show signal voids on images obtained with a non–flow-sensitive sequence. Axial T2, post-contrast T1, and time-resolved MR angiography images show T2 hyperintense infiltrative mass with multiple flow voids within, showing heterogeneous enhancement (see **Fig. 6**). There are areas of high T2 signal within hemangiomas often with characteristic appearance including circular representing vessels seen en face or cavernous spaces and linear or serpentine from vessels seen longitudinally.[86] These serpentine vascular

channels and fat overgrowth can be identified in almost 90% of hemangiomas and are pathognomonic.[87]

Intermediate and Malignant Vascular Tumors

Kaposiform hemangioendotheliomas are intermediate locally-aggressive tumors that commonly affect the deep soft-tissues in children (**Fig. 8**). They are composed of a lobular proliferation of capillaries with endothelial spindle cells and lymphatic vessels. Kaposiform hemangioendotheliomas occur in various locations, mostly affect infants, and exhibit intense heterogeneous enhancement. More than half of the cases show highly infiltrative and locally invasive with ill-defined margins.[88]

Hemangioendothelioma arises from vascular endothelial cells and has intermediate aggressiveness between that of hemangioma and angiosarcoma.[87] This neoplasm has different subtypes. Epithelioid hemangioendothelioma is a rare, low-grade malignant vascular endothelial neoplasm that, despite the label implying its intermediate behavior, has an overall metastatic rate of approximately 15%.[70] Angiosarcomas are malignant vascular neoplasms that usually originate in deep soft tissues.[51] Chronic lymphedema predisposes to angiosarcoma and can be present in approximately 10% of cases.[51] In contrast to hemangioma, the aggressive counterparts do not have fat overgrowth and are not solely composed of vascular channels or spaces.[87] These lesions usually have nonspecific imaging appearances, being hypoechoic or hyperechoic on US and showing nonspecific MR imaging appearances with intermediate intensity on T1-weighted and intermediate-to-high signal on T2-weighted MR images.

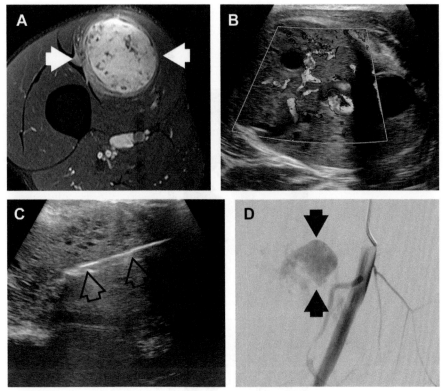

Fig. 8. Low-grade vascular and spindle cell neoplasm in a 29-year-old man. (*A*) Axial T2 image showed a hyperintense intramuscular mass (*white arrows*) within the anterior thigh. (*B*) Transverse pre-procedure color Doppler ultrasound image shows a circumscribed ovoid heterogeneously hyperechoic mass with tubular serpentine anechoic portions compatible with vascular channels and marked vascular flow. (*C*) A relatively nonvascular mass region was targeted for biopsy (needle, hollow *black arrows*). The sampled tissue consists of prominent thin-walled vascular proliferation with marked bland-looking fibrous stroma, which is collagenized. Immunohistochemistry was positive for ERG and CD34 highlighting vessels. Preoperative angiography (*D*) was performed via catheterization of the right superficial femoral artery. Subtraction image confirming a hypervascular mass (*black arrows* in D), which was preoperatively embolized before surgical removal.

On a practical level, US can identify hypervascular lesions with arterial (high-flow feeding vessels), which can be useful for the surgeon before surgical excision. This can allow for preoperative angiography with embolization, thereby reducing intraoperative bleeding (**Fig.8**).

PERICYTIC AND PERIVASCULAR TUMORS

These lesions share a distinctive perivascular growth pattern, with a cell shape resembling pericytes, that is, contractile smooth muscle cells around vessels.[70] This category includes glomus tumor, myopericytoma including myofibroma and angioleiomyoma. Tumors in this group are mostly benign with rare malignant variants such as malignant glomus tumor. Diffuse variants such as glomangiomatosis and myofibromatosis can be associated with significant local morbidity.[70]

The normal glomus body regulates heat and represents a specialized form of arteriovenous anastomosis. Glomus tumors are composed of cells resembling the modified smooth muscle of normal glomus body. The majority of glomus tumors occur in the nailbed of distal extremities (**Fig. 9**).[4,89] Malignant glomus tumors typically occur in deep soft tissues. Most have NOTCH gene rearrangements, BRAF V600 E mutations, or both.[4] On US, a small hypoechoic subungual mass can show a prominent Doppler vascularity signal. MR imaging usually shows a small T2 hyperintense unencapsulated tumor in the nailbed with intense post-contrast enhancement. Extrinsic bone erosion of the underlying bone can be present in 22% to 60% of cases.[90]

Angioleiomyomas are benign tumors composed of well-differentiated perivascular smooth muscle cells and a conglomerate of thick-walled vessels. They are typically small (<2 cm) and located in

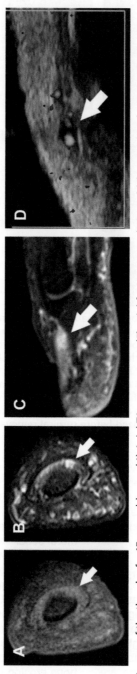

Fig. 9. Glomus tumor of the thumb of a 45-year-old man. (A) Axial T1 pre-contrast, (B) axial fat-suppressed T2, and (C) sagittal T1 fat-suppressed post-contrast MR images show a focal T2 hyperintense nodular mass (white arrows) along the radial aspect of the nail bed. (D) Corresponding longitudinal power Doppler ultrasond image shows a small hypoechoic nodule (white arrow) with internal vascularity (D).

the subcutaneous tissue of extremities. US typically shows a solid, ovoid, well-defined, and relatively homogeneous hypoechoic mass.[91] Doppler shows prominent hypervascularity, which can be associated with feeding vessels. MR imaging shows a well-defined, round to oval, subcutaneous, or dermal mass with a similar to or slightly hyperintense T1 and hyperintense T2 signal to that of skeletal muscle. A low-signal fibrous pseudocapsule has been described.[92]

SMOOTH MUSCLE TUMORS

This group includes leiomyoma and leiomyosarcoma. Smooth muscle is widely distributed throughout the body, though leiomyomas rarely occur outside the uterus and gastrointestinal tract.[93,94] On MR imaging, leiomyomas usually show a hypointense T2 signal due to densely packed cellular architecture.[5] On the other hand, Leiomyosarcomas are generally large heterogeneous masses most commonly seen in the retroperitoneum.

A new entity was added to the recent WHO classification called smooth muscle tumor of uncertain differentiation (STUMP). STUMP is considered an EBV infection-associated smooth muscle neoplasm with uncertain malignant behavior, usually occurring in patients with immunodeficiency.[4]

SKELETAL MUSCLE TUMORS

Rhabdomyomas are benign neoplasms of skeletal muscle differentiation which can be divided into cardiac and extracardiac types. Rhabdomyosarcoma is the malignant counterpart which is the most common soft-tissue sarcoma in children with a mean age of 5 years, presenting as an aggressive STM. It has four major histologic subtypes: embryonal, alveolar, pleomorphic and spindle cell/sclerosing.

Embryonal represents the most common round-to-spindle cell subtype in children younger than 10 years. Alveolar accounts for 25% of cases with a peak incidence in 10 to 25 years (**Fig. 10**). Embryonal are usually more homogeneous, whereas alveolar and pleomorphic often show areas of necrosis, with pleomorphic showing ring-like enhancement.[5] Sonography shows a heterogeneous well-defined irregular mass with low to intermediate echogenicity.

PERIPHERAL NERVE SHEATH TUMORS

Peripheral nerve sheath tumors (PNST) are an exception because they arise from the ectoderm (neuroectoderm) as opposed to the other soft-tissue tumors and sarcomas that arise from mesenchymal/mesodermal cells. They are classified separately as neurogenic tumors in the WHO classification, comprising benign and malignant forms.

Neurofibroma and schwannoma (ie, neurilemomas) are the most common benign forms, accounting for 10% of benign soft-tissue tumors. These are fusiform ovoid encapsulated lesions often longitudinally associated with a nerve, demonstrating a myxoid appearance and 'target sign'. They can be difficult to distinguish radiologically; however, the schwannoma may be seen to be eccentric to and separable from the nerve, whereas the neurofibroma is intrinsic to the nerve. The "split fat sign" occurs due to a preserved surrounding rim of normal fat as the tumor enlarges (**Fig. 11**).

Benign PNSTs are typically T1 isointense to muscle and T2 hyperintense, but signal characteristics are not specific. The "target sign" is more common in neurofibromas than schwannomas and indicates a central area of low T2 signal corresponding to fibrocollagenous tissue and an outer area of high T2 signal of myxomatous tissue. Contrast enhancement in benign PNSTs is variable. Diffusion-weighted imaging is useful in the evaluation and preoperative planning by delineating healthy versus pathologic fascicles.[40,41] The Neuropathy Score Reporting and Data System (NS-RADS) may be included to standardize MR imaging reporting.[95]

On US, PNSTs are often hypoechoic with posterior acoustic enhancement. There may be a target appearance with hyperechoic center and hypoechoic periphery or a pseudocystic appearance.[96] Intrinsic blood flow on color Doppler and peripheral nerve continuity suggest the diagnosis (see **Fig. 11**).

Malignant PNSTs account for 2% to 10% of soft-tissue sarcomas and are associated with type 1 neurofibromatosis in up to 50% of cases. They can be difficult to differentiate from their benign counterparts; however, the malignant variants are typically larger with ill-defined margins, rapid growth, and central necrosis. They usually arise within the deep soft-tissues with a predilection for proximal extremities and paraspinal region. Conventional markers like S100 protein and SOX10 are only focally positive in up to 50% of cases, and loss of trimethylation of lysine 27 of histone H3 on immunohistochemistry is relatively specific for malignancy.[4]

TUMORS OF UNCERTAIN DIFFERENTIATION

In the new WHO classification, the "undifferentiated/unclassified tumors" category was removed

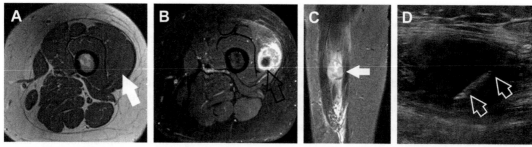

Fig. 10. Rhabdomyosarcoma in a 12-year-old girl. Axial T1 (*A*), contrast-enhanced fat-suppressed T1 (*B*), and sagittal STIR (*C*) MR images show an intramuscular left thigh mass in the left vastus lateralis muscle (*arrows*). The mass is T1 isointense to muscle with peripheral contrast enhancement and a central area without enhancement (hollow *black arrow* in B), suggesting an area of necrosis. There is abnormal perilesional enhancement in a fusiform fashion involving the muscle fibers of the vastus lateralis muscle (*C*). Longitudinal ultrasound-guided biopsy image (*D*) shows intralesional placement of the needle. Histopathological evaluation showed alveolar subtype solid variant rhabdomyosarcoma featuring sheets and nests of intermediate-sized, round to variably rhabdoid cells embedded in a fibromuscular stroma.

and merged into the "tumors of uncertain differentiation". Angiomyolipoma has been introduced in the benign group, epithelioid angiomyolipoma into the intermediate category, and NTRK rearranged spindle cell neoplasm is now categorized

within the malignant tumors. Several tumors in this category have characteristic imaging features and preferences for certain locations.

Myxomas appear as T2 bright intramuscular masses showing variable contrast enhancement

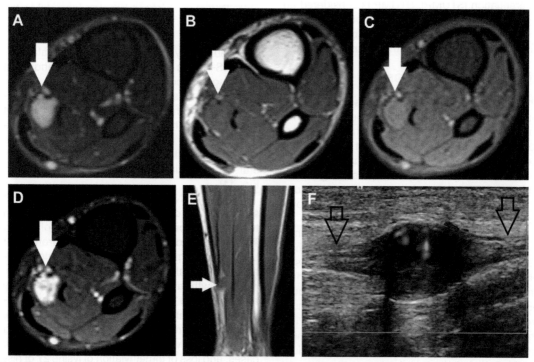

Fig. 11. Peripheral nerve sheath tumor in a 63-year-old man. Axial (*A*) fat-suppressed T2, (*B*) T1, fat-suppressed T1 pre-contrast (*C*), and fat-suppressed T1 post-contrast (*D*) MR images show a fusiform mass (*white arrows*) longitudinally associated with the tibial nerve. The lesion is T1 isointense to muscle, heterogeneously T2 hyperintense, and enhances avidly after the contrast administration. Coronal T1 MR image (*E*) demonstrating the "split fat sign" (*white arrow*). Sagittal ultrasound image with power Doppler (*F*) shows a hypoechoic, vascular fusiform mass in continuity with the posterior tibial nerve proximally and distally (hollow *black arrows*). The mass was excised. Histopathological examination showed a Schwannoma. Immunohistochemistry showed the mass to be S100 positive, Sox10 positive and Ki-67 variable (5%–15%).

(Fig. 12). Synovial sarcoma, often seen in older children and young adults, derives its name from the fact that it microscopically resembles synovium; however, it stains for epithelial markers such as epithelial membrane antigen and cytokeratin and is often found in many locations without synovium (Fig. 13). Undifferentiated pleomorphic sarcoma has no pathognomic features but presents as a heterogeneous mass in the extremities, usually in elderly patients.

UPS usually presents as a rounded or ovoid mass that heterogeneously enhances and contains areas of necrosis. As seen in the related myxofibrosarcoma, UPS may have an infiltrative border with tail-like extensions at imaging. These tumor extensions are believed to account for the high propensity to recur locally.[97] US often shows a well-defined oval shape mildly heterogeneous hypoechoic mass with mild internal vascularity on Doppler images.

COMMON TUMOR MIMICS AND MISCELLANEOUS MASSES

US and MR imaging can aid in differentiating common tumor mimics, particularly ganglia, hematoma, and myositis ossificans, from true neoplasms.

Ganglia

Ganglia commonly occur in the hands, wrists, feet, and ankles, frequently arising from joint capsules, bursae, ligaments, and tendons. Histopathologically, ganglion cysts are lined by a capsule composed of flat spindle cells and do not have a synovial lining. Ganglion cysts differ from synovial cysts, which are true synovial membrane herniations of joint capsules. Although ganglia are attached to the joint capsule in most cases, they are not always seen to communicate with the joint. Sometimes, it may be hard to distinguish a true ganglion from a degenerative periarticular cystic lesion.

On MR imaging and US, lesions typically appear as round or ovoid masses that are uni- or multiloculated, with smooth or slightly lobulated surfaces, often in close proximity to a joint or tendon. Ganglia may be associated with a track extending toward the joint and may have pericystic edema. US may show a circumscribed homogeneously anechoic cyst or more "complex" contents such as septations and internal soft-tissue echogenicity. They are usually T2 hyperintense and either isointense or slightly T1 hypointense to muscle, although a higher proteinaceous content may increase the T1 signal. A thin rim of contrast enhancement with thin low signal-enhancing septae may be seen.

Hematomas

The radiological appearance of hematomas varies with age. Acute hematomas less than a few days old are typically iso- or hypointense to muscle on T1-and T2-weighted MR imaging. Subacute hematomas are usually T1 hyperintense due to methemoglobin. Chronic hematomas are T1 and T2 hyperintense but can have a prominent hypointense rim representing a wall of collagenous fibrous tissue and hemosiderin.

Sonographically, hematomas may initially appear highly echogenic and semisolid as fibrin and erythrocytes form multiple acoustic interfaces. As the clot liquefies and the hematoma becomes increasingly anechoic, a network of fibrin strands and septations can be seen occasionally. Fluid levels may represent separations between anechoic serum and echogenic cellular components. An organizing hematoma may develop a well-defined capsule. As hematomas resolve, a fibrous scar may remain.[98] Persistent hematomas may calcify peripherally.

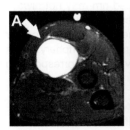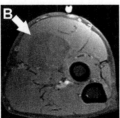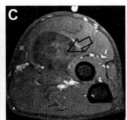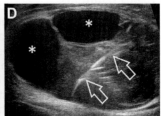

Fig. 12. Intramuscular myxoma in a 67-year-old man. Axial (A) T2, (B) fat-suppressed T1 pre-contrast, and (C) fat-suppressed T1 post-contrast MR images show a multilobular T2 hyperintense mass (arrows) centered in the proximal volar forearm between the brachioradialis, supinator and pronator teres muscles. The MR images show heterogeneously enhancing, ill-defined internal soft-tissue components (black hollow arrow in C). (D) Longitudinal ultrasound image demonstrating anechoic fluid components (*) and an echogenic component targeted for needle placement (white hollow arrows). The anechoic cystic component was also aspirated for cytology (not shown).

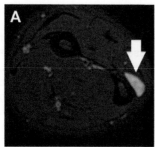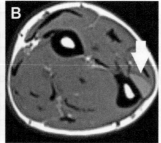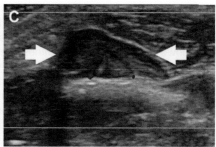

Fig. 13. Synovial sarcoma in a 14-year-old girl. Axial (*A*) fat-suppressed T2 and (*B*) T1 MR images show a well-circumscribed oval mass (*white arrows*) in the posteromedial mid-forearm. The mass shows heterogeneously increased T2 signal intensity, T1 signal intensity greater than muscle, and abuts the posterior cortex of the ulna. (*C*) Longitudinal ultrasound image with Doppler confirms the presence of internal vascularized soft-tissue (*white arrows*). Following a percutaneous biopsy, histopathological examination showed hypercellular spindle cells with a monotonous appearance and considerable cellular overlap with molecular fusion SEQer studies showing the presence of SS18-SSX2 fusion, characteristic of synovial sarcoma.

It is important to be vigilant for hematomas arising from underlying tumors. Therefore, any hematoma with nodular areas of soft-tissue enhancement should be followed to complete resolution to exclude an underlying lesion, especially in the absence of antecedent trauma. The differential diagnosis for internal enhancement includes enhancing fibrovascular tissue in an organizing hematoma.

Fat Necrosis

Trauma to the subcutaneous adipose tissue may cause initial swelling, edema, and hemorrhage that progresses to atrophy and fat necrosis, often with the development of a palpable mass. On US, fat necrosis appears as a poorly defined hyperechoic focus containing hypoechoic infarcted areas of fat or an isoechoic area with a hypoechoic halo. MR imaging tends to show a central globular high signal intensity with a variable low-signal rim and peripheral contrast enhancement. Other patterns such as amorphous, cloudlike stranding and a serpentine appearance may be encountered.[99]

Myositis Ossificans

Myositis ossificans is a benign ossifying STM occurring in muscle, most often after known or unknown trauma of varying intensity. MR imaging and US appearances depend on the stage of evolution. Ossification is rarely seen on radiographs in the first few weeks of the immature inflammatory phase. The mature phase is characterized by a centripetal ossification pattern, starting peripherally and progressing centrally in a zonal pattern. The ossification evolves from faint irregular flocular densities to dense calcifications and, ultimately, to a rim of mature lamellar bone and central osteoid matrix.

The MR appearances vary based on histologic states. Early lesions are poorly defined and isointense on T1-weighted images, heterogeneously T2 hyperintense, and have diffuse surrounding soft-tissue edema. Sonographically, a well-defined ovoid intramuscular hypoechoic mass is usually seen with circumscribed borders.[100]

Early-stage myositis ossificans without mineralization can enhance and be mistaken for a neoplastic mass (**Fig. 14**). On US, central decreased echogenicity is associated with an outer lamellar hyperechoic ill-defined rim often without a clear zonal demarcation and no calcification. Internal low signal regions may not be recognized as calcification or ossification, so it is important to consider myositis ossificans in the differential diagnosis and to assess for the characteristic zonal pattern of mineralization on radiographs or CT. In the immature state, serial radiographs or CT may be necessary to document the beginning of ossification.

With maturation, internal vascularity diminishes, and a hyperechoic rim develops with rim ossification causing posterior acoustic shadowing. However, the superficial calcified rim may not always completely obscure the deep boundary. This contrasts with sarcomas, where the necrotic center typically calcifies first but not the periphery.[101] As peripheral calcification develops, a corresponding low signal becomes evident.

RADIOLOGICAL APPROACH FOR SOFT-TISSUE MASS EVALUATION USING ULTRASOUND AND MR IMAGING

A proposed combined approach for the characterization of masses is presented in **Fig. 15**. Some descriptors are common to both modalities, including margin definition, presence of

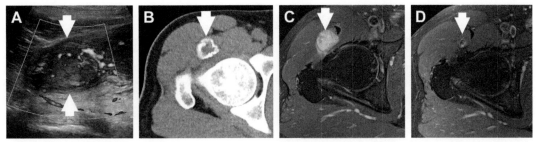

Fig. 14. Myositis Ossificans in a 37-year-old man with a history of trauma. (*A*) Transverse ultrasound image with power Doppler shows a heterogeneous hypervascular intramuscular mass (*white arrows*) centered within the proximal right rectus femoris. Subsequent axial CT image (*B*) confirms the characteristic appearance with peripheral ossification (*white arrow*). (*C*) Axial post-contrast T1 image demonstrating marked enhancement of the mass (*white arrow*), with near-complete resolution (*white arrow*) 4 months later (*D*).

necrosis, perilesional edema, involvement of osseous or neurovascular structures, and compartmental localization. Certain masses show internal heterogeneity with necrosis, calcification, and macroscopic fat, which can be identified with both modalities. Internal vascularity can be ascertained with contrast enhancement on MR imaging or Doppler US and should be described. Internal homogeneity or heterogeneity is described with echogenicity and echotexture on US and T1 and T2 signal intensities on MR imaging (**Fig. 16**).

A systematic approach for evaluating STMs is recommended to aid diagnosis where this is a characteristic appearance and narrow the differential diagnosis where there are indeterminate characteristics.[1] An approach using signal, location, age, multiplicity, and matrix has been proposed.[102] US can be incorporated into these paradigms to aid diagnosis.

FUTURE DIRECTIONS
Shear Wave Elastography

Shear wave elastography uses external compression to determine tissue strain and lesion stiffness.[103,104] The soft-tissues are transiently deformed using acoustic radiation to measure dynamic displacement and estimate mechanical properties. Quantitative and qualitative shear

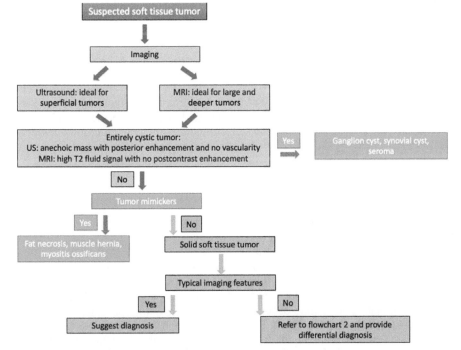

Fig. 15. Combined approach for using US and MR imaging to evaluate soft-tissue masses.

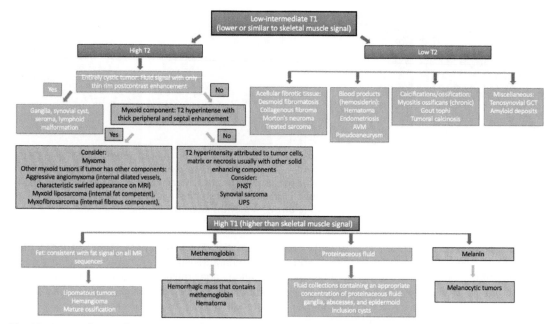

Fig. 16. Approach to soft-tissue masses based on T1 and T2 MR imaging signal characteristics.

wave elastography has been evaluated for the characterization of masses, although its role has yet to be established.[9,10,105] There may be a potential role for mass characterization alongside other US techniques, such as B and Doppler modes, and in conjunction with MR imaging.

Artificial Intelligence

There is interest in how deep learning can be incorporated to augment the sonographic work-up of masses.[95] Early work has suggested that convolutional neural network models can be trained to classify benign and malignant STMs with US and to differentiate commonly observed benign masses, specifically lipomas, benign PNSTs, and vascular malformations. A trained convolutional neural network was capable of differentiating between benign and malignant STMs depicted on US images, with performance matching that of experienced musculoskeletal radiologists.[106,107]

Radiomics

"Radiomics" uses complex pattern recognition tools for high-throughput extraction of quantitative features, resulting in the conversion of images into data mines that can be used for decision support.[108] Radiomics may evaluate tumor characteristics such as genetic, molecular, cellular and histologic data, extrapolating to a macroscopic scale.[109] Early work has suggested that radiomics may predict malignancy in soft-tissue lipomatous tumors on routine MR images.[110]

Ultrasound-MR imaging Fusion

Previously acquired MR images can be fused with US in real-time, which can be used for diagnostic and therapeutic purposes. Ultrasound-MR imaging fusion has shown particular potential for the biopsy of lesions that may be poorly delineated on US images alone, with added accuracy afforded by real-time registration.[111]

SUMMARY

STMs are commonly encountered in clinical practice with a wide range of benign and malignant etiologies. US and MR imaging have evolved to play an important complementary role in the identification and evaluation of these masses as well as in planning percutaneous biopsy, surgical excision, and surveillance. Radiologists should be familiar with the updated WHO classification for STMs and the features pertaining to the various categories.

CLINICS CARE POINTS

- When evaluating soft-tissue masses for the presence of internal vascularization, targeted ultrasound can be used as an adjunct to non-contrast MR imaging, avoiding intravenous contrast administration.

- Where T2 signal hyperintense lesions are identified on MR imaging, focused ultrasound can confirm the cystic nature of the internal contents.

- Ultrasonography should be considered for characterization of superficial soft-tissue masses due to its high axial and spatial resolution, allowing evaluation of tissue echotexture, lesion margins, and vascularity.

- MR imaging provides excellent anatomic detail of deeper soft-tissue masses with respect to compartmental location, soft-tissue contrast, neurovascular involvement, and resolution of deep structures.

DISCLOSURE

The authors have no disclosures.

REFERENCES

1. Wu JS, Hochman MG. Soft-tissue tumors and tumorlike lesions: a systematic imaging approach. Radiology 2009;253(2):297–316.
2. Porrino J, Al-Dasuqi K, Irshaid L, et al. Update of pediatric soft-tissue tumors with review of conventional MRI appearance-part 1: tumor-like lesions, adipocytic tumors, fibroblastic and myofibroblastic tumors, and perivascular tumors. Skeletal Radiol 2022;51(3):477–504.
3. Siegel RL, Miller KD, Jemal A. Cancer statistics, 2018. CA Cancer J Clin 2018;68(1):7–30.
4. Bansal A, Goyal S, Goyal A, et al. WHO classification of soft-tissue tumours 2020: An update and simplified approach for radiologists. Eur J Radiol 2021;143:109937.
5. Walter SS, Fritz J. MRI of Muscular Neoplasms and Tumor-like Lesions: A 2020 World Health Organization Classification-based Systematic Review. Semin Roentgenol 2022;57(3):252–74.
6. Lakkaraju A, Sinha R, Garikipati R, et al. Ultrasound for initial evaluation and triage of clinically suspicious soft-tissue masses. Clin Radiol 2009;64(6): 615–21.
7. Goldman LH, Perronne L, Alaia EF, et al. Does Magnetic Resonance Imaging After Diagnostic Ultrasound for Soft-tissue Masses Change Clinical Management? J Ultrasound Med 2021;40(8): 1515–22.
8. Nagano S, Yahiro Y, Yokouchi M, et al. Doppler ultrasound for diagnosis of soft-tissue sarcoma: efficacy of ultrasound-based screening score. Radiol Oncol 2015;49(2):135–40.
9. Tavare AN, Alfuraih AM, Hensor EMA, et al. Shear-Wave Elastography of Benign versus Malignant Musculoskeletal Soft-Tissue Masses: Comparison with Conventional US and MRI. Radiology 2019; 290(2):410–7.
10. Winn N, Baldwin J, Cassar-Pullicino V, et al. Characterization of soft-tissue tumours with ultrasound, shear wave elastography and MRI. Skeletal Radiol 2020;49(6):869–81.
11. DiDomenico P, Middleton W. Sonographic evaluation of palpable superficial masses. Radiol Clin North Am 2014;52(6):1295–305.
12. Khodarahmi I, Fritz J. The Value of 3 Tesla Field Strength for Musculoskeletal Magnetic Resonance Imaging. Invest Radiol 2021;56(11):749–63.
13. Ahlawat S, Fritz J, Morris CD, et al. Magnetic resonance imaging biomarkers in musculoskeletal soft-tissue tumors: Review of conventional features and focus on nonmorphologic imaging. J Magn Reson Imaging 2019;50(1):11–27.
14. Del Grande F, Rashidi A, Luna R, et al. Five-Minute Five-Sequence Knee MRI Using Combined Simultaneous Multislice and Parallel Imaging Acceleration: Comparison with 10-Minute Parallel Imaging Knee MRI. Radiology 2021;299(3): 635–46.
15. Del Grande F, Guggenberger R, Fritz J. Rapid Musculoskeletal MRI in 2021: Value and Optimized Use of Widely Accessible Techniques. AJR Am J Roentgenol 2021;216(3):704–17.
16. Khodarahmi I, Rajan S, Sterling R, et al. Heating of Hip Arthroplasty Implants During Metal Artifact Reduction MRI at 1.5- and 3.0-T Field Strengths. Invest Radiol 2021;56(4):232–43.
17. Fritz J, Ahlawat S, Fritz B, et al. 10-Min 3D Turbo Spin Echo MRI of the Knee in Children: Arthroscopy-Validated Accuracy for the Diagnosis of Internal Derangement. J Magn Reson Imaging 2019;49(7):e139–51.
18. Fritz J, Fritz B, Zhang J, et al. Simultaneous Multislice Accelerated Turbo Spin Echo Magnetic Resonance Imaging: Comparison and Combination With In-Plane Parallel Imaging Acceleration for High-Resolution Magnetic Resonance Imaging of the Knee. Invest Radiol 2017;52(9):529–37.
19. Fritz J, Guggenberger R, Del Grande F. Rapid Musculoskeletal MRI in 2021: Clinical Application of Advanced Accelerated Techniques. AJR Am J Roentgenol 2021;216(3):718–33.
20. Lin D, Fritz J. AI-Driven Ultra-Fast Super-Resolution MRI: 10-Fold-Accelerated Musculoskeletal Turbo Spin Echo MRI Within Reach. Invest Radiol 2022. https://doi.org/10.1097/RLI.0000000000000928.
21. de Castro Luna R, Kumar NM, Fritz J, et al. MRI evaluation of soft-tissue tumors: comparison of a fast, isotropic, 3D T2-weighted fat-saturated sequence with a conventional 2D T2-weighted fat-saturated sequence for tumor characteristics, resolution, and acquisition time. Eur Radiol 2022. https://doi.org/10.1007/s00330-022-08937-7.

22. Luna R, Fritz J, Del Grande F, et al. Determination of skeletal tumor extent: is an isotropic T1-weighted 3D sequence adequate? Eur Radiol 2021;31(5):3138–46.

23. Dalili D, Isaac A, Rashidi A, et al. Image-guided Sports Medicine and Musculoskeletal Tumor Interventions: A Patient-Centered Model. Semin Musculoskelet Radiol 2020;24(3):290–309.

24. Del Grande F, Delcogliano M, Guglielmi R, et al. Fully Automated 10-Minute 3D CAIPIRINHA SPACE TSE MRI of the Knee in Adults: A Multicenter, Multireader, Multifield-Strength Validation Study. Invest Radiol 2018;53(11):689–97.

25. Fritz J, Fritz B, Thawait GG, et al. Three-Dimensional CAIPIRINHA SPACE TSE for 5-Minute High-Resolution MRI of the Knee. Invest Radiol 2016; 51(10):609–17.

26. Fritz J, Raithel E, Thawait GK, et al. Six-Fold Acceleration of High-Spatial Resolution 3D SPACE MRI of the Knee Through Incoherent k-Space Undersampling and Iterative Reconstruction-First Experience. Invest Radiol 2016;51(6):400–9.

27. Samim M, Khodarahmi I, Burke C, et al. Postoperative Musculoskeletal Imaging and Interventions Following Hip Preservation Surgery, Deformity Correction, and Hip Arthroplasty. Semin Musculoskelet Radiol 2022;26(3):242–57.

28. Ahlawat S, Stern SE, Belzberg AJ, et al. High-resolution metal artifact reduction MR imaging of the lumbosacral plexus in patients with metallic implants. Skeletal Radiol 2017;46(7):897–908.

29. Fritz J, Ahlawat S, Demehri S, et al. Compressed Sensing SEMAC: 8-fold Accelerated High Resolution Metal Artifact Reduction MRI of Cobalt-Chromium Knee Arthroplasty Implants. Invest Radiol 2016;51(10):666–76.

30. Fritz J, Fishman EK, Corl F, et al. Imaging of limb salvage surgery. AJR Am J Roentgenol 2012; 198(3):647–60.

31. Fritz J, Fritz B, Thawait GK, et al. Advanced metal artifact reduction MRI of metal-on-metal hip resurfacing arthroplasty implants: compressed sensing acceleration enables the time-neutral use of SEMAC. Skeletal Radiol 2016;45(10):1345–56.

32. Fritz J, Lurie B, Miller TT. Imaging of hip arthroplasty. Semin Musculoskelet Radiol 2013;17(3): 316–27.

33. Fritz J, Lurie B, Miller TT, et al. MR imaging of hip arthroplasty implants. Radiographics 2014;34(4): E106–32.

34. Fritz J, Lurie B, Potter HG. MR Imaging of Knee Arthroplasty Implants. Radiographics 2015;35(5): 1483–501.

35. Khodarahmi I, Isaac A, Fishman EK, et al. Metal About the Hip and Artifact Reduction Techniques: From Basic Concepts to Advanced Imaging. Semin Musculoskelet Radiol 2019;23(3):e68–81.

36. Fayad LM, Parekh VS, de Castro Luna R, et al. A Deep Learning System for Synthetic Knee Magnetic Resonance Imaging: Is Artificial Intelligence-Based Fat-Suppressed Imaging Feasible? Invest Radiol 2021;56(6):357–68.

37. Kumar NM, Fritz B, Stern SE, et al. Synthetic MRI of the Knee: Phantom Validation and Comparison with Conventional MRI. Radiology 2018;289(2):465–77.

38. Fritz J. T2 Mapping without Additional Scan Time Using Synthetic Knee MRI. Radiology 2019; 293(3):631–2.

39. Eck BL, Yang M, Elia J, et al. Quantitative MRI for Evaluation of Musculoskeletal Disease: Imaging Cartilage and Muscle Composition, Joint Inflammation and Biomechanics in Osteoarthritis. Invest Radiol 2022. https://doi.org/10.1097/RLI.0000000000000909.

40. Mazal AT, Ashikyan O, Cheng J, et al. Diffusion-weighted imaging and diffusion tensor imaging as adjuncts to conventional MRI for the diagnosis and management of peripheral nerve sheath tumors: current perspectives and future directions. Eur Radiol 2019;29(8):4123–32.

41. Yun JS, Lee MH, Lee SM, et al. Peripheral nerve sheath tumor: differentiation of malignant from benign tumors with conventional and diffusion-weighted MRI. Eur Radiol 2021;31(3):1548–57.

42. Chhabra A, Ashikyan O, Slepicka C, et al. Conventional MR and diffusion-weighted imaging of musculoskeletal soft-tissue malignancy: correlation with histologic grading. Eur Radiol 2019;29(8):4485–94.

43. Soldatos T, Ahlawat S, Montgomery E, et al. Multiparametric Assessment of Treatment Response in High-Grade Soft-Tissue Sarcomas with Anatomic and Functional MR Imaging Sequences. Radiology 2016;278(3):831–40.

44. Costa FM, Martins PH, Canella C, et al. Multiparametric MR Imaging of Soft-tissue Tumors and Pseudotumors. Magn Reson Imaging Clin N Am 2018; 26(4):543–58.

45. Choi JH, Ro JY. The 2020 WHO Classification of Tumors of Soft-tissue: Selected Changes and New Entities. Adv Anat Pathol 2021;28(1):44–58.

46. Gaskin CM, Helms CA. Lipomas, lipoma variants, and well-differentiated liposarcomas (atypical lipomas): results of MRI evaluations of 126 consecutive fatty masses. AJR Am J Roentgenol 2004; 182(3):733–9.

47. Nardo L, Abdelhafez YG, Acquafredda F, et al. Qualitative evaluation of MRI features of lipoma and atypical lipomatous tumor: results from a multicenter study. Skeletal Radiol 2020;49(6):1005–14.

48. Gupta P, Potti TA, Wuertzer SD, et al. Spectrum of Fat-containing Soft-Tissue Masses at MR Imaging: The Common, the Uncommon, the Characteristic, and the Sometimes Confusing. Radiographics 2016;36(3):753–66.

49. Kransdorf MJ, Bancroft LW, Peterson JJ, et al. Imaging of fatty tumors: distinction of lipoma and well-differentiated liposarcoma. Radiology 2002; 224(1):99–104.

50. Burt AM, Huang BK. Imaging review of lipomatous musculoskeletal lesions. Sicot j 2017;3:34.

51. Goldblum JR, Folpe AL, Weiss SW. Enzinger & Weiss's soft-tissue tumors. Seventh edition. Philadelphia, PA: Elsevier; 2020.

52. Rahmani G, McCarthy P, Bergin D. The diagnostic accuracy of ultrasonography for soft-tissue lipomas: a systematic review. Acta Radiol Open 2017;6(6). 2058460117716704.

53. Van Treeck BJ, Fritchie KJ. Updates in spindle cell/pleomorphic lipomas. Semin Diagn Pathol 2019; 36(2):105–11.

54. Kransdorf MJ. Malignant soft-tissue tumors in a large referral population: distribution of diagnoses by age, sex, and location. AJR Am J Roentgenol 1995;164(1):129–34.

55. Brisson M, Kashima T, Delaney D, et al. MRI characteristics of lipoma and atypical lipomatous tumor/well-differentiated liposarcoma: retrospective comparison with histology and MDM2 gene amplification. Skeletal Radiol 2013;42(5):635–47.

56. Rosa F, Martinetti C, Piscopo F, et al. Multimodality imaging features of desmoid tumors: a head-to-toe spectrum. Insights Imaging 2020;11(1):103.

57. Dahn I, Jonsson N, Lundh G. DESMOID TUMOURS. A SERIES OF 33 CASES. Acta Chir Scand 1963;126:305–14.

58. Musgrove JE, Mc DJ. Extra-abdominal desmoid tumors; their differential diagnosis and treatment. Arch Pathol (Chic) 1948;45(4):513–40.

59. Murphey MD, Ruble CM, Tyszko SM, et al. From the archives of the AFIP: musculoskeletal fibromatoses: radiologic-pathologic correlation. Radiographics 2009;29(7):2143–73.

60. Vandevenne JE, De Schepper AM, De Beuckeleer L, et al. New concepts in understanding evolution of desmoid tumors: MR imaging of 30 lesions. Eur Radiol 1997;7(7):1013–9.

61. Kransdorf MJ, Murphey MD. Soft-tissue tumors: post-treatment imaging. Radiol Clin North Am 2006;44(3):463–72.

62. Walker EA, Petscavage JM, Brian PL, et al. Imaging features of superficial and deep fibromatoses in the adult population. Sarcoma 2012;2012:215810.

63. Romero JA, Kim EE, Kim CG, et al. Different biologic features of desmoid tumors in adult and juvenile patients: MR demonstration. J Comput Assist Tomogr 1995;19(5):782–7.

64. Kirchgesner T, Tamigneaux C, Acid S, et al. Fasciae of the musculoskeletal system: MRI findings in trauma, infection and neoplastic diseases. Insights into Imaging 2019;10(1):47.

65. Kransdorf MJ, Meis-Kindblom JM. Dermatofibrosarcoma protuberans: radiologic appearance. AJR Am J Roentgenol 1994;163(2):391–4.

66. Demicco EG, Wagner MJ, Maki RG, et al. Risk assessment in solitary fibrous tumors: validation and refinement of a risk stratification model. Mod Pathol 2017;30(10):1433–42.

67. Salas S, Resseguier N, Blay JY, et al. Prediction of local and metastatic recurrence in solitary fibrous tumor: construction of a risk calculator in a multicenter cohort from the French Sarcoma Group (FSG) database. Ann Oncol 2017;28(8): 1979–87.

68. Rosado-de-Christenson ML, Abbott GF, McAdams HP, et al. From the archives of the AFIP: Localized fibrous tumor of the pleura. Radiographics 2003;23(3):759–83.

69. Ginat DT, Bokhari A, Bhatt S, et al. Imaging features of solitary fibrous tumors. AJR Am J Roentgenol 2011;196(3):487–95.

70. Sbaraglia M, Bellan E, Dei Tos AP. The 2020 WHO Classification of Soft-tissue Tumours: news and perspectives. Pathologica 2021;113(2):70–84.

71. Weiss SW, Enzinger FM. Malignant fibrous histiocytoma: an analysis of 200 cases. Cancer 1978;41(6): 2250–66.

72. Ushijima M, Hashimoto H, Tsuneyoshi M, et al. Giant cell tumor of the tendon sheath (nodular tenosynovitis). A study of 207 cases to compare the large joint group with the common digit group. Cancer 1986;57(4):875–84.

73. Savage RC, Mustafa EB. Giant cell tumor of tendon sheath (localized nodular tenosynovitis). Ann Plast Surg 1984;13(3):205–10.

74. Kitagawa Y, Ito H, Amano Y, et al. MR imaging for preoperative diagnosis and assessment of local tumor extent on localized giant cell tumor of tendon sheath. Skeletal Radiol 2003;32(11):633–8.

75. Wang C, Song RR, Kuang PD, et al. Giant cell tumor of the tendon sheath: Magnetic resonance imaging findings in 38 patients. Oncol Lett 2017; 13(6):4459–62.

76. Karasick D, Karasick S. Giant cell tumor of tendon sheath: spectrum of radiologic findings. Skeletal Radiol 1992;21(4):219–24.

77. Wan JM, Magarelli N, Peh WC, et al. Imaging of giant cell tumour of the tendon sheath. Radiol Med 2010;115(1):141–51.

78. Middleton WD, Patel V, Teefey SA, et al. Giant cell tumors of the tendon sheath: analysis of sonographic findings. AJR Am J Roentgenol 2004; 183(2):337–9.

79. Dorwart RH, Genant HK, Johnston WH, et al. Pigmented villonodular synovitis of synovial joints: clinical, pathologic, and radiologic features. AJR Am J Roentgenol 1984;143(4):877–85.

80. Murphey MD, Rhee JH, Lewis RB, et al. Pigmented villonodular synovitis: radiologic-pathologic correlation. Radiographics 2008;28(5):1493–518.

81. Al-Nakshabandi NA, Ryan AG, Choudur H, et al. Pigmented villonodular synovitis. Clin Radiol 2004;59(5):414–20.

82. Fletcher CD. The evolving classification of soft-tissue tumours - an update based on the new 2013 WHO classification. Histopathology 2014; 64(1):2–11.

83. Hawnaur JM, Whitehouse RW, Jenkins JP, et al. Musculoskeletal haemangiomas: comparison of MRI with CT. Skeletal Radiol 1990;19(4):251–8.

84. Dubois J, Soulez G, Oliva VL, et al. Soft-tissue venous malformations in adult patients: imaging and therapeutic issues. Radiographics 2001; 21(6):1519–31.

85. Dubois J, Garel L, David M, et al. Vascular soft-tissue tumors in infancy: distinguishing features on Doppler sonography. AJR Am J Roentgenol 2002;178(6):1541–55.

86. Murphey MD, Fairbairn KJ, Parman LM, et al. From the archives of the AFIP. Musculoskeletal angiomatous lesions: radiologic-pathologic correlation. Radiographics 1995;15(4):893–917.

87. Kransdorf MJ, Murphey MD. Imaging of Soft-Tissue Musculoskeletal Masses: Fundamental Concepts. Radiographics 2016;36(6):1931–48.

88. Ryu YJ, Choi YH, Cheon JE, et al. Imaging findings of Kaposiform Hemangioendothelioma in children. Eur J Radiol 2017;86:198–205.

89. Trehan SK, Athanasian EA, DiCarlo EF, et al. Characteristics of glomus tumors in the hand not diagnosed on magnetic resonance imaging. J Hand Surg Am 2015;40(3):542–5.

90. Mathis WH Jr, Schulz MD. Roentgen diagnosis of glomus tumors. Radiology 1948;51(1):71–6.

91. Smith J, Wisniewski SJ, Lee RA. Sonographic and clinical features of angioleiomyoma presenting as a painful Achilles tendon mass. J Ultrasound Med 2006;25(10):1365–8.

92. Yoo HJ, Choi JA, Chung JH, et al. Angioleiomyoma in soft-tissue of extremities: MRI findings. AJR Am J Roentgenol 2009;192(6):W291–4.

93. Lubbers PR, Chandra R, Markle BM, et al. Case report 421: Calcified leiomyoma of the soft-tissues of the right buttock. Skeletal Radiol 1987;16(3):252–6.

94. McCarthy AJ, Chetty R. Benign Smooth Muscle Tumors (Leiomyomas) of Deep Somatic Soft-tissue. Sarcoma 2018;2018:2071394.

95. Chhabra A, Deshmukh SD, Lutz AM, et al. Neuropathy Score Reporting and Data System (NS-RADS): MRI Reporting Guideline of Peripheral Neuropathy Explained and Reviewed. Skeletal Radiol 2022;51(10):1909–22.

96. Reynolds DL Jr, Jacobson JA, Inampudi P, et al. Sonographic characteristics of peripheral nerve sheath tumors. AJR Am J Roentgenol 2004; 182(3):741–4.

97. Alpert JS, Boland P, Hameed M, et al. Undifferentiated pleomorphic sarcoma: indolent, tail-like recurrence of a high-grade tumor. Skeletal Radiol 2018; 47(1):141–4.

98. Chambers G, Kraft J, Kingston K. The role of ultrasound as a problem-solving tool in the assessment of paediatric musculoskeletal injuries. Ultrasound 2019;27(1):6–19.

99. Chan LP, Gee R, Keogh C, et al. Imaging features of fat necrosis. AJR Am J Roentgenol 2003; 181(4):955–9.

100. Abate M, Salini V, Rimondi E, et al. Post traumatic myositis ossificans: Sonographic findings. J Clin Ultrasound 2011;39(3):135–40.

101. Peetrons P. Ultrasound of muscles. Eur Radiol 2002;12(1):35–43.

102. Boccalini S, Si-Mohamed SA, Lacombe H, et al. First In-Human Results of Computed Tomography Angiography for Coronary Stent Assessment With a Spectral Photon Counting Computed Tomography. Invest Radiol 2022;57(4):212–21.

103. Kolb M, Ekert K, Schneider L, et al. The Utility of Shear-Wave Elastography in the Evaluation of Myositis. Ultrasound Med Biol 2021;47(8):2176–85.

104. Kolb M, Peisen F, Ekert K, et al. Shear Wave Elastography for Assessment of Muscular Abnormalities Related to Systemic Sclerosis. Acad Radiol 2021;28(8):1118–24.

105. Pass B, Jafari M, Rowbotham E, et al. Do quantitative and qualitative shear wave elastography have a role in evaluating musculoskeletal soft-tissue masses? Eur Radiol 2017;27(2):723–31.

106. Fritz J, Kijowski R, Recht MP. Artificial intelligence in musculoskeletal imaging: a perspective on value propositions, clinical use, and obstacles. Skeletal Radiol 2022;51(2):239–43.

107. Wang B, Perronne L, Burke C, et al. Artificial Intelligence for Classification of Soft-Tissue Masses at US. Radiol Artif Intell 2021;3(1):e200125.

108. Gillies RJ, Kinahan PE, Hricak H. Radiomics: Images Are More than Pictures, They Are Data. Radiology 2016;278(2):563–77.

109. Fritz B, Yi PH, Kijowski R, et al. Radiomics and Deep Learning for Disease Detection in Musculoskeletal Radiology: An Overview of Novel MRI- and CT-Based Approaches. Invest Radiol 2022. https://doi.org/10.1097/RLI.0000000000000907.

110. Leporq B, Bouhamama A, Pilleul F, et al. MRI-based radiomics to predict lipomatous soft-tissue tumors malignancy: a pilot study. Cancer Imaging 2020;20(1):78.

111. Burke CJ, Bencardino J, Adler R. The Potential Use of Ultrasound-Magnetic Resonance Imaging Fusion Applications in Musculoskeletal Intervention. J Ultrasound Med 2017;36(1):217–24.

Imaging of Rheumatological Disorders

Thomas M. Armstrong, FRCR[a,*], Andrew J. Grainger, FRCR[b], Emma Rowbotham, FRCR[c,d]

KEYWORDS

• MR imaging • Ultrasound • Rheumatology • Rheumatoid arthritis • Whole-body MR imaging

KEY POINTS

• Both ultrasound (US) and MR imaging add diagnostic information that is superior to clinical examination alone.
• US and MR imaging can detect subclinical synovitis and therefore help early diagnosis.
• Both US and MR imaging as well as computed tomography can detect erosions that may be occult on radiographs.
• Both US and MR imaging are useful for monitoring treatment response and detecting subclinical synovitis in patients in remission.
• MR imaging is useful in assessing deeper structures such as the spine and can image many joints simultaneously using whole-body MR imaging.

INTRODUCTION

In recent years, imaging has become integral to the diagnosis and management of rheumatological disorders. The continued progress of treatment options has meant that early diagnosis is crucial in ensuring the best outcome for patients. Therefore, an understanding of the core imaging features of rheumatological conditions at both the early and chronic stages is of paramount importance. Many of these conditions share particular imaging features due to common endpoints in the way the disease processes affect the joints. Together with clinical examination and blood markers, imaging is essential in making a diagnosis early in the disease process, allowing both optimal treatment planning and disease monitoring.

Conventional radiographs remain the most common initial investigation in the assessment of rheumatological conditions and still play a crucial role in assessing radiological patterns of disease. However, many changes within the bones, such as erosions and joint space loss, are not seen until more advanced stages of disease (**Fig. 1**), by which time the structural changes are usually irreversible. MR imaging and ultrasound imaging are therefore used to detect early signs of disease that are not yet visible on plain radiographs and that may be subclinical. In turn, this will often lead to both early diagnosis and early therapeutic intervention, and this helps to modulate and slow the eventual irreversible structural changes, leading to better patient outcomes and improved day-to-day function.

Both MR imaging and ultrasound add important diagnostic information not only in differentiating between different patterns of disease but also in assessing disease activity. It is therefore important for the radiologist to be aware of the relative merits and pitfalls of both these modalities in the context of assessing rheumatological conditions. For the purposes of this review article, the authors focus on the cornerstone diagnoses within rheumatology, namely rheumatoid arthritis (RA), spondyloarthritis (SpA), crystal arthropathies as well as both primary and erosive osteoarthritis. The

[a] Royal Free Hospitals NHS Foundation Trust, Pond Street, London NW3 2QG, UK; [b] Radiology Department, Cambridge University Hospitals NHS Foundation Trust, Addenbrookes Hospital, Cambridge, Cambridgeshire CB2 0QQ, UK; [c] Chapel Allerton Hospital, Leeds Teaching Hospitals NHS Trust, Leeds, UK; [d] NIHR Biomedical Research Centre Leeds, Chapel Allerton Hospital Leeds, LS4 7SA, UK
* Corresponding author.
E-mail address: thomas.armstrong1@nhs.net

Magn Reson Imaging Clin N Am 31 (2023) 309–320
https://doi.org/10.1016/j.mric.2023.01.008

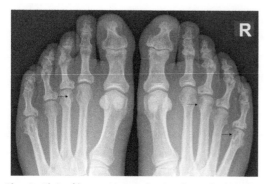

Fig. 1. Plain film erosions—dorsi-palmar (DP) radiograph of the feet in a patient with known rheumatoid arthritis. Note the multifocal erosions either side of multiple metatarsophalangeal joints (*arrows*).

authors also outline key comparators between MR imaging and ultrasound in the assessment of rheumatological conditions, with specific detail on individual conditions.

Ultrasound Versus MR Imaging—"The Principles"

It is important to address the relative strengths and weaknesses of both ultrasound and MR imaging when imaging the various manifestations of rheumatological disorders, not only in terms of their diagnostic efficacy but also in terms of ease of access, interobserver interpretation, cost, and patient satisfaction. It is important for any modality used in rheumatology to be able to image the main tissue components affected with a high degree of accuracy, but in particular the detection of synovitis and erosions and cartilage assessment are crucial.

Ultrasound is relatively inexpensive, does not use ionising radiation, and also offers the musculoskeletal radiologist the capability to assess the patient's anatomy (and pathology) in real time with the option of dynamic imaging and also contralateral side comparison. The addition of power Doppler increases the sensitivity of the imaging for synovial inflammation when compared with color doppler and is often preferred for this reason. Positive power Doppler signal has been shown to correlate well with clinical disease activity within a particular joint and can be used as a quantitative indication of synovial inflammation[1] (**Fig. 2**). In early disease synovitis may be the only imaging feature of active disease when radiographs remain normal.

Ultrasound is heavily operator dependent both in terms of diagnostic clinical experience and the technical acquisition of optimal images. These factors tend to have impact on ultrasound more

markedly than MR imaging and can significantly affect the diagnostic sensitivity and specificity. From a technical point of view when compared with MR imaging, ultrasound has a smaller field of view, which can create challenges when using it as a general screening tool over a large body area. However, the smaller field of view of ultrasound also offers advantages in allowing high-resolution imaging. The inability of ultrasound to detect bone marrow edema, internal bone structure, and to image inaccessible areas of anatomy such as the metacarpal and metatarsal heads are disadvantages of this imaging modality in rheumatological assessment.

MR imaging is free from ionising radiation, which makes it beneficial in comparison to both radiography and computed tomography (CT) imaging, particularly in younger patients, and this modality does allow a consistently reproducible set of images to be acquired that are less operator dependent than ultrasound. In general, MR allows assessment of a large field of view to be imaged, with the added ability to image the entire joint including the intraarticular cartilage. In terms of disadvantages, MR imaging in general will take longer to acquire and require patients to lie still for the duration of the study; it does not routinely allow dynamic assessment of joints although cine imaging can be acquired, and the imaging of multiple joints is much more time-consuming and may become uncomfortable for the patient. The risks associated with MR imaging mainly include localized tissue heating and the possibility of ferromagnetic components being attracted

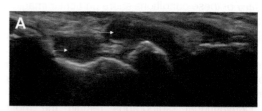

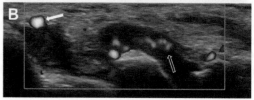

Fig. 2. Power Doppler ultrasound—(*A*) Longitudinal ultrasound of the wrist demonstrating hypoechoic synovial hyperplasia of the radiocarpal and intercarpal joints (*arrows*). (*B*) Power Doppler imaging reveals hypervascularity of the synovium (*open arrow*) consistent with active synovitis. Normal vasculature outside the synovium is also seen and should not be interpreted as pathology (*solid arrow*).

toward the magnetic field.[2] From an imaging point of view, magnetic components such as joint replacement can cause marked artifact, which in turn reduces the diagnostic efficacy of the images despite the advance of techniques such as metal artifact reduction sequences.

Whole-body MR imaging (WB-MR imaging), although not routinely used in clinical practice at present, allows widespread assessment of the axial and appendicular skeleton in one sitting. This technique is currently used in the assessment of patients with myeloma but is also gaining momentum for imaging of rheumatological disease and will be hugely beneficial in early disease where there are few clinical signs and where the pattern of disease is crucial in determining an early diagnosis.

Ultrasound Versus MR Imaging

Bone and erosions

Ultrasound is limited in its ability to image bone; bone edema in particular cannot be detected. Although erosion or enthesitis can be demonstrated on ultrasound, the cortical outline can be challenging to assess with this modality. Assessment of the bone and the erosive patterns and locations can add extremely useful diagnostic information in the context of rheumatological disorders.

MR imaging is superior in the assessment of bone and is sensitive for marrow edema (with fluid sensitive sequences such as proton density fat-saturated [PD FS] or short tau inversion recovery), which is seen as a feature of osteitis in inflammatory arthritis; this also occurs at the sites of tendon, ligament, or joint capsular attachments to bone as a feature of enthesitis in the SpA (**Fig. 3**) including psoriasis. This information may be occult on conventional radiographs, and ultrasound does not allow thorough assessment of the cortex or demonstrate the underlying cancellous bone.

Although ultrasound is often not the first-line imaging tool for osseous erosions, which are well seen on radiographs (see **Fig. 1**), the multiplanar capabilities of ultrasound mean it is more sensitive than radiographs for detecting erosion, especially early erosions.[3] MR imaging is also superior to radiographs for detecting early erosions; however, its use may be limited by ionising radiation; CT remains the gold standard for established erosive change due to its superior resolution[3,4] (**Fig. 4**). At present, when comparing MR imaging and ultrasound in erosion detection, there is conflicting evidence as to superiority in detection of erosions, mainly depending on joint location. In one study from 2004 Magnani and colleagues showed

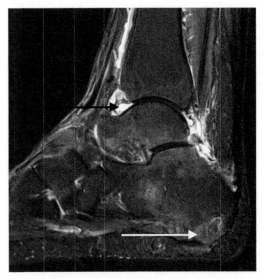

Fig. 3. Enthesitis. Sagittal PD FS image of the hind foot showing marked bone marrow edema within the calcaneus at the site of plantar fascia origin (*white arrow*). There is also evidence of erosive change here as well as synovitis at the tibiotalar joint (*black arrow*). There is periarticular bone marrow edema around the ankle also in this patient with inflammatory arthropathy.

ultrasound to be superior to MR imaging in the detection of erosions at the metacarpophalangeal joints.[5] Hoving and colleagues, however, reported that MR imaging had greater sensitivity for detection of erosions of the hand and wrist compared with ultrasound[6]; however, it is important to remember that both ultrasound and MR imaging remain superior to plain film radiographs in terms of detection of erosions.[3] A study by Hodgson and colleagues assessing markers of disease activity on MR imaging suggested postcontrast T1

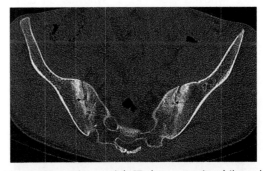

Fig. 4. CT erosion—axial CT demonstrating bilateral erosions of the sacroiliac (SI) joints in this patient with ankylosing spondylitis. Note the ability to clearly demarcate the defects in the cortex (*arrows*), which may be challenging at times to see on MR imaging given the degree of surrounding bony sclerosis.

images were the optimum sequence for assessing peripheral joint erosion size in RA.[7] Unlike the assessment of synovial volume that has been extensively researched with MR imaging, the quantification of bone erosions has however been less well assessed.

Cartilage

The assessment of articular cartilage damage and loss in rheumatology is an important disease sequalae that affects joint function and often contributes to symptoms, particularly in weight-bearing joints. Ultrasound is limited in the extent to which the chondral surfaces can be assessed due to its inability to penetrate bone. As a result, articular cartilage can only be assessed in certain locations. As such, it does not provide a complete overview but can be useful in some areas such as the trochlear cartilage (**Fig. 5**) of the knee and the posterior humeral cartilage deep to the infraspinatus but, as with most of the joints, ultrasound is incapable of assessing the entirety of the knee or shoulder articular surfaces.

MR imaging has an excellent capability to resolve cartilage and assess for chondral damage, particularly using PD FS sequences and high-strength magnets. Unlike ultrasound, MR imaging is able to assess the entirety of the chondral surface and differentiate between partial and full-thickness chondral loss, chondral fissuring, blistering, and delamination in addition to very early chondropathy such as chondral swelling and heterogeneity, all of which have implications in determining treatment options.

Synovium and soft tissues

Although bone edema, erosions, and chondral damage are important manifestations of the rheumatological disorders, it is often the synovium and ability of imaging to detect synovial hyperplasia, active synovitis (see **Fig. 2** synovitis on ultrasound), and enthesitis that allows these conditions

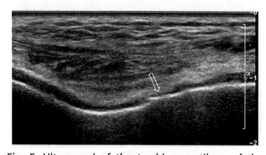

Fig. 5. Ultrasound of the trochlear cartilage of the knee. Transverse ultrasound image of the knee in a patient with established osteoarthritis. The lateral trochlear cartilage is thinned and irregular (*void arrow*) in comparison to the medial aspect.

to be detected at their earliest stage. Many of the imaging and clinic research papers focus on the ability to detect early inflammatory lesions, before development of chondral damage or erosive changes, which are usually irreversible changes.

Synovitis

Ultrasound has excellent resolution when it comes to imaging the synovium and assessing for frond-like synovial proliferation, hyperemia, joint capsule thickening, pannus formation, and associated joint effusion. There remains incomplete agreement on the optimal imaging parameters and the use of intravenous contrast agents, which again is clouded with the rapid advances in imaging resolution and microvascular imaging on ultrasound that has arisen over the last decade.[8]

In terms of detecting synovitis, ultrasound relies mainly on the use of power Doppler—able to detect low levels of blood flow and does not require contrast administration. MR imaging, however, relies on the enhancement of the synovium following intravenous contrast administration in order to detect synovitis.[9] OMERACT (Outcomes Measures in Rheumatoid Arthritis Clinical Trials), established in 2002, defines synovitis on ultrasound as "*thickened hypoechoic synovium when compared to subcutaneous fat (although this can be isoechoic or hyperechoic) that is poorly compressible and may exhibit doppler signal*". Power Doppler has been shown to have greater sensitivity than color Doppler and thus is preferred in the assessment of the inflammatory arthropathies.[10] Doppler flow has been shown to correlate well to disease activity and therefore can add useful diagnostic information to assist rheumatology colleagues in optimizing medical care. The detection of synovitis in addition to other findings such as erosions carries important clinical implications and may justify the initiation of more expensive biological drug therapies, particularly when subclinical synovitis is seen on imaging despite medical management.

The OMERACT definition of synovitis on MR imaging is "*thickening of the synovium with a 'greater than normal' enhancement with gadolinium on T1-weighted sequences*"; this has good sensitivity for disease activity; however, when compared with ultrasound MR imaging comes with the downside of contrast administration, which has potential but rare side effects such as nephrogenic systemic fibrosis and brain deposition.[11] Quantitative assessment of the synovium is possible on MR imaging, with some evidence to suggest that increased synovial volume within a joint correlates to increased disease activity. Some studies have shown reduction in synovial volume within 2 weeks of starting methotrexate therapy[12] and thus synovial volume may be an important finding to elicit. However, there is emerging evidence that contrast-enhanced MR imaging of the synovium is a more sensitive marker of disease activity than synovial volume (**Fig. 6**).[7]

In terms of sensitivity relative to clinical assessment, MR imaging shows strong correlation with clinical examination in approximately 60% of joints, but has superior sensitivity, detecting synovitis in clinically asymptomatic joints.[13] In terms of comparison between ultrasound and MR imaging, at least in patients with early inflammatory arthritis, MR imaging is shown to be more sensitive to synovitis than Doppler ultrasound, particularly in the hand and wrist joints.[14] In addition, there is a reported false-negative rate when using power Doppler ultrasound with studies, showing that biopsy of regions with no positive power Doppler

signal were found to have pathologic synovitis present.[15]

Both MR imaging and ultrasound have been shown to be equivalent when assessing fatty muscle atrophy (**Figs. 7 and 8**) as can occur in the shoulder with rotator cuff disease or severe arthropathy and resultant disuse.[16]

Enthesitis

Enthesitis is defined as inflammation at areas of tendon, ligament, fasciae, or joint capsule insertions to the underlying bone (the enthesis organ) and is a key diagnostic component of the inflammatory spondyloarthropathies. It is commonly seen in psoriatic arthritis (PsA) and can often be asymptomatic and therefore overlooked on clinical examination.[17] On ultrasound, there are several different findings in the case of enthesitis; tendon thickening and loss of the usual internal

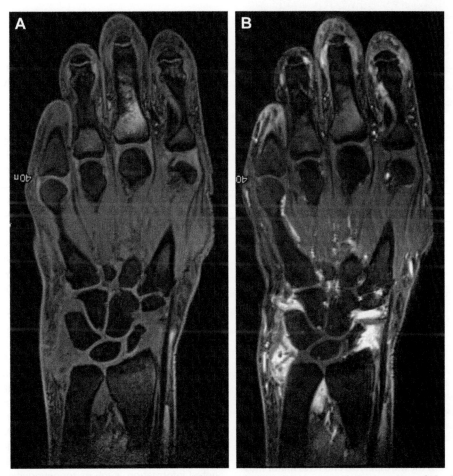

Fig. 6. MR imaging pregadolinium and postgadolinium administration: coronal MR imaging of the hand and wrist in a patient with long-standing rheumatoid arthritis demonstrating precontrast (*A*) and postcontrast (*B*) imaging. Note the extensive synovial hyperplasia with enhancement surrounding the radiocarpal and ulnocarpal joints. This is only appreciated on the postcontrast imaging. There is also erosive change, which is seen on both the precontrast and postcontrast imaging in this patient with established RA.

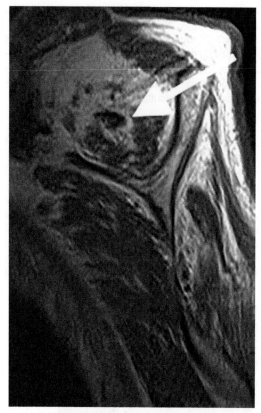

Fig. 7. MR imaging rotator cuff muscle atrophy: sagittal T1-weighted image of the shoulder in a patient with a rotator cuff tear showing atrophy of the supraspinatus (*white arrow*) muscle and of the infraspinatus muscle.

echotexture is seen as well as changes in the adjacent bone such as erosions and enthesophytes (**Fig. 9** Achilles). In 2019, Mathew and colleagues validated a heel score MR imaging model for the

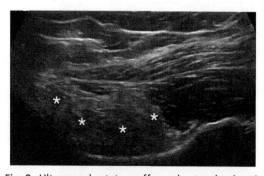

Fig. 8. Ultrasound rotator cuff muscle atrophy: longitudinal view of the infraspinatus and teres minor muscles. The patient had a large rotator cuff tear involving both the supraspinatus and infraspinatus muscles with subsequent hyperechoic replacement of muscle in keeping with fat atrophy change (*asterisk*).

assessment of enthesitis, which used the OMER-ACT definition described earlier and included the assessment of signal abnormality within the Achilles tendon, any evidence of retrocalcaneal bursitis, calcaneal erosive change, and underlying bone edema among others.[18] However, there remains debate about which entheses should be included in a routine assessment in a suspected case of PsA as particularly at the Achilles tendon, as age, body mass index, and regular physical exercise have all been associated with structural damage on ultrasound in PsA.[19] Ultrasound scoring systems for ultrasound are used in clinical practice to aid diagnostic classification—the most common of which is the Glasgow Ultrasound Enthesitis Scoring System (GUESS).[20] As stated previously, the ability of MR imaging to detect osteitis in SpA separates it from ultrasound in this clinical context.

Ultrasound Versus MR Imaging—Imaging-Specific Conditions

Rheumatoid arthritis

RA is a predominantly joint-based inflammatory polyarthropathy affecting approximately 1% of the global population.[10] It is arguably the area of rheumatology that is the most widely researched, as it has implications for a huge population around the world, both in terms of patient outcome and also health economics. The increased awareness of the role of imaging in rheumatology, and in particular in RA, has seen the emergence of the European League Against Rheumatism (EULAR) recommendations for the use of medical imaging in RA, as well as SpA and osteoarthritis.[21] Ultrasound and MR imaging both have a pivotal role in the assessment of RA, particularly in the detection of early disease that may not yet be apparent clinically as well as in disease monitoring.

Periarticular osteitis (bone edema) has been shown to correlate closely with subsequent progression to erosive change and carries a poor prognostic functional outcome[22]; therefore, MR imaging in these patients has the potential advantage over ultrasound in early disease if this is the only active finding. Ultrasound has been shown to be superior to clinical examination in the detection of minimal synovitis in RA with both MR imaging and US being useful in the quantification of synovial volume. Ultrasound can add helpful targeted information, such as tenosynovitis and tendinopathic change. Erosive bony change can occur in individuals without inflammatory arthritis (eg, osteoarthritis [OA]) who may be asymptomatic, and therefore, it is important to take MR and

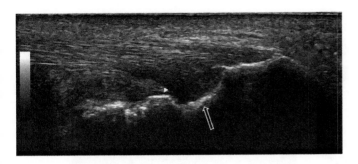

Fig. 9. Enthesitis: longitudinal ultrasound of the distal Achilles tendon shows thickening of the distal tendon with loss of the fibrillar pattern within the distal fibers (*white arrow*) as well as cortical destruction in keeping with erosive change to the posterior calcaneus (*void arrow*).

ultrasound findings in the correct clinical and biochemical context. Ultrasound has also been shown to improve the certainty of an RA diagnosis above clinical criteria and can be used to predict progression, assess treatment response, and monitor disease activity.[21]

Overall, both MR imaging and ultrasound show good evidence of superiority over clinical examination alone for disease detection and have a role in diagnosis, treatment response, and monitoring in clinical remission.

Spondyloarthritides

The SpA category comprises several inflammatory conditions centered around the axial skeleton with other systemic manifestations and organ involvement. They include ankylosing spondylitis, psoriatic spondyloarthropathy, enteropathic spondyloarthropathy, and reactive arthritis (formerly Reiter disease) in addition to undifferentiated types.

Both ultrasound and MR imaging are valuable modalities in the assessment of SpA and are often both used; however, given the nature of the deeper spinal and sacroiliac osseous disease, MR imaging plays the central role in diagnostic and monitoring imaging of the axial skeleton. The ability of MR imaging to detect early erosions particularly at the sacroiliac joints is further enhanced with the advent of T1 imaging with 3-dimensional volumetric sequences (eg, VIBE) (**Fig. 10**). Detection of early changes on MR imaging is a useful predictor in patients with nonradiographic disease who will progress to radiographically apparent disease (by the modified New York criteria).[21] Later in the disease process it is important to be aware of the phenomenon termed "backfill" where there is high intraarticular high signal seen filling up the excavated bone erosions (**Fig. 11**)—a feature that has been shown to have a high diagnostic value for axial SpA with a high specificity.[23] If treated early, regression of spinal inflammatory change has been shown to occur in as little as 6 weeks after antitumor necrosis factor treatment.[24]

Assessment of peripheral joints, in particular enthesitis, can be performed by either modality, and ultrasound can play a role in patients with focal peripheral joint or entheseal pain, which may be the first manifestation of the disease.

Recently in 2020, Kaeley and colleagues highlighted the importance of using ultrasound in differentiating the varying types of inflammatory arthropathy in order to initiate early treatment.[25] Although clinical, laboratory, and radiographic tests are usually sufficient for differentiating these diseases in the latter stages, early disease can be more challenging and thus ultrasound is important in detecting early, often subclinical disease.

Psoriatic arthritis

PsA presents as a heterogenous, often asymmetric, inflammatory arthropathy with a wide spectrum of changes that can make diagnosis challenging. Skin psoriasis is not a prerequisite for diagnosis, with 10% to 15% developing joint pain before skin manifestation.[26] In the hands clinical confusion can occur between early presentations of psoriatic arthritis and erosive osteoarthritis, whereas psoriatic arthritis can also occasionally mimic RA, particularly oligoarthropathic or palindromic types.

Ultrasound can visualize the peripheral joints such as the distal interphalangeal joints and proximal interphalangeal joints as well as the entheses in order to assess for inflammatory changes (see **Fig. 9**). Ultrasound has been demonstrated as superior to clinical examination in the assessment of the lower limb entheses such as the Achilles and can detect entheseal abnormality in clinically asymptomatic individuals.[17]

Martel and colleagues showed that erosions in PsA tend to occur in the "bare" area between the chondral surface and adjacent joint capsule within the interphalangeal or metacarpophalangeal and metatarsophalangeal joints; this differs with most of the cases of erosive osteoarthritis, where erosions tended to occur in the

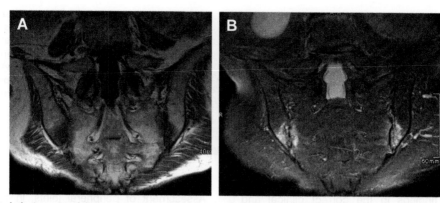

Fig. 10. Ankylosing spondylitis—coronal T1 (*A*) and coronal STIR (*B*) MR imaging sequences demonstrating active sacroiliitis of the anterior inferior aspects of the SI joints bilaterally. Note the high signal edema in (*B*) and corresponding low signal on the T1 in (*A*). The symmetric involvement, as in this case, is most classic of ankylosing. STIR, short tau inversion recovery.

subchondral bone, which can help to differentiate from PsA.[27]

Osteoarthritis and erosive (inflammatory) osteoarthritis

OA is the most prevalent musculoskeletal disease in developed countries with huge financial implications for health care budgets.[28] Conventional radiographs remain the mainstay modality for assessment of this condition demonstrating the classic features of asymmetric joint space loss, subchondral sclerosis, cyst formation, and osteophytosis (**Fig. 12** OA). Haugen and colleagues reviewed both MR imaging and ultrasound of the hands in patients with known OA and revealed that ultrasound allowed for assessment of these features with the additional merit of assessing for associated synovitis or degenerative erosions that may be occult on radiographs.[28] Mancarella

and colleagues demonstrated increased synovial hyperplasia, effusion, and hypervascularity in patients with erosive osteoarthritis on ultrasound when compared with nonerosive osteoarthritis.[29]

MR imaging has the added benefit of multiplanar imaging of the joints and soft tissues, allowing for a more comprehensive assessment of the cartilage, synovium, osseous erosions, and osteophytosis. Baker and colleagues demonstrated an association between knee pain in the context of OA changes and severity of synovitis on contrast-enhanced MR imaging.[30] Enhancement is also seen in patients without radiographic evidence of OA, with normal synovial enhancement seen in asymptomatic patients. It must therefore be taken in context of other findings such as synovial thickening or joint effusion.

The spectrum of disease was reviewed by Marshall and colleagues in 2015, who highlighted

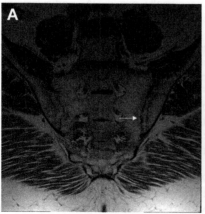
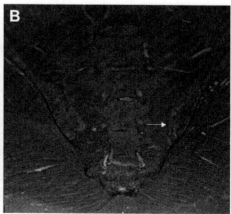

Fig. 11. Ankylosing spondylitis backfill—coronal T1 (*A*) and coronal STIR (*B*) sequences demonstrating erosions being filled (so-called backfill) with high T1 signal granulation tissue, which does not fat suppress on the fat-saturated sequence (*arrows*) proving this is not fat metaplasia.

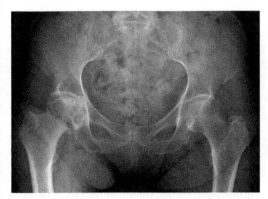

Fig. 12. Osteoarthritis of the hip—anteroposterior (AP) radiograph of the pelvis demonstrating asymmetric joint space loss, subchondral sclerosis, and subchondral cyst formation at the right hip in keeping with severe osteoarthritis.

the similar frequency of joint involvement and pattern of distribution in erosive OA and more severe nonerosive OA; as such, they suggested that erosive OA may be a sequalae of severe OA rather than a distinct pathologic entity.[31]

Crystal arthropathy

The crystal arthropathies comprise a group of disorders characterized by crystal deposition in one or more joints. Urate deposition in gout and calcium pyrophosphate dihydrate deposition disease (CPPD) are the most common. Pyrophosphate crystal disease may present acutely as pseudogout. Gout is the most common inflammatory arthropathy affecting men in the developed world.[32]

Conventional radiographs remain an important modality in differentiating between gout and CPPD, with an important feature being the presence of chondrocalcinosis, for instance in the

triangular fibrocartilage complex or menisci in cases of CPPD. Another very important difference is the predilection for the metacarpophalangeal joints and the patellofemoral joints in cases of CPPD as well as the fact that joint space is preserved in cases of gout until the final stages of the disease. Both conditions may demonstrate tophi, although this is much more common in cases of gout.

MR imaging is useful in the assessment of gout and can demonstrate the volume and location of tophaceous disease. T1 sequences classically show intermediate signal soft tissue deposits, for example, within the quadriceps, patella, and popliteus tendon and at the popliteus hiatus (**Fig. 13**), which seem to be preferentially involved in cases of gout involving the knee.[32]

As with other inflammatory arthropathies both ultrasound and MR imaging can demonstrate erosions, synovial hyperplasia, and synovitis in addition to a joint effusion in cases of acute gout and CPPD (**Fig. 14**). Occasionally floating aggregates of hyperechoic monosodium urate (MSU) crystals (microtophi) can be seen within the joint, and this has been termed a "snowstorm" appearance.[33] The sonographic finding of MSU crystals on the hyaline cartilage gives rise to a hyperechoic layer overlaying the hypoechoic cartilage beneath, sometimes referred to as the "double contour sign."[34] However, this is no longer considered a sign specific to gout and can also be seen in cases of CPPD.[35]

As in other areas of rheumatology, an advantage of MR imaging over ultrasound is in the assessment of deeper structures including intraosseous tophi formation (**Fig. 15** T1), and MR imaging has an established role in imaging of tophaceous gout of the spine that can affect the facet joints. In

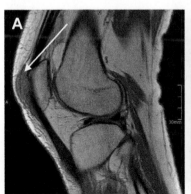
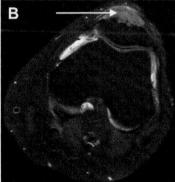
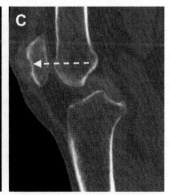

Fig. 13. Gout of the knee. (*A*) T1 sagittal and (*B*) PD FS axial imaging of the knee. (*C*) Sagittal CT of the knee in a patient with known gout. There is tophus formation seen superficial to the patellar (*white arrow*) with erosive change to the underlying cortex (*dashed arrow*)—this is best seen on the CT due to the superior resolution of bone.

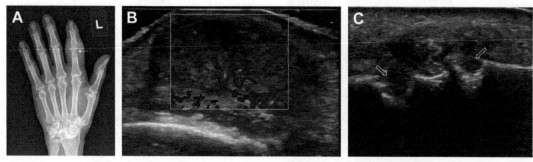

Fig. 14. Gout. (A) DP view of the hand demonstrating periarticular punched out erosion in the radial aspect of the proximal phalanx (arrow) with marked soft tissue swelling in this patient with gout. (*B*) Ultrasound of the same finger in the same patient demonstrating focal tophus formation adjacent to the proximal phalanx with associated positive power Doppler signal. (C) Longitudinal ultrasound image of the proximal phalanx with periarticular "punched out" erosions due to gout (open arrows).

particular, because of calcifications, gout should be considered when there is very low-signal periarticular soft tissue surrounding a facet joint.[36]

Whole-body MR imaging

Given the systemic manifestations of many of the rheumatological conditions and widespread joint and tendon involvement, the ability to simultaneously image soft tissue abnormalities at a wide variety of sites along with multiple joints in patients with suspected rheumatological disorders is potentially beneficial. The use of WB-MR imaging for this purpose is promising but is currently largely reserved for the research setting. WB-MR imaging is mostly used for imaging the spondyloarthropathies, allowing for imaging of both the spine and appendicular joints and entheses (**Fig. 16**). Although most published data on WB-MR imaging focuses on SpA, there is emerging data on its use in the assessment of inflammatory muscle diseases and other systemic rheumatic diseases such as systemic lupus erythematosus and systemic sclerosis with its ability to assess for internal organ derangement such as the brain, heart, and lungs in these connective tissue diseases in addition to the musculoskeletal system.[37] At present the main limitation in utilizing whole-body imaging is the time needed to complete the study; however, as the technique evolves, it will become more practical to image patients using this technique, thereby allowing for multiple joint assessments more readily and providing a thorough picture of joint distribution and involvement.

SUMMARY

Both MR imaging and ultrasound play a valid role in the imaging of rheumatological disorders;

however, it must be carefully interpreted in light of the clinical history. They have relative merits

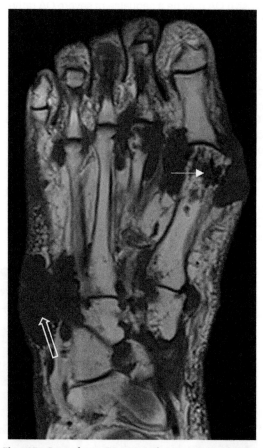

Fig. 15. Gout foot. T1 coronal MR image demonstrating widespread tophi formation (*open arrow*) particularly seen throughout the midfoot and forefoot with intraosseous extension into the first metatarsal head (*arrow*).

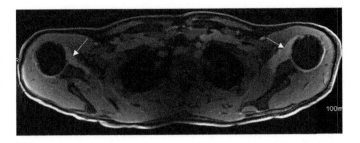

Fig. 16. Whole-body MR imaging. Large field-of-view axial WB-MR image VIBE DIXON sequence postgadolinium demonstrating inflammatory synovitis bilaterally with synovial hyperplasia within both glenohumeral joints in a patient with RA (*arrows*).

as described, and limitations must be kept in mind. Both conventional radiography and CT also add important information in certain cases and should not be forgotten, such as dual-energy CT in the imaging of gout. The best approach is likely to be a combined one with the merits of both modalities, particularly in the assessment of early disease with careful consideration to the distribution of disease. Rheumatological disorders and their imaging interpretation can be nuanced, and diagnostic decisions should be made on a case-by-case basis with a musculoskeletal imaging expert in addition to rheumatology colleagues' input. With increased awareness of the relative merits and limitations of the modalities discussed, it is hoped that the reader has gained further insight into this fascinating yet complex area of medical practice.

CLINICS CARE POINTS

- Both ultrasound and MR imaging add diagnostic information that is superior to clinical examination alone.
- Ultrasound and MR imaging can detect subclinical synovitis and therefore help early diagnosis.
- Both ultrasound and MR imaging, as well as CT can detect erosions that may be occult on radiographs.
- Both ultrasound and MR imaging are useful for *monitoring* treatment response and detecting subclinical synovitis in patients in remission.
- Early diagnosis on imaging allows timely drug modification of the disease process with the aim of lowering burden of disease and slowing progression.
- MR imaging is useful in assessing deeper structures such as the spine and can image many joints simultaneously using WB-MR imaging.

- Ultrasound has the additional capability of combined clinical assessment and dynamic assessment at the time of scanning that can help to formulate more complete clinical understanding in complex or atypical disease patterns.

DISCLOSURE

The authors declare no financial or other conflicts of interest.

REFERENCES

1. Newman JS, Adler RS, Bude RO, et al. Detection of soft-tissue hyperemia: value of power Doppler sonography. Am J Roentgenol 1994;163(2):385–9.
2. Dill T. Contraindications to magnetic resonance imaging. Heart 2008;94(7):943–8.
3. Wakefield RJ, Gibbon WW, Conaghan PG, et al. The value of sonography in the detection of bone erosions in patients with rheumatoid arthritis: a comparison with conventional radiography. Arthritis Rheum 2000 Dec;43(12):2762–70.
4. Perry D, Stewart N, Benton N, et al. Detection of erosions in the rheumatoid hand; a comparative study of multidetector computerized tomography versus magnetic resonance scanning. J Rheumatol 2005 Feb;32(2):256–67.
5. Magnani M, Salizzoni E, Mulè R, et al. Ultrasonography detection of early bone erosions in the metacarpophalangeal joints of patients with rheumatoid arthritis. Clin Exp Rheumatol 2004;22(6):743–8.
6. Hoving JL, Buchbinder R, Hall S, et al. A comparison of magnetic resonance imaging, sonography, and radiography of the hand in patients with early rheumatoid arthritis. J Rheumatol 2004 Apr;31(4):663–75.
7. Hodgson RJ, O'Connor P, Moots R. MRI of rheumatoid arthritis image quantitation for the assessment of disease activity, progression and response to therapy. Rheumatology 2008 Jan 1;47(1):13–21.
8. Fritz J. Magnetic resonance imaging versus ultrasonography for the diagnosis of synovitis in rheumatoid arthritis. Rheumatology 2018 Jan 1;57(1):5–7.

9. Mathew AJ, Krabbe S, Eshed I, et al. The OMERACT MRI in Enthesitis Initiative: Definitions of Key Pathologies, Suggested MRI Sequences, and a Novel Heel Enthesitis Scoring System. J Rheumatol 2019 Sep;46(9):1232–8.

10. Rowbotham EL, Grainger AJ. Rheumatoid Arthritis: Ultrasound Versus MRI. Am J Roentgenol 2011 Sep;197(3):541–6.

11. Gulani V, Calamante F, Shellock FG, et al. Gadolinium deposition in the brain: summary of evidence and recommendations. Lancet Neurol 2017 Jul; 16(7):564–70.

12. Palmer WE, Rosenthal DI, Schoenberg OI, et al. Quantification of inflammation in the wrist with gadolinium-enhanced MR imaging and PET with 2-[F-18]-fluoro-2-deoxy-D-glucose. Radiology 1995; 196(3):647–55.

13. Tamai M, Kawakami A, Iwamoto N, et al. Comparative study of the detection of joint injury in early-stage rheumatoid arthritis by MRI of wrist and finger joints and physical examination. Arthritis Care Res 2010;63(3):436–9.

14. Navalho M, Resende C, Rodrigues AM, et al. Bilateral Evaluation of the Hand and Wrist in Untreated Early Inflammatory Arthritis: A Comparative Study of Ultrasonography and Magnetic Resonance Imaging. J Rheumatol 2013;40(8):1282–92.

15. Andersen M, Ellegaard K, Hebsgaard JB, et al. Ultrasound colour Doppler is associated with synovial pathology in biopsies from hand joints in rheumatoid arthritis patients: a cross-sectional study. Ann Rheum Dis 2014;73(4):678–83.

16. Khoury V, Cardinal É, Brassard P. Atrophy and Fatty Infiltration of the Supraspinatus Muscle: Sonography Versus MRI. Am J Roentgenol 2008;190(4):1105–11.

17. Balint PV. Ultrasonography of entheseal insertions in the lower limb in spondyloarthropathy. Ann Rheum Dis 2002;61(10):905–10.

18. Mathew AJ, Østergaard M. Magnetic Resonance Imaging of Enthesitis in Spondyloarthritis, Including Psoriatic Arthritis—Status and Recent Advances. Front Med 2020;30:7.

19. KAELEY GS, D'AGOSTINO MA, GRASSI W, et al. GRAPPA 2011: Proceedings from the Ultrasound Imaging Module. J Rheumatol 2012;39(11):2211–3.

20. Balint PV. Inflamed retrocalcaneal bursa and Achilles tendonitis in psoriatic arthritis demonstrated by ultrasonography. Ann Rheum Dis 2000;59(12): 931–4.

21. Bara X, Conaghan PG, D-Agostino M-A, et al. Imaging in rheumatoid arthritis, psoriatic arthritis, axial spondyloarthritis, and osteoarthritis: An international viewpoint on the current knowledge and future research priorities. Eur J Rheumatol 2019;6(1):37–45.

22. McQueen FM, Ostendorf B. What is MRI bone oedema in rheumatoid arthritis and why does it matter? Arthritis Res Ther 2006;8(6):222.

23. Laloo F, Herregods N, Varkas G, et al. MR signal in the sacroiliac joint space in spondyloarthritis: a new sign. Eur Radiol 2017;27(5):2024–30.

24. Rudwaleit M. Magnetic resonance imaging of the spine and the sacroiliac joints in ankylosing spondylitis and undifferentiated spondyloarthritis during treatment with etanercept. Ann Rheum Dis 2005; 64(9):1305–10.

25. Kaeley GS, Bakewell C, Deodhar A. The importance of ultrasound in identifying and differentiating patients with early inflammatory arthritis: a narrative review. Arthritis Res Ther 2020;22(1):1.

26. Coates LC, Helliwell PS. Psoriatic arthritis: state of the art review. Clin Med 2017;17(1):65–70.

27. Martel W, Stuck K, Dworin A, et al. Erosive osteoarthritis and psoriatic arthritis: a radiologic comparison in the hand, wrist, and foot. Am J Roentgenol 1980; 134(1):125–35.

28. Haugen IK, Bøyesen P. Imaging modalities in hand osteoarthritis - status and perspectives of conventional radiography, magnetic resonance imaging, and ultrasonography. Arthritis Res Ther 2011;13(6): 248.

29. Mancarella L, Magnani M, Addimanda O, et al. Ultrasound-detected synovitis with power Doppler signal is associated with severe radiographic damage and reduced cartilage thickness in hand osteoarthritis. Osteoarthr Cartil 2010;18(10):1263–8.

30. Baker K, Grainger A, Niu J, et al. Relation of synovitis to knee pain using contrast-enhanced MRIs. Ann Rheum Dis 2010;69(10):1779–83.

31. Marshall M, Nicholls E, Kwok W-Y, et al. Erosive osteoarthritis: a more severe form of radiographic hand osteoarthritis rather than a distinct entity? Ann Rheum Dis 2015;74(1):136–41.

32. Girish G, Glazebrook KN, Jacobson JA. Advanced Imaging in Gout. Am J Roentgenol 2013;201(3): 515–25.

33. Rettenbacher T, Ennemoser S, Weirich H, et al. Diagnostic imaging of gout: comparison of high-resolution US versus conventional X-ray. Eur Radiol 2008;18(3):621–30.

34. Thiele RG, Schlesinger N. Diagnosis of gout by ultrasound. Rheumatology 2007;46(7):1116–21.

35. Löffler C, Sattler H, Peters L, et al. Distinguishing Gouty Arthritis from Calcium Pyrophosphate Disease and Other Arthritides. J Rheumatol 2015 Mar; 42(3):513–20.

36. Hsu CYTF, Shih T, Huang K-M, Chen P-Q, et al. Tophaceous Gout of the Spine: MR Imaging Features. Clin Radiol 2002;57(10):919–25.

37. Weckbach S. Whole-Body MRI for Inflammatory Arthritis and Other Multifocal Rheumatoid Diseases. Semin Musculoskelet Radiol 2012;16(05):377–88.

MR Imaging–Ultrasonography Correlation of Acute and Chronic Foot and Ankle Conditions

Benjamin Fritz, MD[a,b], Jan Fritz, MD[c,*]

KEYWORDS

- MR imaging • Ultrasonography • Injury • Ankle • Foot

KEY POINTS

- Foot and ankle sports injuries range among the most common sports injuries.
- Acute ligamentous injuries are most common, followed by fractures, tendon tears, and osteochondral injuries.
- Common chronic and overuse injuries include osteochondral and articular cartilage defects, tendinopathies, stress fractures, and neuropathies.
- Ultrasonography is well-suited for evaluating superficial tendons, ligaments, and muscles.
- MR imaging is best for deeper-located soft tissue structures, articular cartilage, and cancellous bone.

INTRODUCTION

Foot and ankle injuries are common musculoskeletal disorders, broadly categorized as traumatic and overuse injuries and chronic conditions. The ankle is the second most frequently injured joint after the knee; however, in some team sports, the ankle has the highest injury prevalence.[1] In the acute setting, ligamentous injuries are most common, whereas fractures, osseous avulsion injuries, tendon and retinaculum tears, and osteochondral injuries are less common. The most common chronic and overuse injuries include osteochondral and articular cartilage defects, tendinopathies, stress fractures, impingement syndromes, and neuropathies. Common forefoot conditions include traumatic and stress fractures, metatarsophalangeal and plantar plate injuries and degenerations, intermittent bursitis, and perineural fibrosis.

DIAGNOSTIC IMAGING

Based on indications derived by clinical examination, radiographs are often the first-line imaging modality, whereas MR imaging is a second-line examination for further evaluation of soft tissue structures and problem-solving of indeterminate radiographic findings.

Ultrasound (US) may be used as a first-line imaging modality as point-of-care examinations in the office or bedside, as a portable sideline examination during sports events, or as a second-line

a Department of Radiology, Balgrist University Hospital, Forchstrasse 340, Zurich 8008, Switzerland; b Faculty of Medicine, University of Zurich, Zurich, Switzerland; c Division of Musculoskeletal Radiology, Department of Radiology, New York University Grossman School of Medicine, 660 1st Avenue, 3rd Floor, Room 313, New York, NY 10016, USA
* Corresponding author.
E-mail address: jan.fritz@nyulangone.org
Twitter: JanFritzMSK (J.F.)

Magn Reson Imaging Clin N Am 31 (2023) 321–335
https://doi.org/10.1016/j.mric.2023.01.009

examination in the case of negative radiographs or for problem-solving of indeterminate radiographic findings.

US is readily available; usually cheaper than MR imaging; and, similar to MR imaging, does not require the use of ionizing radiation. An additional advantage of US is the ability for dynamic observation of tendon and joint movements and stress testing. The invention of portable handheld US devices, which allow the connection of a transducer to a smartphone or tablet device, further improved the portability and utility.

US is limited to visualizing superficial structures around the foot and ankle, whereas most intraarticular and marrow spaces are not accessible because of cortical bone representing an impenetrable barrier to US waves. In contrast, MR imaging can visualize the foot and ankle in a single session, including all aspects of the articular cartilage, the ligamentous and tendinous structures, and bone marrow.

Clinical MR imaging examinations are often performed with an emphasis on proton density–weighted or T2-weighted fast and turbo spin echo pulse sequences, which may be obtained without and with fat suppression. This combination of cartilage and fluid-sensitive pulse sequences allows detecting and characterizing soft tissue injuries around the foot and ankle. An additional T1-weighted pulse sequence can increase the accuracy of bone marrow assessment, specifically in the infection setting and occasionally increase the conspicuity of fractures. Intravenous contrast agent application is useful for inflammation, infection, and neoplasms and may aid in the detection of tendon disorders. MR imaging examinations of high diagnostic quality may be obtained with modern 0.55-, 1.5-, and 3.0-T scanners.[2,3] Surface coils, which may have the shape of a boot, improve image quality, signal, and fat suppression.[4] Various metal artifact reduction techniques reduce image artifacts induced by orthopedic implants.[5–7] Modern pulse sequence acceleration techniques, deep learning–based image reconstruction, and artificial intelligence–driven superresolution permit high-quality MR imaging examinations within 5 minutes of acquisition time.[4,8–14] Artificial intelligence–based disease detection algorithms are promising tools to increase the diagnostic performance of detecting foot and ankle injuries.[15]

Most MR imaging examinations of the foot and ankle consist of two-dimensional pulse sequences in three orthogonal planes, permitting visualization of all anatomic structures. However, oblique ligaments and tendons and curved articular surfaces are difficult to visualize. These limitations are overcome with pulse sequences aligned to the structure of interest, such as the peroneal tendons and anterior tibiofibular ligament.[4,16–19]

Modern three-dimensional (3D) fast and turbo spin echo pulse sequences permit the acquisition of proton density–weighted and T2-weighted isotropic high spatial resolution data sets in less than 5 minutes.[16] Those datasets are used for multiplanar and curved planar reformations along any nonlinear structure to improve visualization, detect abnormalities, and overcome the limitations of two-dimensional MR imaging.[17]

Because of tremendous improvements in the time speed of MR imaging, the examination time of a clinical MR imaging and systematic US examination of the ankle are similar, in the range of 20-minute room time at the authors' institutions.

US of the ankle is usually performed with high-frequency transducers of 9 MHz to 20 MHz. Higher frequency transducers are beneficial for improving the detail of evaluated structures. Although penetration depth decreases with increasing frequency, a high penetration depth of the US waves is usually not required in the ankle because most structures of interest are usually close to the subcutaneous tissue or within a depth of 3 to 4 cm.

Compared with MR imaging, dynamic US is particularly beneficial for assessing joint stability in ligament tears and tendon continuity in the setting of tears and retinaculum disorders.

LIGAMENTS

Ligaments are strong, fibered, soft tissue structures primarily composed of collagen (mainly type I), proteoglycan, and water.[20] Ligaments around the foot and ankle usually connect two bones and serve as primary joint stabilizers with either intra- or extra-articular location. Many, often small and short, ligaments exist between the various hindfoot and midfoot joints. In most parts, these ligaments span a single joint between adjacent bones; however, at the ankle, some also span over two joints, such as the calcaneofibular ligament stabilizing the tibiotalar and the subtalar joint.

On MR imaging, intact ligaments usually appear as tubular or bandlike structures with hypointense signal on all pulse sequences. Some ligaments can also appear as striated, partially hyperintense structures on non-fat-suppressed pulse sequences because of fibrofatty portions, most notably the tibiotalar and deltoid ligaments.[17]

On US, ligaments appear as fibrillar or bandlike, hyperechogenic structures with sharp borders.[21] Anisotropy occurs if the transducer and the insonating beam are not perpendicular to the tendon orientation and can help to differentiate ligaments, particularly surrounding hyperechogenic fatty tissue (**Fig. 1**).[22]

Ligament disorders are frequent and the most common acute traumatic injury at the foot and ankle. Acute ligament injuries are categorized into microscopic interstitial tears and macroscopic partial-thickness and full-thickness tears. Injured ligaments heal with scar remodeling of the original fibers, which may result in reconstituting sufficient ligament capacity or ligamentous insufficiency with resulting joint instability.

The ankle is stabilized by three ligament complexes: the lateral, medial (deltoid), and syndesmotic ligaments. The lateral collateral ligament complex is most frequently injured, comprising more than 60% of all acute ligament injuries of the ankle.[23] Inversion trauma mechanisms are most common, during which the anterior talofibular ligament tears first, followed by the calcaneofibular ligament and the posterior talofibular ligament.[24] Concomitant low-grade injuries of the deep layers of the medial collateral ligament complex are frequent.[25]

The medial collateral ligament complex is injured in about 10% to 16% of acute traumatic ankle injuries in athletes, most frequently after forced ankle eversion.[26,27] Isolated injuries of the medial collateral ligament complex are rare, whereas most tears occur in conjunction with lateral collateral or syndesmotic ligament injuries.[28]

The syndesmosis is the least commonly injured ligament complex of the ankle, most frequently occurring in contact sports, such as football, wrestling, and ice hockey.[29] High ankle sprains are the clinical correlate. The robust ligament complex is the main stabilizer of the distal tibiofibular joint, preventing the dissociation of the tibial plafond under axial loading. Injuries often result in longer recovery periods and may result in chronic ankle instability in case of inadequate healing.[29,30]

On MR imaging, acutely injured ligaments demonstrate increased signal on proton density–weighted and T2-weighted MR images, usually with periligamentous fluid. The degree of cross-sectional fiber disruption can usually be well visualized in larger ligaments; however, ligament visualization in more than one contrast and plane may be necessary for diagnosis if standard two-dimensional MR imaging is applied. Isotropic 3D MR imaging data sets can be aligned to the oblique ligament orientations and improve ligament tear detection accuracy.[17]

On US, an acutely injured ligament usually demonstrates thickening, diffuse hypoechogenicity, and some degree of surrounding fluid.[31] Fiber disruptions are visualized as gaps or discontinuities. Dynamic US can directly visualize superphysiologic joint space opening on applying varus or valgus stress. Ligament healing typically results in varying degrees of ligament fiber scarring, presenting as variable ligament caliber, hypointense signal on MR images, and hypoechogenicity on US.

On US examination, ligaments should be evaluated in perpendicular cross-sectional and longitudinal planes. Aligning the US probe perpendicular to

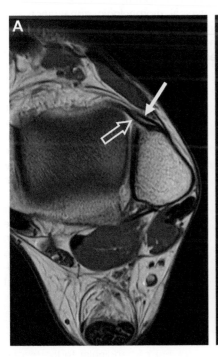
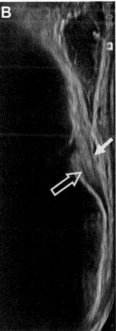

Fig. 1. A 29-year-old healthy woman. (A) Axial proton density–weighted MR image of the ankle shows the anterior talofibular ligament, which has a two-bundled appearance with a hypointense superficial (*solid arrow*) and a hypointense deep (*open arrow*) component. (B) On ultrasonography, the anatomy of the anterior talofibular ligament correlates well with the MR imaging, visualizing the two-bundled anatomy with the superficial (*solid arrow*) and the deep (*open arrow*) portions with the typical striated appearance in high detail.

the long ligament axis allows for a detailed cross-sectional assessment of superficially located ligaments.

Clinically important and well-visualizable ligaments with US and MR imaging are the anterior talofibular ligament and calcaneofibular ligament of the lateral collateral ligament complex, the superficial and deep layers of the medial ligament complex, and the anterior tibiofibular ligament of the syndesmotic complex (**Fig. 2**). The posterior talofibular and the syndesmotic interosseous and posterior tibiofibular ligaments are more difficult to image with US, often representing indications for MR imaging.

The often-small ligaments of the midfoot and forefoot, such as the dorsal talonavicular ligament, are assessable with US using high-frequency probes because of their superficial location. Deeper located ligaments at the plantar arch, such as the spring ligament complex, bifurcate ligament, and interosseous ligament of the sinus tarsi, are not reliably assessable with US, representing indications for MR imaging.

TENDONS

Tendons connect muscles to the bone, transmitting muscle strength to the joints to facilitate movements. At the foot and ankle, tendons act as static and dynamic joint stabilizers. Similar to ligaments, tendons are primarily composed of type I collagen, proteoglycans, and water. Parallel-oriented fibrils and wavy-oriented bundles highly organize tendons. Tendons are either covered by a tendon sheath or surrounded by a paratenon. Both are distinct histologic entities that reduce tendon friction and facilitate the gliding of tendons against surrounding tissues. Retinacula are fibrous sheaths that act like sliding channels, often where tendon directions change, for tendon stabilization and prevention of dislocation during force transmission.

On MR imaging, healthy tendons are hypointense on all MR imaging weightings and appreciable as tubular or flat structures. Because of their anatomy with tightly packed, parallel fibers and bundles, tendons are prone to the magic angle effect, which results in increased tendon signal on MR images with short echo times, as used with T1-weighted and proton density–weighted turbo and fast spin echo pulse sequences. On US, tendons are sharply bordered, hyperechoic structures with well-visible parallel fibers. Strong anisotropy effects are common for all tendons if the US probe is not perpendicular oriented to the tendons.

Achilles Tendon

The Achilles tendon is the thickest tendon of the ankle. Because of its superficial location and almost perfectly straight orientation, the Achilles tendon is easy to find and visualize on US. There is no tendon sheath around the Achilles tendon, but a looser organized paratenon providing tendon nutrition.[32] Achilles tendinopathy describes a common, noninflammatory spectrum of tendon degeneration, with contributing pathomechanisms including a decreased blood supply and hypoxia. Conceptually, insertional and noninsertional midsubstance tendinopathy may be differentiated.

The prototypical morphologic appearance of noninsertional, midsubstance tendinopathy of the Achilles tendon is similar to MR and US images. The Achilles tendon midsubstance appears as

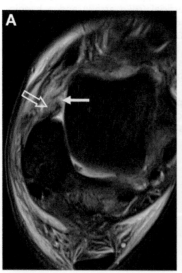
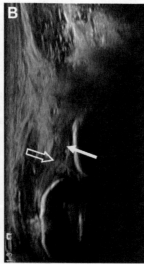

Fig. 2. A 17-year-old male soccer player with supination trauma of the ankle. (*A*) Axial proton density–weighted MR image with fat suppression shows a full-thickness tear of the anterior talofibular ligament with a fluid-filled gap (*solid arrow*). The torn ligament is hyperintense and thickened (*open arrow*). (*B*) On ultrasonography, the torn anterior talofibular ligament is thickened with a partly wavy appearance of the torn ligament fibers (*open arrow*). The fluid-filled gap is hypoechogenic (*solid arrow*).

fusiform thickening, typically located 2 to 6 cm proximal to the distal calcaneal insertion. On cross-sectional axial and anteroposterior longitudinal images, thickening of the short-axis tendon diameter greater than 7 mm and a loss of the normal concavity of the anterior tendon margin represent the two cardinal findings (**Fig. 3**). Disease progression can result in central or superficial longitudinal partial-thickness tears, presenting on MR and US images as fluid-filled fiber defects.

Partial- and full-thickness cross-sectional midsubstance Achilles tendon tears are often the result of acute trauma, usually superimposed on preexisting tendinopathy and degenerative partial-thickness longitudinal tears. The resulting gap and degree of proximal and distal tendon retraction are accurately measured on MR and US images. In addition, MR imaging and US accurately assess the tissue quality and degree of degeneration of the torn tendon ends. Accurate measurements and morphologic descriptions can help plan surgical repair and the necessity for crafting. Dynamic US examination further allows the visualization of the approximation of the torn tendon ends during plantar flexion of the foot, which has prognostic value for conservative treatment and bracing.

Insertional or distal Achilles tendinopathy (**Fig. 4**) is a chronic overuse condition frequently found in runners and dancers and is also associated with wearing high heel shoes.[33] A posterosuperior boney prominence at the calcaneus, the so-called Haglund deformity, is a common association and thought to represent a predisposing factor for the development of insertional Achilles tendinopathy.[34] Distention and fluid accumulation psoriatic arthritis–associated retrocalcaneal bursitis is a differential diagnostic consideration, especially when debris is present within the distended bursa. Haglund deformities, fluid amount, and internal debris within the retrocalcaneal bursa is assessed with MR imaging and US. The localized inflammatory activity of retrocalcaneal bursitis is assessed with Doppler US and contrast enhancement on MR imaging. Some cases present additionally with adventitial retro-Achilles tendon bursitis.

Long Flexor, Extensor, and Peroneal Tendons

The anteriorly located extensor tendons, the medially located long flexor tendons, and the laterally located peroneal tendons constitute the three other tendon groups about the ankle. The proximal attachments and muscle bellies are located around the proximal tibia and fibula, whereas the tendons are attached distally in the midfoot and forefoot. The combined functions of the three tendon groups are essential for dorsal extension, eversion, and inversion or combined movements. The peroneal and long flexor tendons are crucial for stabilizing the longitudinal and sagittal arch of the hindfoot by functioning as dynamic and static stabilizers.[35,36]

The dynamic and static stabilizing functions are facilitated by complex tendon anatomies and courses around the ankle with many changes in direction for force vectors, stabilized by retinacula

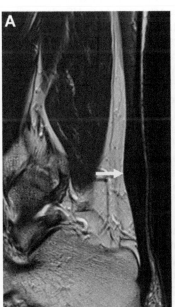
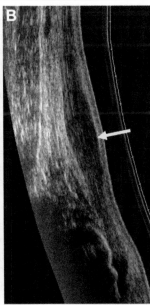

Fig. 3. A 34-year-old man with painful Achilles tendon. (*A*) Sagittal T2-weighted MR image of the left hindfoot shows fusiform thickening of the Achilles tendon midsubstance (*arrow*), indicative of degenerative tendinopathy without tear. (*B*) Longitudinal panoramic ultrasonographydemonstrates fusiform hypoechoic thickening of the Achilles tendon (*arrow*) with a fine internal longitudinal striated pattern, representing the highly organized tendon microstructure with intact fibers.

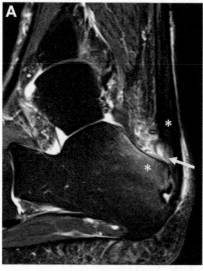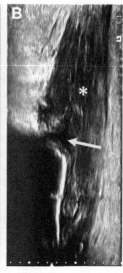

Fig. 4. A 58-year-old man with painful distal Achilles tendon. Sagittal fat-suppressed T2-weighted MR image (*A*) and corresponding ultrasonography image (*B*) of the distal Achilles tendon show severe insertional tendinopathy, characterized by tendon thickening (*white asterisks*) and calcaneal-sided partial-thickness tear with fluid-distended and inflamed retrocalcaneal bursa (*arrows*). MR imaging additionally demonstrates bone marrow edema pattern of the posterosuperior calcaneus (*yellow asterisk in A*).

and bone structures. For instance, around the malleoli, the force vector directions of the posterior tibial tendon and the peroneal tendons demonstrate changes of 40° to 50°.[17] On MR imaging, multiple imaging planes and on US, multiple probe orientations are necessary to fully visualize the tendons and follow their entire course around the foot and ankle. For MR imaging, isotropic 3D data sets can be interactively aligned along the tendon courses and aid the longitudinal and axial visualization perpendicular to the spatial tendon orientation.[17]

For MR imaging, axial oblique plane orientations and plane angulations of about 45° at the level of the malleoli have been evaluated to improve the visualization of the flexor and peroneal tendons.

The magic angle effect may interfere with accurately diagnosing tendinopathy and partial-thickness tears based on tendon signal intensities when using pulse sequences with short echo times. The magic angle effect results in hyperintense tendon signals in structures with a highly organized longitudinal microanatomy if oriented with an angle of approximately 55° to the z-axis of the external main B0 magnetic field of the MR imaging scanner. This direction is typically horizontal in horizontal bore scanners, whereas in C-shaped MR scanners, this direction is typically vertical. On clinical MR images, increased signal intensity caused by the magic angle effect occurs regularly within segments of the flexor and peroneal tendons near the malleoli or in the peroneal longus tendon near the cuboid bone. On US images, strong anisotropy effects are found similarly within the ankle tendons. Strict perpendicular probe orientation to the tendons on long- and short-axis views reduces anisotropy. Short-axis

inspection of the entire tendon course may be most important.

Acute injuries of ankle tendons present on a spectrum ranging from internal interstitial tears to partial-thickness cross-sectional and longitudinal tears to complete tendon tears with possible retraction (**Fig. 5**). Additional retinacular tears with tendon displacement and bowstring may occur in acute injury. Chronic injuries of the ankle tendons mainly include degenerative tendinopathy and scarring of the retinacula. Lower-grade tendon tears and attritional degenerative tendinopathy may similarly lead to caliber irregularities, tendon thinning, or tendon thickening with increased signal on all common MR imaging pulse sequences and hypoechogenicity on US, depending on their acuity, stage of healing, and remodeling.

Interstitial tears typically describe the lowest grade of tendon tears and are, by definition, confined to the internal tendon substance without surface extension. Interstitial tears may be cross-sectional, longitudinal, or complex.

Partial tendon tears may occur as partial-thickness cross-sectional fiber defects or longitudinal partial splits of the tendon substance. Tendon splits are frequent within segments of the peroneal tendons between the fibula tip and the peroneal tubercle, although frequently asymptomatic (**Fig. 6**).

Complete or full-thickness tears describe discontinuity of all fibers, usually associated with a variable amount of retraction, depending on the location, integrity of retinacula, and amount of scarring in tethering around the tendon.

Supraphysiologic amounts of peritendinous fluid are signs of tenosynovitis if sharply bordered or paratenonitis if diffuse. On MR imaging,

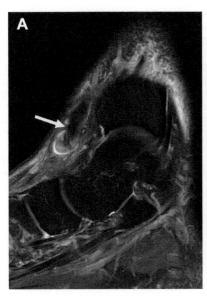
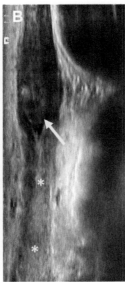

Fig. 5. A 53-year-old man with decreased dorsal extension strength of the foot and ankle. (*A*) Sagittal fat-suppressed T2-weighted MR image shows a full-thickness tear of the anterior tibial tendon with retraction of the thickened tendon to the level of the tibiotalar joint line (*arrow*). (*B*) On ultrasonography, the retracted and thickened tendon (*arrow*) is similarly well visualized at the level of the tibiotalar joint line with empty tendon sheath distal to the tendon stump (*asterisks*).

increased peritendinous contrast enhancement indicates hyperperfusion, which may be seen in tendon injury, tenosynovitis, and paratenonitis, which may also be visualized on Doppler sonography. Tendon dislocations and subluxations may be constant or intermittent, best assessed with dynamic US if intermittent (**Fig. 7**).

Compared with ligament injuries, acute injuries of ankle tendons are less common. However, chronic degenerative tendinopathy and partial tears are frequent findings that increase with age. Tenosynovitis is common in patients with rheumatologic disorders.

PLANTAR FASCIA

The plantar fascia is a strong ligamentous structure predominantly composed of type I collagen fibers, extending from the calcaneus to the metatarsal heads along the plantar aspect of the

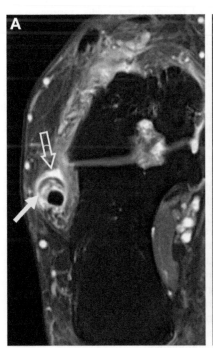
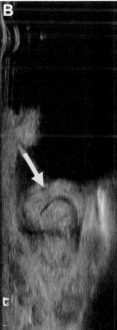

Fig. 6. A 57-year-old woman with lateral ankle pain. (*A*) Axial oblique fat-suppressed contrast-enhanced T1-weighted MR image shows a degenerated peroneus brevis split tear (*solid arrow*) with surrounding tenosynovitis (*open arrow*). (*B*) On ultrasonography, the thickened and torn peroneus brevis tendon is hyperechoic (*arrow*).

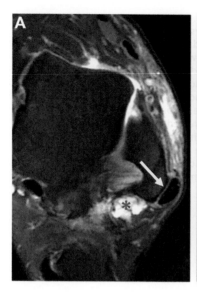
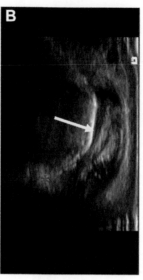

Fig. 7. A 54-year-old man with lateral ankle pain and snapping sensation. Axial proton density–weighted MR image with fat suppression (*A*) and the ultrasonography image (*B*) show laterally dislocated peroneal tendons (*arrows*) with empty retromalleolar groove (*asterisks*), indicating a superior peroneal retinaculum tear.

foot. The plantar fascia is an important stabilizer of the longitudinal arch of the foot composed of the medial, central, and lateral cords. The central cord is the strongest and most frequently abnormal, whereas the medial cord is the thinnest and only rarely abnormal.[37] Because of its superficial location and interposition of only the heel fat pad between the skin and the fascia, the plantar fascia is exquisitely well evaluated with US.

The normal plantar fascia is hyperechogenic on US with a striated, longitudinal pattern.[38] On MR imaging, all aspects of the plantar fascia are easily demonstrated as a hypointense structure on all common pulse sequences. Because of its straight course, the magic angle usually does not occur on MR images; however, anisotropy effects occur on US images. For both imaging modalities, the anteroposterior sagittal longitudinal and axial cross-sectional planes are sufficient to detect and accurately describe the spectrum of abnormalities.

Plantar Fasciitis

Plantar fasciitis may be more accurately described as plantar fasciopathy because of a lack of inflammatory cells.[39] Either term describes the most common painful heel condition characterized by the formation of enthesophytes, thickening and remodeling, and tears of the calcaneal fascial attachment with surrounding soft tissue inflammation and occasionally calcaneal osseous stress reactions and fractures.[40] The central cord is most commonly involved. Although not fully understood, repetitive stress, microtearing, and tissue remodeling are implicated in the pathoetiology.

On US and MR images, the early spectrum of plantar fasciitis presents with fusiform thickening and perifascial edema (**Fig. 8**). In addition, a loss of the fibrillar matrix of the fascia is seen on US, whereas hyperintense signal alterations on all common pulse sequences are typical appearances for MR imaging. Plantar fasciitis frequently presents with hyperemia on Doppler US and increased contrast-enhancement MR imaging. Bone marrow edema pattern of the calcaneus adjacent to the plantar fascia attachment is suggestive of symptomatic plantar fasciitis; however, only detectable with MR imaging (see **Fig. 8**).[37] Plantar bony spur formation at the calcaneal attachment of the plantar fasciitis, representing mineralized enthesophytes, is frequently associated with plantar fasciitis. Those bony spurs typically form close to the inferior calcaneal nerve, which may be compressed, leading to Baxter neuropathy with atrophying fat infiltration of the abductor digiti minimi muscle bulk. In advanced stages of plantar fasciitis, partial and eventually rare complete tears occur, presenting as often fluid-filled tendon defects with variable degrees of retraction on MR and US images.

Traumatic tears of the plantar fascia are rare but can present similar findings as advanced plantar fasciitis with partial tearing. Increased thickness, surrounding edema, loss of fibrillar facia structure, and edema signal of the plantar fascia are additional frequent overlapping findings. However, the location of acute injuries may be more distally on the plantar fascia, approximately 2 to 3 cm distal to the calcaneal attachment, whereas plantar fasciitis typically occurs at the calcaneal attachment.[38] Clinical history describing a trauma with strong force on the plantar fascia often represents the most useful information for differentiation.

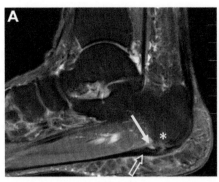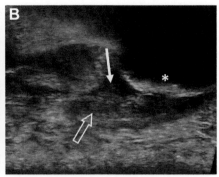

Fig. 8. A 64-year-old woman with plantar fasciitis. (*A*) Sagittal fat-suppressed, proton density–weighted MR image of the ankle shows a thickened and edematous proximal plantar fascia (*open arrow*), calcaneus-sided partial-thickness tear (*solid arrow*), perifascial and heel fat pad edema, and calcaneal bone marrow edema (*asterisk*). (*B*) On ultrasonography, the degenerated plantar fascia is hyperechoic (*open arrow*), and the partial-thickness plantar fascial tear is hypoechogenic (*solid arrow*). The asterisk denotes the plantar aspect of the calcaneus.

Plantar Fibromatosis

Plantar fibromatosis, also called Ledderhose disease, describes a benign nodular proliferation of fibroblasts within the substance of the plantar fascia of unknown cause. Multifocal and bilateral manifestations along the plantar fascia are common.[41] In principle, plantar fibromatosis can occur at any location of the plantar fascia; however, most common locations are around the level of the tarsometatarsal joints. A hallmark sign is a nodular thickening of the plantar fascia, with sizes ranging from a few millimeters to a few centimeters. Small nodules are seen on US and MR images as architectural distortions and surface convexities of the plantar fascia, whereas larger nodules are easily appreciable as masslike lesions. On US, lesions are more often hypoechogenic than hyperechogenic, possibly demonstrating increased Doppler signal. On T2-weighted MR images, plantar fibromatosis lesions are hyperintense, hypointense, or mixed signal intensity. Larger lesions are usually T2 hyperintense with central hypointense septations, often best seen with fat suppression. After intravenous contrast administration, most lesions demonstrate at least segmental or partial contrast enhancement.[42]

Tumor and masslike lesions

Various neoplastic lesions can occur around the foot and ankle, including primary benign, locally aggressive, and malignant bone and soft tissue tumors, metastasic diseases, or hematologic disorders. Except for enchondroma of the metatarsal bones and phalanges, bone tumors in the ankle and foot are rare.

Morton Neuroma

Tumorlike and masslike lesions of the foot are more common. Morton neuroma is a frequent finding in symptomatic and asymptomatic individuals. The expression neuroma is now considered a misnomer because Morton neuromas do not represent true neuromas but nonneoplastic perineural fibrosis of the interdigital nerves of the forefoot at the levels of the metatarsal heads.[43] This process is often accompanied by intermetatarsal bursitis. Instead of Morton neuroma, perineural fibrosis intermetatarsal bursitis complex may describe this entity more accurately.

Mechanical irritation and pressure are presumed contributing factors for this type of degenerative neuropathy. Macroscopically, a Morton neuroma appears as thickening, surface irregularity, and nodularity along the interdigital nerves. Most Morton neuromas are located in the second and third web spaces, interposed between the intermetatarsal heads. Demonstration of displacement of a Morton neuroma from the intermetatarsal to a more plantar position may increase the accuracy of imaging diagnosis for small lesions.

On US, Morton neuromas are maneuvered in a plantar direction by applying dorsal pressure on the webspace and either manually splaying or squeezing the metatarsal heads.[44] A sonographic Mulder test describing a dynamic plantar displacement of Morton neuroma out of the webspace during manual squeezing of the metatarsal heads may increase diagnostic accuracy.[45] On MR imaging, plantar displacement of Morton neuromas is achieved by placing the patient in a prone position on the MR imaging table and forefoot prone into a larger coil, such as a knee coil.[46]

On US, Morton neuromas are nodular, noncompressible, hypoechogenic lesions, which are usually distinguishable from the surrounding hyperechogenic plantar fatty tissue (**Fig. 9**).[47] US performed from the plantar aspect of the foot, preferably in the axial plane, often demonstrates Morton neuromas best. Doppler US may not provide additional value.

On MR imaging, Morton neuromas present as nodular masses with hypointense signal on T1- and T2-weighted MR images (see **Fig. 9**). Accompanying intermetatarsal bursitis is easy to identify on fat-suppressed T2-weighted MR images. Although usually not necessary in clinical practice, Morton neuromas demonstrate variable gadolinium enhancement.

A meta-analysis demonstrated for US and MR imaging a similar sensitivity of 90% and 93% for the detection of Morton neuromas, respectively, but a higher specificity of 88% for US in comparison with 68% of MR imaging.[48]

Tenosynovial Giant Cell Tumors

Tenosynovial giant cell tumors are benign soft tissue tumors with a low incidence. However, at the foot and ankle, tenosynovial giant cell tumors are the most common soft tissue tumor.[49] These lesions are of synovial origin and found at tendon sheaths, within joint capsules, and in bursae. Former terms included pigmented villonodular synovitis for intra-articular lesions and giant cell tumor of the tendon sheath for extra-articular peritendinous lesions. Histologically, all these lesions are identical and primarily composed of fibroblasts, multiloculated giant cells, and histiocytes.[50]

On imaging, extra-articular and intra-articular tumors have identical imaging characteristics. On US, tenosynovial giant cell tumors are usually sharply bordered, homogenously hypoechogenic, and sometimes show hyperechogenic foci. On dynamic US, tenosynovial giant cell tumors do not move with adjacent tendons during flexion or extension. Doppler US often shows increased central vascularity.[51] On MR imaging, tenosynovial giant cell tumors are usually T1 and T2 hypointense and demonstrate homogenous enhancement after intravenous contrast administration.[52] Gradient echo MR images with sufficiently long echo time may demonstrate blooming artifacts caused by hemosiderin deposits, which are considered pathognomonic. Bone erosions often occur because of chronic pressure in case of long-standing intra- and extra-articular tumor manifestations. Tenosynovial giant cell tumors typically do not show mineralized deposits on radiographs.

Gout

Gout is classified as inflammatory arthritis because of the chronic deposition of monosodium urate crystals in capsuloligamentous structures and acutely within joints in the setting of an acute gout attack.[53] Gout has a higher incidence in men with a 20:1 ratio.[54] The forefoot joints, particularly the first metatarsophalangeal joint, are frequent locations of uric acid depositions, primarily found in capsuloligamentous structures.

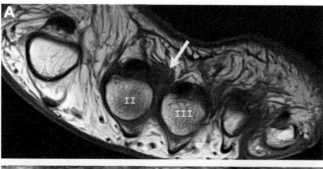

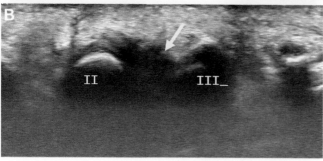

Fig. 9. A 54-year-old woman with second intermetatarsal pain. (*A*) Axial T1-weighted MR image of the forefoot shows a nodular soft tissue mass (*arrow*) plantar to the second (II) and third (III) metatarsal bones (*arrow* in *A*), compatible with Morton neuroma. (*B*) On ultrasonography, Morton neuroma has a hypoechogenic appearance with indistinct margins (*arrow*).

Uncontrolled long-standing gout eventually results in severe joint damage, which classically presents with characteristic punched-out erosions on imaging. In chronic gout, mineralized periarticular or extra-articular uric acid soft tissue deposits may form, also known as tophi, which may resemble neoplastic soft tissue lesions.[55] On US, gout tophi are usually heterogeneously hyperechogenic with poorly defined borders.[56] On MR imaging, the tophi are usually T1 isointense and T2 hypointense to skeletal muscle with varying degrees of gadolinium enhancement (**Fig. 10**).[57] Associated erosions and joint effusions are seen with US and MR imaging. In acute episodes of gouty arthritis, US may demonstrate floating monosodium urate crystals within joint effusions and coating articular cartilage surfaces.

JOINT DISORDERS
Articular Cartilage

Imaging of articular cartilage is a primary MR imaging domain, which can visualize all articular cartilage surfaces of the foot and ankle joints with high spatial and contrast resolution. Because of their typically oblique and curved orientations, cartilage-sensitive pulse sequences, such as proton density–weighted turbo spin echo, are often acquired in three orthogonal planes. Because of substantial advances in the acceleration of MR imaging acquisitions, entire comprehensive foot and ankle MR imaging protocols made nowadays can be acquired in less than 6 minutes.[2,8,9,11,13] Modern 3D fast and turbo spin echo–based sequences are time-efficient alternatives to traditional two-dimensional fast and turbo spin echo pulse sequences, allowing thin slice multiplanar reconstructions because of their small isotropic voxels, which is aligned to joint surfaces in virtually limitless planar and curved orientations.[16]

Osteochondral lesions of the talus may be primary or secondary cartilaginous or osseocartilaginous injuries.[58] In up to 70% of inversion injuries, osteochondral lesions of the talus and capsuloligamentous injuries occur together.[59] Higher-grade osteochondral lesions are diagnosed on radiographs; however, cartilaginous and lower-grade osteochondral lesions are typically occult.

MR imaging is most accurate for diagnosing and classifying osteochondral lesions of the talus. Five MR imaging stages may be differentiated.[60] Depending on symptoms, grade, and size, osteochondral lesions of the talus may require surgical treatment for which MR imaging can provide important detail.[1]

Even though US may detect peripheral cartilage defects that are accessible to US in certain joint positions, most parts of the foot and ankle joints are not accessible to insonation. Locations accessible to US include the anterior aspect of the talar surface in plantar flexion and some aspects of the metatarsophalangeal joints in flexion and extension.

Fracture with cortical extension (**Fig. 11**) and superficially located nerves and nerve lesions (**Fig. 12**) may be diagnosed with MR imaging and US.

Joint Effusion and Synovitis

Joint effusion and synovitis of the talocrural and metatarsophalangeal joints are easily detected with US. MR imaging has a high accuracy for detecting effusion of any foot and ankle joint.

On US images, a joint effusion presents as an anechoic, compressible fluid collection often best seen along joint recesses. Simple joint effusions do not present internal Doppler flow, whereas synovial proliferation may demonstrate internal vascularity. The inflammatory activity of synovitis may be assessed by the degree of Doppler flow within the synovial lining.

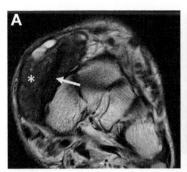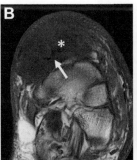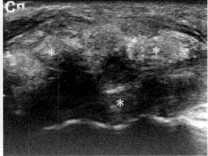

Fig. 10. A 62-year-old man presenting with pain and swelling of the midfoot. Coronal T2-weighted (*A*) and axial oblique T1-weighted (*B*) MR images demonstrate T1 and T2 hypointense tophaceous gout deposits (*asterisk in A and B*) inside and around the anterior tibial tendon (*arrows in A and B*). (*C*) On ultrasonography, the tophaceous gout deposits are heterogeneously hyperechoic (*asterisks*).

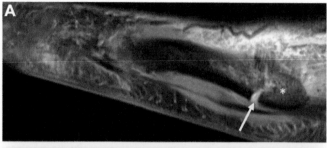

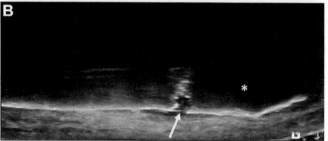

Fig. 11. A 69-year-old woman with lateral foot pain after trauma. (*A*) Sagittal fat-suppressed T2-weighted MR image shows a mildly distracted proximal fifth metatarsal fracture (*arrow*) and a hyperintense linear substance defect (*arrow in A*). (*B*) On ultrasonography, the fracture (*arrow*) demonstrates as hypoechogenic osseous defect of the proximal fifth metatarsal cortex. The asterisk in A and B denotes the base of the fifth metatarsal bone.

On MR imaging, joint effusions typically demonstrate waterlike T2 hyperintense and T1 hypointense signal characteristics. Hemorrhagic components may increase the T1 signal intensity and reduce T2 signal intensity (shading), depending on their protein fraction, number and integrity of erythrocytes, and state of hemoglobin degradation. Synovial proliferations present on MR imaging as many small fronds, may contain internal fat, and demonstrate increasing gadolinium contrast enhancement with increased inflammatory activity.

Plantar Plate Injuries

Plantar plates are fibrocartilaginous structures embedded at the plantar aspect of the capsuloligamentous complex of the metatarsophalangeal joints.[61] Plantar plate injuries usually occur at the distal attachment to the base of the proximal phalanx.[62,63] Full-thickness tears cause various degrees of retraction (**Fig. 13**). Acute injuries are often athletic activity–related because of excessive force to the metatarsophalangeal joint in dorsal extension and consecutive traumatic hyperextension.[62]

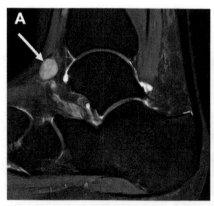
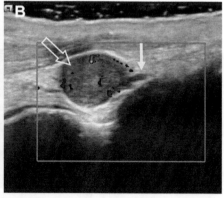

Fig. 12. A 33-year-old woman with painful palpable mass along the dorsum of the talus. (*A*) Sagittal fat-suppressed proton density–weighted MR image shows a well-circumscribed, hyperintense soft tissue mass (*arrow*) with mild central heterogeneity. (*B*) On the corresponding ultrasonography image, the soft tissue mass is hypoechogenic (*open arrow*) with internal color Doppler blood flow and demonstrated nerve continuation (*solid arrow*). Histopathologic examination diagnosed a schwannoma.

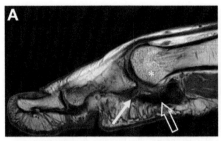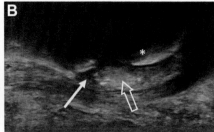

Fig. 13. A 60-year-old woman with first metatarsophalangeal plantar pain. (*A*) Sagittal proton density–weighted MR image of the forefoot shows a full-thickness distal plantar plate tear (*solid arrow*) with mildly retracted plantar plate (*open arrow*) subjacent to the first metatarsal head (*asterisk*). (*B*) On corresponding ultrasonography, the full-thickness plantar plate tear (*solid arrow*) is hypoechoic, and the retracted plantar plate is hyperechogenic (*open arrow*). The first metatarsal head (*asterisk*) is partially visualized.

The intact plantar plate is a slightly hyperechoic structure on US with a longitudinally striated pattern. The thick distal attachment is well visualized in the sagittal longitudinal plane. A well-marginated physiologic central recess at the distal plantar plate can be present and should not be mistaken for tears.[64]

Similar to ligaments, anisotropy may occur during US of the plantar plate. Partial- and full-thickness tears most frequently present as anechoic or hypoechoic substance defects of the plantar plate.

On MR imaging, plantar plates are hypointense on all common pulse sequences and easily distinguishable from the adjacent flexor tendons and metatarsal heads. Defects are usually T2 hyperintense because of fluid of the gap in the plantar plate substance.[65] A tear of the distal plantar plate usually starts at the articular surface and progresses to the plantar surface with increasing tear severity (see **Fig. 13**).[64]

SUMMARY

US and MR imaging are valuable imaging tests for a broad spectrum of foot and ankle conditions. Superficially tendons, ligaments, and muscles are exquisitely well evaluated with US, whereas deeper-located structures, articular cartilage, and cancellous bone are the domain of MR imaging.

CLINICS CARE POINTS

- Superficially tendons, ligaments, and muscles are exquisitely well evaluated with ultrasonography.

- Deeper-located structures, articular cartilage, and cancellous bone are the domain of MR imaging.

- Acute plantar fascia injuries may locate 2 to 3 cm distal to the calcaneal attachment, whereas plantar fasciitis typically occurs at the calcaneal attachment.

- Plantar fasciitis may be more accurately described as plantar fasciopathy because of a lack of inflammatory cells.

- Instead of Morton neuroma, perineural fibrosis intermetatarsal bursitis complex may describe this entity more accurately.

DISCLOSURE

B. Fritz: Nothing to disclose. J. Fritz received institutional research support from Siemens AG, BTG International Ltd, United Kingdom, Zimmer Biomed, DePuy Synthes, QED, and Synthetic MR; is a scientific advisor for Siemens AG, SyntheticMR, GE Healthcare, QED, BTG, ImageBiopsy Lab, Boston Scientific, and Mirata Pharma; and has shared patents with Siemens Healthcare, Johns Hopkins University, and New York University.

REFERENCES

1. Fritz B, Parkar AP, Cerezal L, et al. Sports imaging of team handball injuries. Semin Musculoskelet Radiol 2020;24(3):227–45.
2. Khodarahmi I, Fritz J. The value of 3 Tesla field strength for musculoskeletal magnetic resonance imaging. Invest Radiol 2021;56(11):749–63.
3. Khodarahmi I, Keerthivasan MB, Brinkmann IM, et al. Modern low-field MRI of the musculoskeletal system: practice considerations, opportunities, and challenges. Invest Radiol 2023;58(1):76–87.
4. Kijowski R, Fritz J. Emerging technology in musculoskeletal MRI and CT. Radiology 2023;306(1):6–19.

5. Burke CJ, Khodarahmi I, Fritz J. Postoperative MR imaging of joints: technical considerations. Magn Reson Imaging Clin N Am 2022;30(4):583–600.

6. Umans H, Cerezal L, Linklater J, et al. Postoperative MRI of the ankle and foot. Magn Reson Imaging Clin N Am 2022;30(4):733–55.

7. Murthy S, Fritz J. Metal Artifact Reduction MRI in the Diagnosis of Periprosthetic Hip Joint Infection. Radiology 2022;220134. https://doi.org/10.1148/radiol.220134.

8. Del Grande F, Guggenberger R, Fritz J. Rapid musculoskeletal MRI in 2021: value and optimized use of widely accessible techniques. AJR Am J Roentgenol 2021;216(3):704–17.

9. Del Grande F, Rashidi A, Luna R, et al. Five-minute five-sequence knee MRI using combined simultaneous multislice and parallel imaging acceleration: comparison with 10-minute parallel imaging knee MRI. Radiology 2021;299(3):635–46.

10. Fritz B, Yi PH, Kijowski R, et al. Radiomics and deep learning for disease detection in musculoskeletal radiology: an overview of novel MRI- and CT-based approaches. Invest Radiol 2023;58(1):3–13.

11. Fritz J, Guggenberger R, Del Grande F. Rapid musculoskeletal MRI in 2021: clinical application of advanced accelerated techniques. AJR Am J Roentgenol 2021;216(3):718–33.

12. Fritz J, Kijowski R, Recht MP. Artificial intelligence in musculoskeletal imaging: a perspective on value propositions, clinical use, and obstacles. Skeletal Radiol 2022;51(2):239–43.

13. Lin DJ, Walter SS, Fritz J. Artificial intelligence-driven ultra-fast superresolution MRI: 10-fold accelerated musculoskeletal turbo spin echo MRI within reach. Invest Radiol 2023;58(1):28–42.

14. Fritz J, Fritz B, Zhang J, et al. Simultaneous multislice accelerated turbo spin echo magnetic resonance imaging: comparison and combination with in-plane parallel imaging acceleration for high-resolution magnetic resonance imaging of the knee. Invest Radiol 2017;52(9):529–37.

15. Fritz B, Fritz J. Artificial intelligence for MRI diagnosis of joints: a scoping review of the current state-of-the-art of deep learning-based approaches. Skeletal Radiol 2022;51(2):315–29.

16. Fritz B, Bensler S, Thawait GK, et al. CAIPIRINHA-accelerated 10-min 3D TSE MRI of the ankle for the diagnosis of painful ankle conditions: performance evaluation in 70 patients. Eur Radiol 2019;29(2):609–19.

17. Fritz B, Fritz J, Sutter R. 3D MRI of the ankle: a concise state-of-the-art review. Semin Musculoskelet Radiol 2021;25(3):514–26.

18. Fritz J, Fritz B, Thawait GG, et al. Three-dimensional CAIPIRINHA SPACE TSE for 5-minute high-resolution MRI of the knee. Invest Radiol 2016;51(10):609–17.

19. Kalia V, Fritz B, Johnson R, et al. CAIPIRINHA accelerated SPACE enables 10-min isotropic 3D TSE MRI of the ankle for optimized visualization of curved and oblique ligaments and tendons. Eur Radiol 2017;27(9):3652–61.

20. Asahara H, Inui M, Lotz MK. Tendons and ligaments: connecting developmental biology to musculoskeletal disease pathogenesis. J Bone Miner Res 2017;32(9):1773–82.

21. Brasseur JL, Luzzati A, Lazennec JY, et al. Ultrasono-anatomy of the ankle ligaments. Surg Radiol Anat 1994;16(1):87–91.

22. Hodgson RJ, O'Connor PJ, Grainger AJ. Tendon and ligament imaging. Br J Radiol 2012;85(1016):1157–72.

23. Holmer P, Sondergaard L, Konradsen L, et al. Epidemiology of sprains in the lateral ankle and foot. Foot Ankle Int 1994;15(2):72–4.

24. Brostroem L. Sprained ankles. I. Anatomic lesions in recent sprains. Acta Chir Scand 1964;128:483–95.

25. Klein MA. MR imaging of the ankle: normal and abnormal findings in the medial collateral ligament. AJR Am J Roentgenol 1994;162(2):377–83.

26. Clanton TO, Porter DA. Primary care of foot and ankle injuries in the athlete. Clin Sports Med 1997;16(3):435–66.

27. Kofotolis ND, Kellis E, Vlachopoulos SP. Ankle sprain injuries and risk factors in amateur soccer players during a 2-year period. Am J Sports Med 2007;35(3):458–66.

28. Mengiardi B, Pinto C, Zanetti M. Medial collateral ligament complex of the ankle: MR imaging anatomy and findings in medial instability. Semin Musculoskelet Radiol 2016;20(1):91–103.

29. Mauntel TC, Wikstrom EA, Roos KG, et al. The epidemiology of high ankle sprains in National Collegiate Athletic Association sports. Am J Sports Med 2017;45(9):2156–63.

30. Rammelt S, Zwipp H, Grass R. Injuries to the distal tibiofibular syndesmosis: an evidence-based approach to acute and chronic lesions. Foot Ankle Clin 2008;13(4):611–33. vii-viii.

31. Morvan G, Busson J, Wybier M, et al. Ultrasound of the ankle. Eur J Ultrasound 2001;14(1):73–82.

32. Schweitzer ME, Karasick D. MR imaging of disorders of the Achilles tendon. AJR Am J Roentgenol 2000;175(3):613–25.

33. Pierre-Jerome C, Moncayo V, Terk MR. MRI of the Achilles tendon: a comprehensive review of the anatomy, biomechanics, and imaging of overuse tendinopathies. Acta Radiol 2010;51(4):438–54.

34. Jones DC, James SL. Partial calcaneal ostectomy for retrocalcaneal bursitis. Am J Sports Med 1984;12(1):72–3.

35. Chhabra A, Soldatos T, Chalian M, et al. 3-Tesla magnetic resonance imaging evaluation of posterior

tibial tendon dysfunction with relevance to clinical staging. J Foot Ankle Surg 2011;50(3):320–8.

36. Hatch GF, Labib SA, Rolf RH, et al. Role of the peroneal tendons and superior peroneal retinaculum as static stabilizers of the ankle. J Surg Orthop Adv 2007;16(4):187–91.

37. Ehrmann C, Maier M, Mengiardi B, et al. Calcaneal attachment of the plantar fascia: MR findings in asymptomatic volunteers. Radiology 2014;272(3): 807–14.

38. McNally EG, Shetty S. Plantar fascia: imaging diagnosis and guided treatment. Semin Musculoskelet Radiol 2010;14(3):334–43.

39. Lemont H, Ammirati KM, Usen N. Plantar fasciitis: a degenerative process (fasciosis) without inflammation. J Am Podiatr Med Assoc 2003;93(3):234–7.

40. Riddle DL, Schappert SM. Volume of ambulatory care visits and patterns of care for patients diagnosed with plantar fasciitis: a national study of medical doctors. Foot Ankle Int 2004;25(5):303–10.

41. Fetsch JF, Laskin WB, Miettinen M. Palmar-plantar fibromatosis in children and preadolescents: a clinicopathologic study of 56 cases with newly recognized demographics and extended follow-up information. Am J Surg Pathol 2005;29(8):1095–105.

42. Morrison WB, Schweitzer ME, Wapner KL, et al. Plantar fibromatosis: a benign aggressive neoplasm with a characteristic appearance on MR images. Radiology 1994;193(3):841–5.

43. Wu KK. Morton's interdigital neuroma: a clinical review of its etiology, treatment, and results. J Foot Ankle Surg 1996;35(2):112–9. ; discussion 87-8.

44. Quinn TJ, Jacobson JA, Craig JG, et al. Sonography of Morton's neuromas. AJR Am J Roentgenol 2000; 174(6):1723–8.

45. Torriani M, Kattapuram SV. Technical innovation. Dynamic sonography of the forefoot: the sonographic Mulder sign. AJR Am J Roentgenol 2003;180(4): 1121–3.

46. Weishaupt D, Treiber K, Kundert HP, et al. Morton neuroma: MR imaging in prone, supine, and upright weight-bearing body positions. Radiology 2003; 226(3):849–56.

47. Redd RA, Peters VJ, Emery SF, et al. Morton neuroma: sonographic evaluation. Radiology 1989; 171(2):415–7.

48. Xu Z, Duan X, Yu X, et al. The accuracy of ultrasonography and magnetic resonance imaging for the diagnosis of Morton's neuroma: a systematic review. Clin Radiol 2015;70(4):351–8.

49. Chou LB, Ho YY, Malawer MM. Tumors of the foot and ankle: experience with 153 cases. Foot Ankle Int 2009;30(9):836–41.

50. Fletcher CDM, World Health Organization. International Agency for Research on Cancer. In: WHO classification of tumours of soft tissue and bone. 4th edition. Lyon: IARC Press; 2013. p. 468.

51. Wang Y, Tang J, Luo Y. The value of sonography in diagnosing giant cell tumors of the tendon sheath. J Ultrasound Med 2007;26(10):1333–40.

52. Jelinek JS, Kransdorf MJ, Shmookler BM, et al. Giant cell tumor of the tendon sheath: MR findings in nine cases. AJR Am J Roentgenol 1994;162(4):919–22.

53. Richette P, Bardin T. Gout. Lancet 2010;375(9711): 318–28.

54. Dirken-Heukensfeldt KJ, Teunissen TA, van de Lisdonk H, et al. Clinical features of women with gout arthritis." A systematic review. Clin Rheumatol 2010;29(6):575–82.

55. Sheldon PJ, Forrester DM, Learch TJ. Imaging of intraarticular masses. Radiographics 2005;25(1): 105–19.

56. de Avila Fernandes E, Kubota ES, Sandim GB, et al. Ultrasound features of tophi in chronic tophaceous gout. Skeletal Radiol 2011;40(3):309–15.

57. Yu JS, Chung C, Recht M, et al. MR imaging of tophaceous gout. AJR Am J Roentgenol 1997; 168(2):523–7.

58. Berndt AL, Harty M. Transchondral fractures (osteochondritis dissecans) of the talus. J Bone Joint Surg Am 1959;41-A:988–1020.

59. Hannon CP, Smyth NA, Murawski CD, et al. Osteochondral lesions of the talus: aspects of current management. Bone Joint Lett J 2014;96-B(2): 164–71.

60. Mintz DN, Tashjian GS, Connell DA, et al. Osteochondral lesions of the talus: a new magnetic resonance grading system with arthroscopic correlation. Arthroscopy 2003;19(4):353–9.

61. Deland JT, Lee KT, Sobel M, et al. Anatomy of the plantar plate and its attachments in the lesser metatarsal phalangeal joint. Foot Ankle Int 1995;16(8): 480–6.

62. Gregg JM, Schneider T, Marks P. MR imaging and ultrasound of metatarsalgia: the lesser metatarsals. Radiol Clin North Am 2008;46(6):1061–78. vi-vii.

63. Umans HR, Elsinger E. The plantar plate of the lesser metatarsophalangeal joints: potential for injury and role of MR imaging. Magn Reson Imaging Clin N Am 2001;9(3):659–69, xii.

64. McCarthy CL, Thompson GV. Ultrasound findings of plantar plate tears of the lesser metatarsophalangeal joints. Skeletal Radiol 2021;50(8):1513–25.

65. Umans H, Srinivasan R, Elsinger E, et al. MRI of lesser metatarsophalangeal joint plantar plate tears and associated adjacent interspace lesions. Skeletal Radiol 2014;43(10):1361–8.

Moving?

Make sure your subscription moves with you!

To notify us of your new address, find your **Clinics Account Number** (located on your mailing label above your name), and contact customer service at:

Email: **journalscustomerservice-usa@elsevier.com**

800-654-2452 (subscribers in the U.S. & Canada)
314-447-8871 (subscribers outside of the U.S. & Canada)

Fax number: **314-447-8029**

Elsevier Health Sciences Division
Subscription Customer Service
3251 Riverport Lane
Maryland Heights, MO 63043

*To ensure uninterrupted delivery of your subscription, please notify us at least 4 weeks in advance of move.

Printed and bound by CPI Group (UK) Ltd, Croydon, CR0 4YY

08/05/2025

01864717-0011